CONTAGIOUS DISEASES
SOURCEBOOK

FIFTH EDITION

Health Reference Series

CONTAGIOUS DISEASES SOURCEBOOK

FIFTH EDITION

Provides Basic Consumer Health Information about Diseases Spread from Person to Person through Direct Physical Contact, Airborne Transmission, Sexual Contact, or Contact with Blood or Other Body Fluids, Including Pneumococcal, Staphylococcal, and Streptococcal Diseases; Colds; Influenza; Lice; Measles; Mumps; Tuberculosis; and Others

Along with Information about Self-Care and Over-the-Counter Medications, Antibiotics and Drug Resistance, Disease Prevention, and Vaccines; a Glossary; and a Directory of Resources for More Information

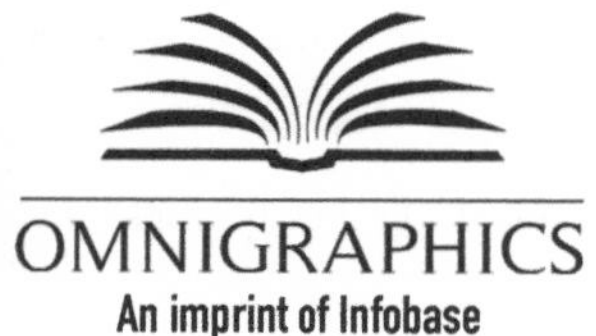

OMNIGRAPHICS
An imprint of Infobase

* * *

OMNIGRAPHICS
An imprint of Infobase
132 W. 31st St.
New York, NY 10001
www.infobase.com
James Chambers, *Editorial Director*

* * *

ISBN 978-0-7808-2088-3
E-ISBN 978-0-7808-2089-0

Library of Congress Cataloging-in-Publication Data

Names: Chambers, James (Editor), editor.

Title: Contagious diseases sourcebook: basic consumer health information about diseases spread from person to person through direct physical contact, airborne transmissions, sexual contact, or contact with blood or other body fluids, including pneumococcal, staphylococcal, and streptococcal diseases, colds, influenza, lice, measles, mumps, tuberculosis, and others, along with information about self-care and over-the-counter medications, antibiotics and drug resistance, disease prevention, and vaccines, a glossary, and a directory of resources for more information / edited by James Chambers.

Description: Fifth edition. | New York, NY: Omnigraphics, an imprint of Infobase, [2023] | Series: Health reference series | Revised edition of: Contagious diseases sourcebook / Angela L. Williams, managing editor. Fourth edition. [2019]. | Includes bibliographical references and index. | Summary: "Provides basic consumer health information about the transmission and treatment of diseases spread from person to person, along with facts about prevention, self-care, and drug resistance. Includes index, glossary of related terms, and other resources"-- Provided by publisher.

Identifiers: LCCN 2023033864 (print) | LCCN 2023033865 (ebook) | ISBN 9780780820883 (library binding) | ISBN 9780780820890 (ebook)

Subjects: LCSH: Communicable diseases--Popular works.

Classification: LCC RC113 .C664 2023 (print) | LCC RC113 (ebook) | DDC 362.1969--dc23/eng/20230817 Classification: LCC RG525 .P675 2023 (print) | LCC RG525 (ebook) | DDC 618.2--dc23/eng/20230706
LC record available at https://lccn.loc.gov/2023033864
LC ebook record available at https://lccn.loc.gov/2023033865

This book is printed on acid-free paper meeting the ANSI Z39.48 Standard. The infinity symbol that appears above indicates that the paper in this book meets that standard.

Printed in the United States

Table of Contents

Part 3. Bacterial Contagious Diseases

Part 4. Parasitic and Fungal Contagious Diseases

Part 5. Self-Care and Treatment for Contagious Diseases

Part 6. Prevention and Control Measures for Contagious Diseases

Part 7. Additional Help and Information

Preface

ABOUT THIS BOOK

Contagious diseases occur when microbes—bacteria, viruses, and fungi—are passed from person to person. Vaccination programs and other prevention measures have been successful in reducing the number of new cases of many contagious diseases. However, in many industrialized countries where communicable disease mortality has greatly decreased over the past century, the resurgence of old communicable diseases, the emergence of new ones, and the evolution of antimicrobial resistance continue to present a challenge. Infectious diseases remain a major public health concern in the United States and around the world.

Contagious Diseases Sourcebook, Fifth Edition provides updated information about microbes that spread from person to person and the diseases they cause, including influenza, lice infestation, pneumonia, staphylococcal and streptococcal infections, tuberculosis, and others. The types of diagnostic tests and treatments available from medical professionals are explained, and self-care practices for familiar symptoms—such as fever and sore throat that often accompany the common cold—are described. Other topics addressed include antibiotic resistance, personal hygiene, and recommendations and possible side effects of vaccination. The book concludes with a glossary of related terms and a directory of additional resources.

HOW TO USE THIS BOOK

This book is divided into parts and chapters. Parts focus on broad areas of interest. Chapters are devoted to single topics within a part.

Part 1: Introduction to Microbes and Contagious Diseases provides information about various types of microbes and the diverse range of infections they can cause. It explains how the immune system responds to these germs and the mechanisms through which diseases can be transmitted from one person to another. It also describes the risk of infectious diseases through blood transfusion.

Part 2: Viral Contagious Diseases provides information about the origins, transmission, symptoms, diagnosis, treatment, and preventive measures for a range of diseases caused by viruses. These include well-known illnesses such as chickenpox, mumps, gonorrhea, hepatitis, influenza, measles, polio, rubella, among others.

Part 3: Bacterial Contagious Diseases explains in detail the diseases and infections caused by bacteria. It covers a spectrum of conditions including bacterial meningitis, chancroid, Hansen disease, diphtheria, syphilis, pneumonia, salmonellosis, streptococcal infections, tuberculosis, and more.

Part 4: Parasitic and Fungal Contagious Diseases provides information about contagious diseases caused by parasites and fungi, including conditions such as amebiasis, cryptosporidiosis, lice infestation, pinworms, scabies, giardiasis, trichomoniasis, and various fungal infections.

Part 5: Self-Care and Treatment for Contagious Diseases discusses commonly used remedies for prevalent illnesses and disease symptoms. Facts about the appropriate usage of over-the-counter (OTC) medications, antibiotics, antivirals, and other prescription medicines are included, along with a chapter highlighting potential risks associated with drug interactions. The part concludes with information about probiotics, herbal and dietary supplements, and various forms of complementary and alternative medicine.

Part 6: Prevention and Control Measures for Contagious Diseases begins with information about personal hygiene practices. It proceeds to emphasize the vital role of vaccines in impeding disease spread. Information about vaccine recommendations for children, adolescents, and adults is included. Moreover, it addresses challenges related to vaccines, the vaccine adverse event reporting system, and the impacts of vaccine misinformation.

Part 7: Additional Help and Information provides a glossary of terms related to contagious diseases and a directory of resources for additional information.

BIBLIOGRAPHIC NOTE

This volume contains documents and excerpts from publications issued by the following U.S. government agencies: Centers for Disease Control and Prevention (CDC); HIV.gov; National Center for Complementary and Integrative Health (NCCIH); National Heart, Lung, and Blood Institute

(NHLBI); National Institute of Allergy and Infectious Diseases (NIAID); National Institute on Aging (NIA); National Institute on Drug Abuse (NIDA); National Institutes of Health (NIH); *NIH News in Health*; Office of Adolescent Health (OAH); Office of Disease Prevention and Health Promotion (ODPHP); Office of Population Affairs (OPA); Office on Women's Health (OWH); U.S. Department of Health and Human Services (HHS); and U.S. Food and Drug Administration (FDA).

It also contains original material prepared by Infobase and reviewed by medical consultants.

ABOUT THE *HEALTH REFERENCE SERIES*

The *Health Reference Series* is designed to provide basic medical information for patients, families, caregivers, and the general public. Each volume provides comprehensive coverage on a particular topic. This is especially important for people who may be dealing with a newly diagnosed disease or a chronic disorder in themselves or in a family member. People looking for preventive guidance, information about disease warning signs, medical statistics, and risk factors for health problems will also find answers to their questions in the *Health Reference Series*. The *Series*, however, is not intended to serve as a tool for diagnosing illness, in prescribing treatments, or as a substitute for the physician–patient relationship. All people concerned about medical symptoms or the possibility of disease are encouraged to seek professional care from an appropriate health-care provider.

A NOTE ABOUT SPELLING AND STYLE

Health Reference Series editors use *Stedman's Medical Dictionary* as an authority for questions related to the spelling of medical terms and *The Chicago Manual of Style* for questions related to grammatical structures, punctuation, and other editorial concerns. Consistent adherence is not always possible, however, because the individual volumes within the *Series* include many documents from a wide variety of different producers, and the editor's primary goal is to present material from each source as accurately as is possible. This sometimes means that information in different chapters or sections may follow other guidelines and alternate spelling authorities. For example, occasionally a copyright holder may require that eponymous terms be shown in possessive forms (Crohn's disease vs. Crohn disease) or that British spelling norms be retained (leukaemia vs. leukemia).

MEDICAL REVIEW

Infobase contracts with a team of qualified, senior medical professionals who serve as medical consultants for the *Health Reference Series*. As necessary, medical consultants review reprinted and originally written material for currency and accuracy. Medical consultation services are provided to the *Health Reference Series* editors by:

Dr. Vijayalakshmi, MBBS, DGO, MD

Dr. Senthil Selvan, MBBS, DCH, MD

Dr. K. Sivanandham, MBBS, DCH, MS (Research), PhD

HEALTH REFERENCE SERIES UPDATE POLICY

The inaugural book in the *Health Reference Series* was the first edition of *Cancer Sourcebook* published in 1989. Since then, the *Series* has been enthusiastically received by librarians and in the medical community. In order to maintain the standard of providing high-quality health information for the layperson, the editorial staff felt it was necessary to implement a policy of updating volumes when warranted.

Medical researchers have been making tremendous strides, and it is the purpose of the *Health Reference Series* to stay current with the most recent advances. Each decision to update a volume is made on an individual basis. Some of the considerations include how much new information is available and the feedback we receive from people who use the books. If there is a topic you would like to see added to the update list, or an area of medical concern you feel has not been adequately addressed, please write to: custserv@infobaselearning.com.

Part 1 | Introduction to Microbes and Contagious Diseases

Chapter 1 | **Understanding Microbes**

Chapter Contents

Section 1.1 | What Are Microbes?

Microbes are tiny organisms—too tiny to see without a microscope, yet they are abundant on Earth. They live everywhere—in air, soil, rock, and water. Some live happily in searing heat, while others thrive in freezing cold. Some microbes need oxygen to live, but others do not. These microscopic organisms are found in plants and animals, as well as in the human body.

Some microbes cause disease in humans, plants, and animals. Others are essential for a healthy life, and we could not exist without them. Indeed, the relationship between microbes and humans is delicate and complex. Most microbes belong to one of four major groups: bacteria, viruses, fungi, or protozoa. A common word for microbes that cause disease is "germs." Some people refer to disease-causing microbes as "bugs." "I have got the flu bug," for example, is a phrase you may hear during the wintertime to describe an influenza virus infection.

Since the 19th century, we have known microbes cause infectious diseases. Near the end of the 20th century, researchers began to learn that microbes also contribute to many chronic diseases and conditions. Mounting scientific evidence strongly links microbes to some forms of cancer, coronary artery disease (CAD), diabetes, multiple sclerosis, and chronic lung diseases.

BACTERIA

Microbes belonging to the bacteria group are made up of only one cell. Under a microscope, bacteria look like balls, rods, or spirals. Bacteria (refer to Figure 1.1) are so small that a line of 1,000 could fit across the eraser of a pencil. Life in any form on Earth could not exist without these tiny cells. Scientists have discovered fossilized remains of bacteria that date back more than 3.5 billion years, placing them among the oldest living things on Earth. Bacteria can inhabit a variety of environments, including extremely hot and cold areas.

- Psychrophiles, or cold-loving bacteria, can live in the subfreezing temperature of the Arctic.

- Thermophiles are heat-loving bacteria that can live in extreme heat, such as in the hot springs in Yellowstone National Park.
- Extreme thermophiles, or hyperthermophiles, thrive at 235 °F (112.8 °C) near volcanic vents on the ocean floor.

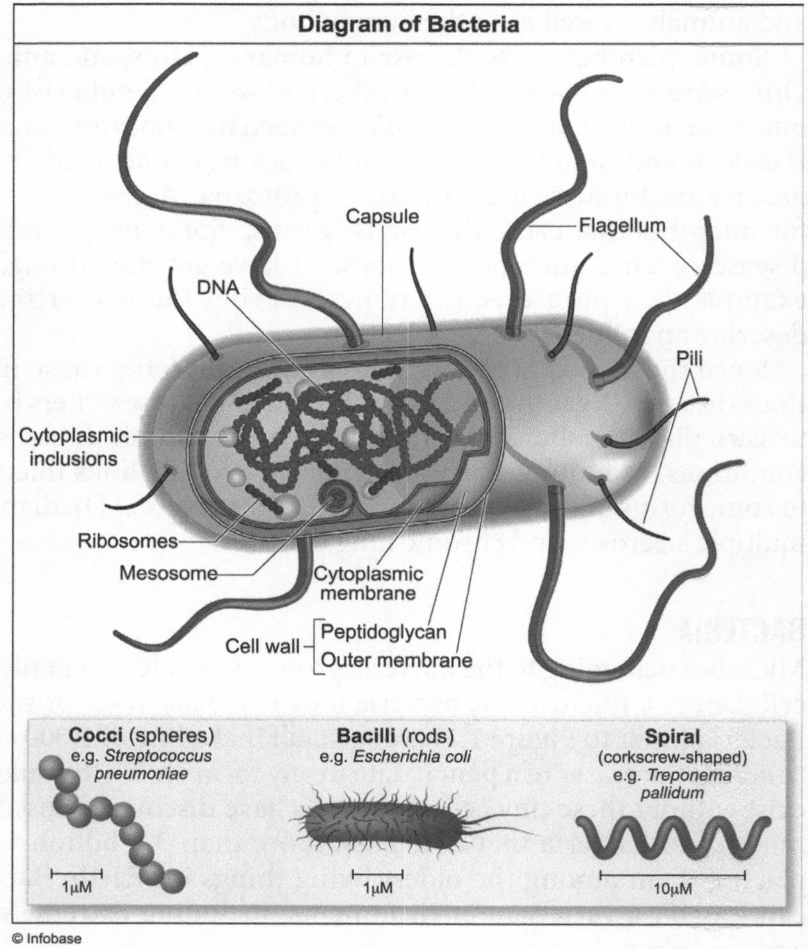

Figure 1.1. Bacteria

Infobase

Many bacteria prefer the milder temperature of the healthy human body. Like humans, some bacteria (aerobic bacteria) need oxygen to survive. Others (anaerobic bacteria), however, do not. Amazingly, some can adapt to new environments by learning to survive with or without oxygen. Like all living cells, each bacterium requires food for energy and building materials. There are countless numbers of bacteria on Earth—most are harmless, and many are even beneficial to humans. In fact, less than 1 percent of bacteria cause diseases in humans. For example, harmless anaerobic bacteria, such as *Lactobacillus acidophilus*, live in our intestines, where they help digest food, destroy disease-causing microbes, fight cancer cells, and give the body needed vitamins. Healthy food products, such as yogurt, sauerkraut, and cheese, are made using bacteria. Some bacteria produce poisons called "toxins," which can also make us sick.

VIRUSES

Viruses are among the smallest microbes, much smaller even than bacteria. Viruses are not cells. They consist of one or more molecules of deoxyribonucleic acid (DNA) or ribonucleic acid (RNA), which contain the virus's genes surrounded by a protein coat. Viruses can be rod-shaped, sphere-shaped, or multisided. Some viruses look like tadpoles.

Unlike most bacteria, most viruses do cause disease because they invade living, normal cells, such as those in your body. They then multiply and produce other viruses like themselves. Each virus is very particular about which cell it attacks. Various human viruses specifically attack particular cells in your body's organs, systems, or tissues, such as the liver, respiratory system, or blood.

Although different types of viruses behave differently, most survive by taking over the machinery that makes a cell work. Briefly, when a piece of a virus, called a "virion," comes in contact with a cell it likes, it may attach to special landing sites on the surface of that cell. From there, the virus may inject molecules into the cell, or the cell may swallow the virion. Once inside the cell, viral molecules, such as DNA or RNA, direct the cell to make new virus offspring. That is how a virus infects a cell.

Viruses can even "infect" bacteria. These viruses, called "bacteriophages," may help researchers develop alternatives to antibiotic medicines for preventing and treating bacterial infections. Many viral infections do not result in disease. For example, by the time most people in the United States become adults, they have been infected by cytomegalovirus (CMV). Most of these people, however, do not develop CMV-disease symptoms. Other viral infections can result in deadly diseases, such as acquired immunodeficiency syndrome (AIDS) or Ebola hemorrhagic fever.

FUNGI

A fungus is actually a primitive plant. Fungi can be found in the air, in soil, on plants, and in water. Thousands, perhaps millions, of different types of fungi exist on Earth. The most familiar ones to us are mushrooms, yeast, mold, and mildew. Some live in the human body, usually without causing illness. Fungal diseases are called "mycoses." Mycoses can affect your skin, nails, body hair, internal organs such as your lungs, and body systems such as your nervous system. *Aspergillus fumigatus*, for example, can cause aspergillosis, a fungal infection in your respiratory system.

Some fungi have made our lives easier. Penicillin and other antibiotics, which kill harmful bacteria in our bodies, are made from fungi. Other fungi, such as certain yeasts, can also be helpful. For example, when a warm liquid, such as water, and a food source are added to certain yeasts, the fungus ferments. The process of fermentation is essential for making healthy foods, such as breads and cheeses.

PROTOZOA

Protozoa are a group of microscopic one-celled animals. Protozoa can be parasites or predators. In humans, protozoa usually cause disease. Some protozoa, such as plankton, live in water environments and serve as food for marine animals, such as some kinds of whales. Protozoa can also be found on land in decaying matter and in soil, but they must have a moist environment to survive. Termites would not be able to do such a good job of digesting wood without these microorganisms in their guts.

Malaria is caused by a protozoan parasite. Another protozoan parasite, *Toxoplasma gondii*, causes toxoplasmosis in humans. This is an especially troublesome infection in pregnant women because of its effects on the fetus and in people with human immunodeficiency virus (HIV) infection or other immune deficiency disorders.[1]

Section 1.2 | **Microbial Infections**

Germs (microbes) are a part of everyday life and are found in the air, soil, and water and in and on our bodies. Some germs are helpful; others are harmful. Many germs live in and on our bodies without causing harm, and some even help us stay healthy. Only a small portion of germs are known to cause infection.

HOW DO INFECTIONS OCCUR?

An infection occurs when germs enter the body, increase in number, and cause a reaction in the body. The following are the three things that are necessary for an infection to occur:

- **Source**. Places where infectious agents (germs) live (e.g., sinks, surfaces, and human skin).
- **Susceptible person**. A way for germs to enter the body.
- **Transmission**. A way germs are moved to the susceptible person.

Source

A source is an infectious agent or germ and refers to a virus, bacteria, or other microbe. In health-care settings, germs are found in many places. People are one source of germs, including:

- patients
- health-care workers
- visitors and household members

[1] "Understanding Microbes in Sickness and in Health," National Institute of Allergy and Infectious Diseases (NIAID), January 2006. Available online. URL: https://irp-cdn.multiscreensite.com/562d25c6/files/uploaded/Understanding%20Microbes_In%20Sickness%20and%20in%20Health_2006.pdf. Accessed July 4, 2023.

People can be sick with symptoms of an infection or colonized with germs (not having symptoms of an infection but able to pass the germs to others).

Germs are also found in the environment. The following are examples of environmental sources of germs:

- dry surfaces in patient care areas (e.g., bed rails, medical equipment, countertops, and tables)
- wet surfaces, moist environments, and biofilms (e.g., cooling towers, faucets and sinks, and equipment such as ventilators)
- indwelling medical devices (e.g., catheters and intravenous (IV) lines)
- dust or decaying debris (e.g., construction dust or wet materials from water leaks)

Susceptible Person

A susceptible person is someone who is not vaccinated or otherwise immune, or a person with a weakened immune system which is a way for the germs to enter the body. For an infection to occur, germs must enter a susceptible person's body and invade tissues, multiply, and cause a reaction whereas a healthy immune system helps fight infection. Devices, such as IV catheters and surgical incisions, can provide an entryway. When patients are sick and receive medical treatment in health-care facilities, the following factors can increase their susceptibility to infection:

- Patients who have underlying medical conditions, such as diabetes, cancer, and organ transplantation, are at increased risk for infection because often these illnesses decrease the immune system's ability to fight infection.
- Certain medications used to treat medical conditions, such as antibiotics, steroids, and certain cancer-fighting medications, increase the risk of some types of infections.
- Lifesaving medical treatments and procedures used in health care, such as urinary catheters, tubes, and

surgery, increase the risk of infection by providing additional ways that germs can enter the body.

Transmission

Transmission refers to the way germs are moved to the susceptible person. Germs do not move themselves. Germs depend on people, the environment, and/or medical equipment to move in health-care settings. The following are a few general ways that germs travel in health-care settings:

- **Contact.** Germs can be transmitted through touch (e.g., methicillin-resistant *Staphylococcus aureus* (MRSA) or vancomycin-resistant enterococci (VRE)). For example, health-care provider hands can become contaminated by touching germs present on medical equipment or high-touch surfaces, then carry the germs on their hands and spread them to a susceptible person when proper hand hygiene is not performed before touching the susceptible person.
- **Sprays and splashes.** These occur when an infected person coughs or sneezes, creating droplets that carry germs short distances (within approximately 6 feet). These germs can land on a susceptible person's eyes, nose, or mouth and can cause infection (e.g., pertussis or meningitis).
- **Inhalation.** This occurs when germs are aerosolized in tiny particles that survive on air currents over great distances and time and reach a susceptible person. Airborne transmission can occur when infected patients cough, talk, or sneeze germs into the air (e.g., tuberculosis or measles) or when germs are aerosolized by medical equipment or by dust from a construction zone (e.g., nontuberculous mycobacteria or *Aspergillus*).
  - Close-range inhalation occurs when a droplet containing germs is small enough to breathe in but not durable over distance.

- **Sharps injuries**. These can lead to infections (e.g., human immunodeficiency virus (HIV), hepatitis B virus (HBV), and hepatitis C virus (HCV)) when blood-borne pathogens enter a person through a skin puncture by a used needle or sharp instrument.[2]

[2] "How Infections Spread," Centers for Disease Control and Prevention (CDC), January 7, 2016. Available online. URL: www.cdc.gov/infectioncontrol/spread/index.html. Accessed August 18, 2023.

Chapter 2 | **Overview of the Immune System**

Your immune system is a complex network of cells, tissues, and organs. Together they help the body fight infections and other diseases. When germs, such as bacteria or viruses, invade your body, they attack and multiply. This is called an "infection." The infection causes the disease that makes you sick. Your immune system protects you from the disease by fighting off the germs.

WHAT ARE THE PARTS OF THE IMMUNE SYSTEM?

The immune system (refer to Figure 2.1) has many different parts, including:

- your skin, which can help prevent germs from getting into the body
- mucous membranes, which are the moist, inner linings of some organs and body cavities (They make mucus and other substances that can trap and fight germs.)
- white blood cells, which fight germs
- organs and tissues of the lymph system, such as the thymus, spleen, tonsils, lymph nodes, lymph vessels, and bone marrow (They produce, store, and carry white blood cells.)

HOW DOES THE IMMUNE SYSTEM WORK?

Your immune system (refer to Figure 2.2) defends your body against substances it sees as harmful or foreign. These substances are called "antigens." They may be germs, such as bacteria and viruses. They might be chemicals or toxins. They could also be cells that are damaged from things, such as cancer or sunburn.

When your immune system recognizes an antigen, it attacks it. This is called an "immune response." Part of this response is to make antibodies. Antibodies are proteins that work to attack, weaken, and destroy antigens. Your body also makes other cells to fight the antigen.

Afterward, your immune system remembers the antigen. If it sees the antigen again, it can recognize it. It will quickly send out the right antibodies, so in most cases, you do not get sick. This protection against a certain disease is called "immunity."

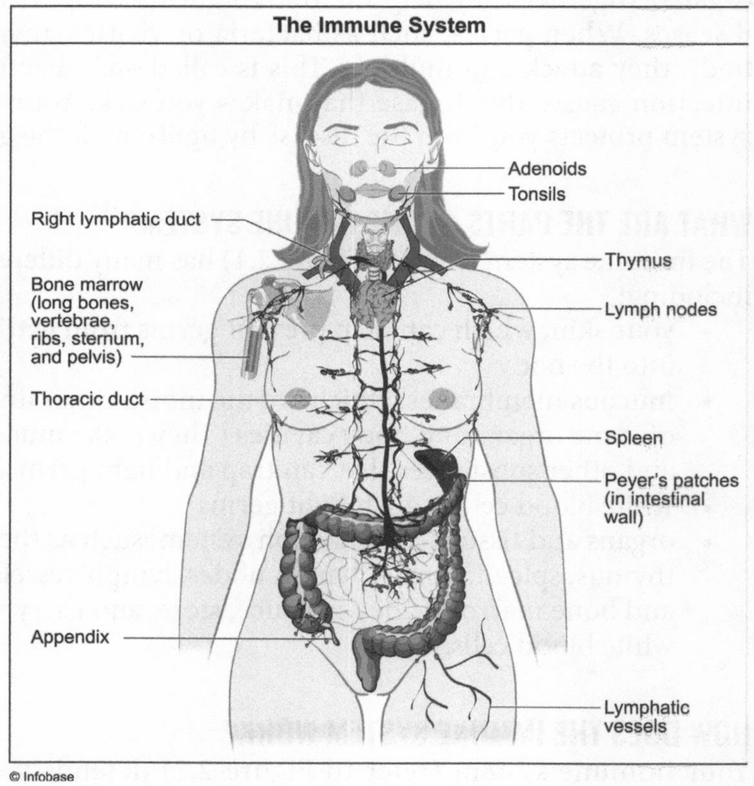

Figure 2.1. Immune System

Infobase

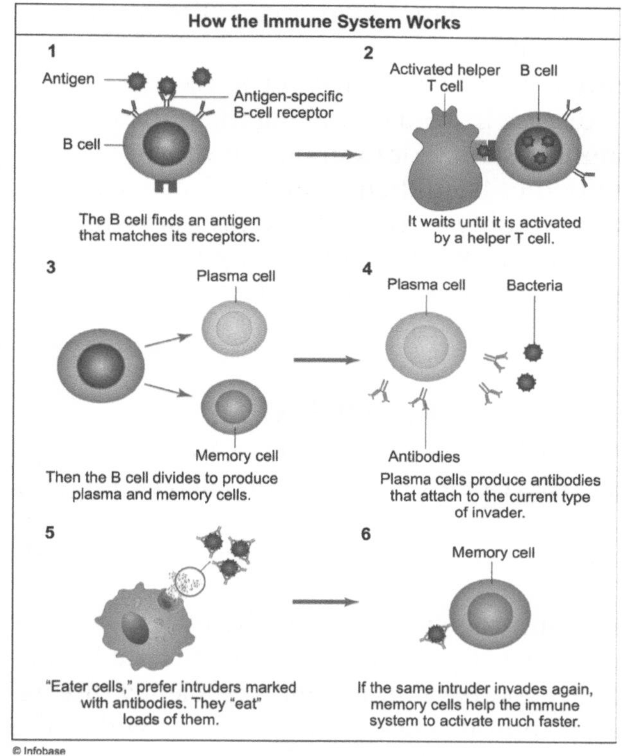
How the Immune System Works
1
Antigen
Antigen-specific B-cell receptor
B cell
The B cell finds an antigen that matches its receptors.
2
Activated helper T cell
B cell
It waits until it is activated by a helper T cell.
3
Plasma cell
Memory cell
Then the B cell divides to produce plasma and memory cells.
4
Plasma cell
Bacteria
Antibodies
Plasma cells produce antibodies that attach to the current type of invader.
5
"Eater cells," prefer intruders marked with antibodies. They "eat" loads of them.
6
Memory cell
If the same intruder invades again, memory cells help the immune system to activate much faster.
© Infobase

Figure 2.2. How the Immune System Works

Infobase

WHAT ARE THE TYPES OF IMMUNITY?

The following are the three different types of immunity:

- **Innate immunity**. This is the protection that you are born with. It is your body's first line of defense. It includes barriers, such as the skin and mucous membranes. They keep harmful substances from entering the body. It also includes some cells and chemicals that can attack foreign substances.
- **Active immunity**. Also called "adaptive immunity," active immunity develops when you are infected with or vaccinated against a foreign substance. Active

immunity is usually long-lasting. For many diseases, it can last your entire life.
- **Passive immunity**. This happens when you receive antibodies to a disease instead of making them through your own immune system. For example, newborn babies have antibodies from their mothers. People can also get passive immunity through blood products that contain antibodies. This kind of immunity gives you protection right away. But it only lasts a few weeks or months.

WHAT CAN GO WRONG WITH THE IMMUNE SYSTEM?

Sometimes, a person may have an immune response even though there is no real threat. This can lead to problems such as allergies, asthma, and autoimmune diseases. If you have an autoimmune disease, your immune system attacks healthy cells in your body by mistake.

Other immune system problems happen when your immune system does not work correctly. These problems include immunodeficiency diseases. If you have an immunodeficiency disease, you get sick more often. Your infections may last longer and can be more serious and harder to treat. They are often genetic disorders.

There are other diseases that can affect your immune system. For example, human immunodeficiency virus (HIV) is a virus that harms your immune system by destroying your white blood cells. If HIV is not treated, it can lead to acquired immunodeficiency syndrome (AIDS). People with AIDS have badly damaged immune systems. They get an increasing number of severe illnesses.[1]

[1] MedlinePlus, "Immune System and Disorders," National Institutes of Health (NIH), August 17, 2020. Available online. URL: https://medlineplus.gov/immunesystemanddisorders.html. Accessed July 18, 2023.

Chapter 3 | Immune System Response to Infection

An immune response is generally divided into innate and adaptive immunity. Innate immunity occurs immediately when circulating innate cells recognize a problem. Adaptive immunity occurs later, as it relies on the coordination and expansion of specific adaptive immune cells. Immune memory follows the adaptive response when mature adaptive cells, highly specific to the original pathogen, are retained for later use.

INNATE IMMUNITY

Innate immune cells express genetically encoded receptors, called "toll-like receptors" (TLRs), which recognize general danger- or pathogen-associated patterns. Collectively, these receptors can broadly recognize viruses, bacteria, fungi, and even noninfectious problems. However, they cannot distinguish between specific strains of bacteria or viruses.

There are numerous types of innate immune cells with specialized functions. They include neutrophils, eosinophils, basophils, mast cells, monocytes, dendritic cells, and macrophages. Their main feature is the ability to respond quickly and broadly when a problem arises, typically leading to inflammation. Innate immune cells are also important for activating adaptive immunity. Innate cells are critical for host defense, and disorders in innate cell function may cause chronic susceptibility to infection.

ADAPTIVE IMMUNITY

Adaptive immune cells are more specialized, with each adaptive B- or T-cell-bearing unique receptors, B-cell receptors (BCRs) and T-cell receptors (TCRs), that recognize specific signals rather than general patterns. Each receptor recognizes an antigen, which is simply any molecule that may bind to a BCR or TCR. Antigens are derived from a variety of sources, including pathogens, host cells, and allergens. Antigens are typically processed by innate immune cells and presented to adaptive cells in the lymph nodes (refer to Figure 3.1).

The genes for BCRs and TCRs are randomly rearranged at specific cell maturation stages, resulting in unique receptors that may potentially recognize anything. Random generation of receptors allows the immune system (refer to Figure 3.2) to respond to new or unforeseen problems. This concept is especially important because environments may frequently change, for instance, when seasons change or a person relocates, and pathogens are constantly evolving to survive. Because BCRs and TCRs are so specific, adaptive cells may only recognize one strain of a particular pathogen,

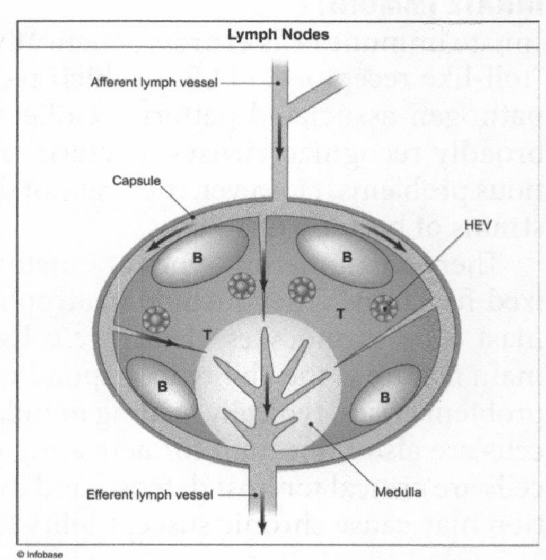

Figure 3.1. Lymph Nodes
Infobase

unlike innate cells, which recognize broad classes of pathogens. In fact, a group of adaptive cells that recognize the same strain will likely recognize different areas of that pathogen.

If a B or T cell has a receptor that recognizes an antigen from a pathogen and also receives cues from innate cells that something is wrong, the B or T cell will activate, divide, and disperse to address the problem. B cells make antibodies, which neutralize pathogens, rendering them harmless. T cells carry out multiple functions, including killing infected cells and activating or recruiting other immune cells. The adaptive response has a system of checks and balances to prevent unnecessary activation that could cause damage to the host. If a B or T cell is autoreactive, meaning its receptor recognizes antigens from the body's own cells, the cell will be deleted. Also, if a B or T cell does not receive signals from innate cells, it will not be optimally activated.

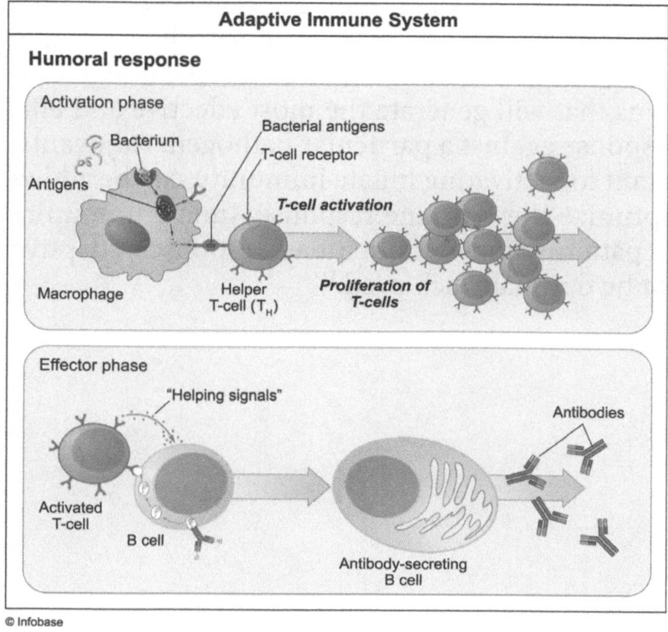

Figure 3.2. Adaptive Immune System

Infobase

Immune memory is a feature of the adaptive immune response. After B or T cells are activated, they expand rapidly. As the problem resolves, cells stop dividing and are retained in the body as memory cells. The next time this same pathogen enters the body, a memory cell is already poised to react and can clear away the pathogen before it establishes itself.

VACCINATION

Vaccination, or immunization, is a way to train your immune system against a specific pathogen. Vaccination achieves immune memory without an actual infection, so the body is prepared when the virus or bacterium enters. Saving time is important to prevent a pathogen from establishing itself and infecting more cells in the body.

An effective vaccine will optimally activate both the innate and adaptive response. An immunogen is used to activate the adaptive immune response so that specific memory cells are generated. Because BCRs and TCRs are unique, some memory cells are simply better at eliminating the pathogen. The goal of vaccine design is to select immunogens that will generate the most effective and efficient memory response against a particular pathogen. Adjuvants, which are important for activating innate immunity, can be added to vaccines to optimize the immune response. Innate immunity recognizes broad patterns, and without innate responses, adaptive immunity cannot be optimally achieved.[1]

[1] "Features of an Immune Response," National Institute of Allergy and Infectious Diseases (NIAID), January 16, 2014. Available online. URL: www.niaid.nih.gov/research/immune-response-features. Accessed August 30, 2023.

Chapter 4 | Transmission of Contagious Diseases

Chapter Contents

MICROBES CAN MAKE US SICK

According to health-care experts, infectious diseases caused by microbes are responsible for more deaths worldwide than any other single cause. They estimate the annual cost of medical care for treating infectious diseases in the United States alone is about $120 billion.

The science of microbiology explores how microbes work and how to control them. It seeks ways to use that knowledge to prevent and treat the diseases microbes cause. The 20th century saw an extraordinary increase in our knowledge about microbes. Microbiologists and other researchers had many successes in learning how microbes cause certain infectious diseases and how to combat those microbes.

Unfortunately, microbes are much better at adapting to new environments than are people. Having existed on Earth for billions of years, microbes are constantly challenging human newcomers with ingenious new survival tactics.

- Many microbes are developing new properties to resist drug treatments that once effectively destroyed them. Drug resistance has become a serious problem worldwide.
- Changes in the environment have put certain human populations in contact with newly identified microbes that cause diseases we have never seen before or those that previously occurred only in isolated populations.
- Newly emerging diseases are a growing global health concern. Since 1976, scientists have identified approximately 30 new pathogens.

MICROBES CAN INFECT US

The following are some of the many different ways you can get infected by germs.

Some Microbes Can Travel through the Air

You can transmit microbes to another person through the air by coughing or sneezing. These are common ways to get viruses that cause colds or the flu or the bacteria that cause tuberculosis (TB). Interestingly, international airplane travel can expose you to germs not common in your own country.

Close Contact Can Pass Germs to Another Person

Scientists have identified more than 500 types of bacteria (refer to Figure 4.1) that live in our mouths. Some keep the oral environment healthy, while others cause problems, such as gum disease. One way you can transmit oral bacteria is by kissing.

Microbes such as human immunodeficiency virus (HIV), herpes simplex virus (HSV), and gonorrhea bacteria are examples of germs that can be transmitted directly during sexual intercourse.

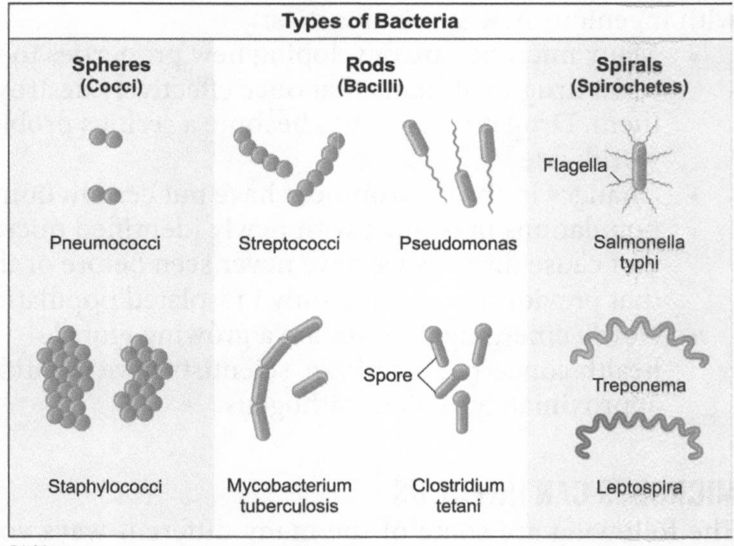

Figure 4.1. Types of Bacteria

Infobase

You Can Pick Up and Spread Germs by Touching Infectious Material

A common way for some microbes to enter the body, especially when caring for young children, is through unintentionally passing feces from hand to mouth or to the mouths of young children. Infant diarrhea is often spread in this way. Day care workers, for example, can pass diarrhea-causing rotavirus or *Giardia lamblia* (protozoa) from one baby to the next between diaper changes and other childcare practices. It is also possible to pick up cold viruses from shaking someone's hand or from touching contaminated surfaces, such as a handrail or telephone.

A Healthy Person Can Carry Germs and Pass Them to Others

The story of "Typhoid Mary" is a famous example from medical history about how a person can pass germs on to others yet not be affected by those germs. The germs, in this case, were *Salmonella typhi* bacteria, which cause typhoid fever and are usually spread through food or water.

In the early 20th century, Mary Mallon, an Irish immigrant, worked as a cook for several New York City families. More than half of the first family she worked for came down with typhoid fever. Through clever deduction, a researcher determined that the disease was caused by the family cook. He concluded that although Mary had no symptoms of the disease, she probably had a mild typhoid infection sometime in the past. Though not sick, she still carried the *Salmonella* bacteria and was able to spread them to others through the food she prepared.

Germs from Your Household Pet Can Make You Sick

You can catch a variety of germs from animals, especially household pets. The rabies virus, which can infect cats and dogs, is one of the most serious and deadly of these microbes. Fortunately, the rabies vaccine prevents animals from getting rabies. Vaccines protect people from accidentally getting the virus from an animal. They also prevent people who already have been exposed to the virus, such as through an animal bite, from getting sick.

Dog and cat saliva can contain any of more than 100 different germs that can make you sick. *Pasteurella* bacteria, the most common, can be transmitted through bites that break the skin causing serious, and sometimes fatal, diseases, such as blood infections and meningitis. Meningitis is an inflammation of the lining of the brain and spinal cord.

Warm-blooded animals are not the only ones that can cause you harm. Pet reptiles, such as turtles, snakes, and iguanas, can give *Salmonella* bacteria to their unsuspecting owners.

You Can Get Microbes from Tiny Critters

Mosquitoes may be the most common insect carriers, also called "vectors," of pathogens. *Anopheles* mosquitoes can pick up *Plasmodium*, which causes malaria, from the blood of an infected person and transmit the protozoan to an uninfected person. Fleas that pick up *Yersinia pestis* bacteria from rodents can then transmit plague to humans. Ticks, which are more closely related to crabs than to insects, are another common vector. The tiny deer tick can infect humans with *Borrelia burgdorferi*, the bacterium that causes Lyme disease, which the tick picks up from mice.

Some Microbes in Food or Water Could Make You Sick

Every year, millions of people worldwide become ill from eating contaminated foods. Although many cases of foodborne illness or "food poisoning" are not reported, the Centers for Disease Control and Prevention (CDC) estimates that there are 76 million cases of such illnesses in the United States each year. In addition, the CDC estimates that 325,000 hospitalizations and 5,000 deaths are related to foodborne diseases each year. Microbes can cause these illnesses, some of which can be fatal if not treated properly.

Poor manufacturing processes or poor food preparation can allow microbes to grow in food and, subsequently, infect the consumer. *Escherichia coli* bacteria sometimes persist in food products, such as undercooked hamburger meat and unpasteurized fruit juice. These bacteria can have deadly consequences for vulnerable people, especially children and the elderly. *Cryptosporidia* are bacteria found in human and animal feces. These bacteria can get into the lake, river, and ocean water from sewage spills, animal waste, and water runoff. Millions can be released from infectious fecal matter. People who drink, swim, or play in infected water can get sick.

People, including babies, with diarrhea caused by *Cryptosporidia* or other diarrhea-causing microbes, such as *Giardia*, can infect others while using swimming pools, water parks, hot tubs, and spas.

Transplanted Animal Organs May Harbor Germs

Researchers are investigating the possibility of transplanting animal organs, such as pig hearts, into people. They, however, must guard against the risk that those organs may also transmit microbes that were harmless to the animal into humans, where they may cause disease.[1]

Section 4.2 | Risk of Infectious Disease from Blood Transfusion

BLOOD TRANSFUSION

A blood transfusion is a common, safe medical procedure in which healthy blood is given to you through an intravenous (IV) line inserted in one of your blood vessels. Blood transfusions replace blood that is lost through surgery or injury. This treatment also provides blood if your body is not making blood properly on its own. The following are the four types of blood products that may be given through blood transfusions:

- whole blood
- red blood cells (RBCs), the blood cells that carry oxygen throughout the body
- platelets, blood cell fragments that help your blood clot
- plasma, the fluid part of the blood

[1] "Understanding Microbes in Sickness and in Health," National Institute of Allergy and Infectious Diseases (NIAID), January 2006. Available online. URL: https://irp-cdn.multiscreensite.com/562d25c6/files/uploaded/Understanding%20Microbes_In%20Sickness%20and%20in%20Health_2006.pdf. Accessed July 18, 2023.

Most of the blood used for transfusions comes from whole blood donations given by volunteer blood donors. Sometimes, people have their own blood collected and stored a few weeks before elective surgery in case it is needed. After a doctor determines that you need a blood transfusion, your blood will be tested to make sure that the blood you are given is a good match. Blood transfusions usually take one to four hours to complete. You will be monitored during and after the procedure. Blood transfusions are usually very safe because donated blood is carefully tested, handled, and stored. However, there is a small chance that your body may have a mild or even a severe reaction to the donor blood. Other complications of blood transfusions may include:

- fever
- heart or lung problems
- alloimmunization, when the body's natural defense system attacks donor blood cells
- rare but serious reactions where donated white blood cells attack your body's healthy tissues

Some people also have health problems from getting too much iron after frequent transfusions. There is also a very small chance of getting an infectious disease, such as hepatitis B or C or human immunodeficiency virus (HIV), through a blood transfusion. For HIV, that chance is less than 1 in 1 million. Scientific research and careful medical controls make the supply of donated blood very safe.[2]

POTENTIAL INFECTIONS OF BLOOD TRANSFUSION

The U.S. blood supply is safer than it has ever been. However, any blood-borne pathogen has the potential to be transmitted by blood transfusion. Transfusion-transmitted infections (TTIs) are infections resulting from the introduction of a pathogen into a person through blood transfusion. A wide variety of organisms, including bacteria, viruses, prions, and parasites, can be

[2] "Treatments for Blood Disorders," National Heart, Lung, and Blood Institute (NHLBI), March 24, 2022. Available online. URL: www.nhlbi.nih.gov/health/blood-bone-marrow-treatments. Accessed July 18, 2023.

transmitted through blood transfusions. The use of a standard donor screening questionnaire, as well as laboratory tests, helps reduce the risk of an infectious organism being transmitted by blood transfusion.

Additionally, the introduction of pathogen reduction technology (PRT) may help further reduce the risk of TTIs. PRT involves treating certain blood products with a pathogen-inactivating agent soon after collection. In addition to potentially limiting the number of TTIs, PRT may also eliminate the need for irradiation to prevent transfusion-associated graft versus host diseases (TA-GVHD) and serologic testing for cytomegalovirus (CMV) for at-risk patients. This technology is approved for apheresis platelets and plasma products.

Bacterial Contamination of Blood Products

Bacterial contamination of blood products, especially in platelets that are stored at room temperature, is the most common infectious risk of blood transfusion, occurring in approximately 1 of 2,000–3,000 platelet transfusions. Transfusion-transmitted sepsis, while less common, can cause severe illness and death. Improved donor screening, as well as improved methods of collection, handling, and storing of blood products, has decreased bacterial contamination in recent years.

- **Gram-positive bacteria.** These bacteria are normally found on the skin, such as *Staphylococcus epidermidis* or *Staphylococcus aureus*, which are the most common bacterial contaminants of blood products. This type of contamination is thought to occur when the bacteria on the skin are passed into the collected blood through the collection needle.
- **Gram-negative bacteria.** These bacteria are a part of the normal flora in the gastrointestinal tract (intestines). These bacteria can move from a person's gastrointestinal tract to their bloodstream, causing infections of varying severity. Contamination of blood products with gram-negative bacteria is thought to occur when blood is collected from donors

who have bacteria in their bloodstream but do not have symptoms of an infection. Examples include *Acinetobacter*, *Klebsiella* (www.cdc.gov/HAI/organisms/organisms.html#k), and *Escherichia coli*. Some gram-negative bacteria are resistant to multiple drugs and are increasingly resistant to many available antibiotics.

- **Anaplasmosis**. It is a tick-borne disease caused by the bacterium *Anaplasma phagocytophilum*. It is transmitted to humans by tick bites, primarily from the black-legged tick and the western black-legged tick, and can be transmitted via blood product from an infected donor. Symptoms of anaplasmosis include fever, headache, chills, and muscle aches.
- **Brucellosis**. It is a disease caused by bacteria from the *Brucella species*, which is transmitted to humans from contact with infected animals, such as sheep, cattle, and dogs. Brucellosis has been previously described to be transmissible via blood product from an infected donor. Symptoms include fever, sweats, headache, and fatigue.
- **Ehrlichiosis**. It is a group of tick-borne diseases caused by bacteria in the *Ehrlichia* species. It is transmitted to humans mainly from the lone star tick and the black-legged tick. Transmission via blood product from an infected donor has previously been documented. Symptoms include fever, chills, headache, and muscle aches.

Parasitic Diseases

Transmission of parasitic infections through blood donation is rare. To help minimize the risk of transfusion-transmitted illnesses, including parasitic infections, donors are asked questions to assist in determining if they are in good health. To reduce the risk of transmitting specific infections (e.g., malaria), donors are asked about recent travel to areas where some infections are more common. The following are examples of parasitic diseases that can be transmitted by blood transfusion:

- **Babesiosis**. It is caused by microscopic parasites that infect RBCs and are spread by certain ticks. In the United

States, tick-borne transmission is most common in particular regions and seasons; it mainly occurs in parts of the Northeast and upper Midwest and usually peaks during the warm months.

- **Chagas disease.** It is caused by the parasite *Trypanosoma cruzi*, which is transmitted to animals and people by insects. *T. cruzi* is found only in the Americas, and transmission of the parasite occurs mainly in rural areas of Latin America, where poverty is widespread. Since 2007, first-time blood donors have been screened for antibodies to *T. cruzi* in the United States, making the risk of transfusion-transmitted *T. cruzi* extremely rare.
- **Leishmaniasis.** It includes two major diseases: cutaneous leishmaniasis and visceral leishmaniasis, caused by more than 20 different leishmanial species. Leishmaniasis is transmitted by the bite of small insects called "sand flies." The distribution of leishmania is worldwide. Several transfusion-transmitted cases of the visceral form of leishmania have been reported.
- **Malaria.** It is a serious and sometimes fatal disease caused by a parasite that commonly infects a certain type of mosquito, which feeds on humans. People who get malaria are typically very sick with high fevers, shaking chills, and flu-like illness. About 1,700 cases of malaria are diagnosed in the United States each year. The vast majority of cases in the United States are in travelers and immigrants returning from countries where malaria transmission occurs, many from sub-Saharan Africa and South Asia.

Viral Diseases

As with bacteria and parasites, viruses that are blood-borne can be transmitted by blood transfusion. Donors are asked questions about their social behavior and health history to help minimize the risk of transfusion-transmitted viral diseases. The following are examples of viral diseases that can be transmitted through transfusion:

- **Chikungunya virus (CHIKV).** It is an arbovirus spread to humans from mosquitoes. CHIKV outbreaks have occurred in Africa, Asia, Europe, the Indian and Pacific Oceans, and the Caribbean. No CHIKV outbreaks have been reported in the United States. Symptoms include fever and joint pain, and there is no vaccine or medicine to prevent or treat CHIKV.

- **Dengue fever (DF).** It is caused by any one of four related viruses transmitted by *Aedes* species mosquitoes. With more than one-third of the world's population living in areas at risk for transmission, dengue infection is a leading cause of illness and death in the tropics and subtropics. As many as 100 million people are infected yearly.
- **Hepatitis A virus (HAV).** Hepatitis A is a contagious liver disease that results from infection with the HAV. Hepatitis A is spread primarily by the fecal–oral route, but transfusion-transmitted HAV infection has been reported. Hepatitis A can range in severity from a mild illness lasting a few weeks to a severe illness lasting several months and, on rare occasions, can cause death.
- **Hepatitis B virus (HBV).** Hepatitis B is a contagious liver disease caused by HBV. In total, 1.2 million Americans are living with chronic hepatitis B, and most are unaware of their infection. Over time, approximately 15–25 percent of people with chronic hepatitis B develop serious liver problems, including liver damage, cirrhosis, liver failure, and liver cancer. Every year, approximately 3,000 people in the United States and more than 600,000 people worldwide die from hepatitis B-related liver disease. Since 1972, the blood supply has been screened for hepatitis B in the United States, making the risk of transfusion-transmitted HBV extremely rare.
- **Hepatitis C virus (HCV).** Hepatitis C is a contagious liver disease caused by HCV. Hepatitis C is the most common chronic blood-borne infection in the United States. In total, 3.2 million Americans are living with chronic hepatitis C, and most are unaware of their infection. Chronic hepatitis C is a serious disease that

can result in long-term health problems, including liver damage, cirrhosis, liver failure, and liver cancer. Since 1992, the blood supply has been screened for hepatitis C in the United States, making the risk of transfusion-transmitted HCV extremely rare.

- **Hepatitis E virus (HEV).** Hepatitis E is a contagious liver disease caused by the HEV. HEV is transmitted via the fecal–oral route, generally through contaminated water in areas with poor sanitation. Though HEV is rare in the United States, it is more common in other countries. Hepatitis E-related liver disease is self-limiting and does not lead to chronic infection.
- **HIV.** It is the cause of acquired immunodeficiency syndrome (AIDS). The Centers for Disease Control and Prevention (CDC) estimates that about 38,500 people in the United States contracted HIV in 2015. This risk of transfusion-transmitted HIV is extremely remote due to the rigorous testing of the U.S. blood supply.
- **Human T-cell lymphotropic virus (HTLV).** It is a viral infection prevalent in Japan, sub-Saharan Africa, the Caribbean Islands, and South America. HTLV can be spread from the mother to the child, through sexual contact, or via infected blood products. Though many infected remain asymptomatic, HTLV can lead to neoplastic diseases, inflammatory syndromes, and opportunistic infections.
- **West Nile virus (WNV).** It is a potentially serious illness. Experts believe WNV is established as a seasonal epidemic in North America that flares up in the summer and continues into the fall. Symptoms of the illness include fever, headache, tiredness, aches, and sometimes rash. Although WNV is most often transmitted by the bite of infected mosquitoes, the virus can also be transmitted through contact with infected animals, their blood, or other tissues.
- **Zika virus (ZIKV).** It is a mosquito-borne arbovirus spread by the *Aedes aegypti* mosquito. ZIKV can

be passed from a pregnant woman to her fetus, and infection during pregnancy can lead to serious birth defects. Symptoms of Zika include fever, rash, headache, joint pain, red eyes, and muscle pain. Transfusion-transmitted cases of ZIKV have been reported.

Prion Diseases

Prion diseases, or transmissible spongiform encephalopathies (TSEs), are a family of rare, progressive neurodegenerative disorders that affect both humans and animals. The causative agent of TSEs is believed to be a prion. A prion is an abnormal, transmissible agent that is able to induce abnormal folding of normal cellular prion proteins in the brain, leading to brain damage and the characteristics signs and symptoms of the disease. Prion diseases are usually rapidly progressive and always fatal. As with viruses, bacteria, and parasites, prions are blood-borne and may be transmitted by blood transfusion.

- **Variant Creutzfeldt-Jakob disease (vCJD).** It is a rare, rapidly progressing neurological disease that causes dementia and death. In 1996, cases of vCJD were first reported in the United Kingdom. Transmission of vCJD in the United Kingdom has been thought to be related to transfusions received years earlier with non-leukoreduced RBCs from healthy donors who became ill with vCJD months to less than four years after the donations. Recipients of blood components from other donors later diagnosed with vCJD remain under surveillance in the United Kingdom and France. The magnitude of the risk of acquiring vCJD from transfusion is uncertain.[3]

[3] "Diseases and Organisms," Centers for Disease Control and Prevention (CDC), September 29, 2022. Available online. URL: www.cdc.gov/bloodsafety/bbp/diseases-organisms.html#anchor_1555502078. Accessed July 18, 2023.

Section 4.3 | Contagious Disease Transmission in Travel Settings

IN-FLIGHT TRANSMISSION OF COMMUNICABLE DISEASES

Communicable diseases can be transmitted during air travel. People who are acutely ill or still within the infectious period for a specific disease should delay their travel until they are no longer contagious. For example, otherwise healthy adults can transmit influenza to others for five to seven days, and transmission of respiratory viruses (e.g., measles) has been documented on commercial aircraft.

Travelers should wash their hands frequently and thoroughly or use an alcohol-based hand sanitizer containing 60 or more percent alcohol, especially after using the airplane lavatory and before eating meals. Some diseases spread by contact with infectious droplets (e.g., when an ill person sneezes or coughs and the secretions or droplets land on another person's face, mouth, nose, or eyes) or when an ill person touches communal surfaces (e.g., door handles and restroom faucets) with contaminated hands. Other people handling the contaminated surfaces can then be inoculated with the contaminant. Practicing good handwashing and respiratory hygiene (covering the mouth with a tissue when coughing or sneezing) can help decrease the risk of infection by direct or indirect contact.

Cabin Ventilation and Air Filtration

Large commercial jet aircraft recirculate 35–55 percent of the air in the cabin, mixed with outside air. The recirculated air passes through high-efficiency particulate air (HEPA) filters that capture 99.97 percent of particles (bacteria, larger viruses or virus clumps, and fungi) greater than or equal to 0.3 µm in diameter. Furthermore, laminar airflow generally circulates in defined areas within the aircraft, thus limiting the radius of distribution of pathogens spread by small-particle aerosols. As a result, the cabin air environment is less conducive to the spread of most infectious diseases than typical environmental systems in buildings.[4]

---

[4] "Air Travel," Centers for Disease Control and Prevention (CDC), May 1, 2023. Available online. URL: wwwnc.cdc.gov/travel/yellowbook/2024/air-land-sea/air-travel#inflight. Accessed July 19, 2023.

PROTECTING TRAVELERS' HEALTH FROM AIRPORT TO COMMUNITY

What if a passenger was sick on your flight? What if that person was later diagnosed with a serious infectious disease and was contagious during your flight? Are you at risk? If you were exposed, how do you protect yourself?

Although the risk of getting a contagious disease on an airplane is low, public health officers sometimes need to find and alert travelers who may have been exposed to a sick passenger on a flight. The search for these travelers is known as a "contact investigation." A contact investigation is one of the ways the Centers for Disease Control and Prevention (CDC) works with partners in the United States and other countries to protect the health of people exposed to an illness during travel and to protect their communities from contagious diseases that are just a flight away.

Answering the Call

A contact investigation often starts with a phone call to a CDC Quarantine Station located at a U.S. International Airport. The caller is a public health official who informs the CDC about a recent air traveler diagnosed with a specific contagious disease. Sometimes, the CDC is notified about a sick traveler while the plane is still in the air or shortly after the plane has landed. However, in most cases, the CDC is notified when a sick traveler seeks treatment at a medical facility. These notifications can be made days, weeks, or even months after the travel. This sick traveler is now referred to as the "index patient."

The caller notifies the CDC because other passengers on the arriving international flights or connecting domestic flights may have been exposed and need to be notified. Or an international partner calls the CDC about exposed U.S. passengers on overseas flights. The passengers exposed to the index patient are called "contacts."

The CDC is responsible for coordinating contact investigations of illness exposures on arriving international flights or flights between states. A single infected traveler can trigger more than one contact investigation if the traveler takes connecting flights to reach a U.S. destination.

A person can be contagious without showing any symptoms while the disease is developing (incubating) in the body. Quarantine public health officers must determine whether the index patient was contagious during a flight. Their decision is based on the disease, history of symptoms, and date of the flight.

Starting the Contact Investigation

If the index patient was contagious during the flight, passengers seated nearby may have been exposed to the disease. The CDC will start a contact investigation to find these passengers.

The CDC requests the flight manifest for passengers seated near the index patient. The flight manifest is a document that contains passengers' names, seat numbers, and contact information. The CDC guards the privacy of passengers by keeping this information secure.

Diseases of Concern during Air Travel

Most flight contact investigations are performed for infectious tuberculosis (TB), measles, rubella (German measles), pertussis (whooping cough), and meningococcal disease (meningitis).

The CDC has developed instructions (protocols) for investigating contagious diseases. The CDC uses these protocols to identify passengers who may have been exposed during a flight. Identifying contacts is based on the disease, how it spreads, and where a passenger was seated in relation to the index patient.

Did You Provide Accurate Information?

Contact information from the flight manifest is often incomplete. The CDC relies on the U.S. Customs and Border Protection (CBP) for help with contact investigations involving international flights. The CBP can often provide more information that fills in the gaps. Remember to provide a current telephone number when making your flight reservations. Otherwise, how will you know if you were exposed if no one can reach you? The CDC staff then combined the information from the CBP and the airline's flight manifest to locate exposed passengers (contacts). At every step, the CDC protects the privacy of this information.

Protecting the Health of Passengers

The CDC provides the exposed passengers' contact information to state and local health departments or ministries of health in the countries where the passengers live. These agencies then try to locate these passengers and inform them about their exposure and what to do.

Exposed passengers (contacts) may be asked whether they are protected against (immune to) the specific disease. They can be immune if they had the disease in the past or have received a vaccine.

Public health officers will educate contacts about how to watch for and report symptoms of the illness being investigated. Contacts who are not immune (e.g., because they have not been vaccinated for the disease) may need to receive preventive drugs or a vaccine to protect them from the disease. Any recommendations will be based on the disease, availability of preventive drugs or vaccines, and the amount of time passed since exposure.

The contact investigation process is how federal agencies and airlines work together to help state and local health departments find exposed passengers. If you are considered a contact of an index patient on an airplane, they will call you. So make sure you leave a number where they can reach you.[5]

CRUISE SHIP TRAVEL AND TRANSMISSION OF COMMUNICABLE DISEASES

Cruise ship travel presents a unique combination of health concerns. Travelers from diverse regions brought together in the often crowded, semi-enclosed shipboard environment can facilitate the spread of person-to-person, foodborne, and waterborne diseases. Outbreaks on ships can be sustained over multiple voyages by crew members who remain onboard or by persistent environmental contamination. Port visits can expose travelers to local diseases and, conversely, be a conduit for disease introduction into shoreside communities.

[5] "Protecting Travelers' Health from Airport to Community: Investigating Contagious Diseases on Flights," Centers for Disease Control and Prevention (CDC), April 3, 2019. Available online. URL: www.cdc.gov/quarantine/contact-investigation.html. Accessed July 19, 2023.

Some people (e.g., those with chronic health conditions or who are immunocompromised, older people, and pregnant people) merit additional considerations when preparing for a cruise. Because travelers at sea might need to rely on a ship's medical capabilities for an extended period, potential cruise passengers with preexisting medical needs should prepare accordingly by calling the cruise line's customer service center to learn what type and level of health-care services are (and are not) available on specific ships.

Cruise Ship Medical Capabilities

Medical facilities on cruise ships can vary widely depending on ship size, itinerary, cruise duration, and passenger demographics. Generally, shipboard medical centers can provide medical care comparable to that of ambulatory care centers; some are capable of providing hospitalization services or renal dialysis. Although no agency officially regulates medical practice aboard cruise ships, the American College of Emergency Physicians (ACEP) published consensus-based guidelines for cruise ship medical facilities in 1995 and updated the guidelines in 2013. ACEP guidelines, which most major cruise lines follow, state that cruise ship medical facilities should be able to provide quality medical care for passengers and crew; initiate appropriate stabilization, diagnostic, and therapeutic maneuvers for critically ill or medically unstable patients; and assist in the medical evacuation of patients in a timely fashion, when appropriate.

Illness and Injury

Cruise ship medical centers deal with a wide variety of illnesses and injuries; approximately 10 percent of conditions reported to cruise ship medical centers are an emergency or require urgent care. Approximately 95 percent of illnesses are treated or managed onboard, with the remainder requiring evacuation and shoreside consultation for dental, medical, or surgical issues. Roughly half of all passengers seeking medical care are aged 65 or over.

Medical center visits are primarily the result of acute illness or injury. The most frequently reported diagnoses include respiratory illnesses (30–40%); injuries from slips, trips, or falls (12–18%); seasickness (10%); and gastrointestinal (GI) illness (10%), and 80 percent of onboard deaths are due to cardiovascular events.

Infectious Disease Outbreaks

The most frequently reported cruise ship outbreaks involve GI infections (e.g., norovirus), respiratory infections (e.g., coronavirus disease 2019 (COVID-19) and influenza), and other vaccine-preventable diseases (VPDs), such as varicella. Although cruise ships do not have public health authority to reduce the risk of introducing communicable diseases, some ships conduct medical screening during embarkation to identify ill passengers, prevent them from boarding, or require isolation if permission to board is given.

Before travel, to help limit the introduction and spread of communicable diseases on cruise ships, prospective cruise ship travelers and their clinicians should consult the CDC Travelers' Health website (https://wwwnc.cdc.gov/travel/) for updates on outbreaks and destination-specific travel health notices. People who become ill with a communicable disease before a voyage should consult their health-care provider and delay their travel until they are no longer contagious. When booking a cruise, travelers should check the trip cancellation policies and consider purchasing trip cancellation insurance.

Travelers who become ill during a voyage should seek care in the ship's medical center; the onboard staff will provide clinical management, facilitate infection-control measures, and take responsibility for reporting potential public health events.

INFECTIOUS DISEASE HEALTH RISKS

Gastrointestinal Illnesses

During 2006–2019, rates of GI illness among passengers on voyages lasting 3–21 days fell from 32.5 to 16.9 cases per 100,000 travel days. Despite the decrease, outbreaks continue to occur. The CDC assists the cruise ship industry in preventing and controlling the introduction, transmission, and spread of GI illnesses on cruise ships.

NOROVIRUS

On cruise ships, more than 90 percent of GI illness outbreaks with a confirmed cause are due to norovirus. Characteristics of norovirus that facilitate outbreaks include a low infective dose, easy person-to-person transmissibility, prolonged viral shedding, absence of long-term immunity, and the ability of the virus to survive routine cleaning procedures. For international cruise ships porting in the United States during 2006–2019, an average of 12 norovirus outbreaks occurred each year.

OTHER SOURCES OF GASTROINTESTINAL ILLNESS

GI outbreaks on cruise ships also have been caused by contaminated food or water; most outbreaks were associated with *Campylobacter*, *Clostridium perfringens*, or enterotoxigenic *Escherichia coli*.

PROTECTIVE MEASURES

Travelers can reduce the risk of acquiring a GI illness on cruise ships by frequently washing hands with soap and water, especially before eating and after using the restroom. Travelers should call the ship's medical center promptly, even for mild symptoms of a GI illness, and strictly follow cruise ship guidance regarding isolation and other infection-control measures.

Respiratory Illnesses

Respiratory illnesses are the most common medical complaint on cruise ships. During the pretravel visit, evaluate whether vaccines or boosters (e.g., COVID-19 and influenza) are needed and emphasize the importance of practicing good respiratory hygiene and cough etiquette while onboard. As with GI illnesses, cruise ship passengers should report respiratory illness to the medical center promptly and follow isolation recommendations as instructed.

CORONAVIRUS DISEASE 2019

Severe acute respiratory syndrome coronavirus 2 (SARS-CoV-2), the virus that causes COVID-19, spreads more easily between people in close quarters, and multiple studies have concluded that transmission rates of SARS-CoV-2 among travelers on ships are much greater than in other settings. Cruise ship COVID-19 outbreaks can tax onboard medical and public health resources. Ship-to-shore medical evacuations to facilities capable of providing higher levels of medical care can present logistical challenges and pose additional risks to ill patients.

Cruise passengers and crew members who are not up-to-date with their COVID-19 vaccines are at increased risk for severe illness, hospitalization, medical evacuation, and death. Since cruising will always pose some risk of SARS-CoV-2 transmission, ensure that people planning cruise ship travel are up-to-date with their vaccinations and assess their likelihood of developing severe COVID-19. For people at increased risk of severe COVID-19 regardless of their vaccination status (e.g., pregnant people and people who are immunocompromised), discuss the potential health hazards associated with cruise ship travel. The CDC has developed recommendations and guidance designed to help cruise ship operators provide a safer and healthier environment for crew members, passengers, port personnel, and communities.

INFLUENZA

Historically, influenza has been among the most often reported VPDs occurring on cruise ships. Because passengers and crew originate from all regions of the globe, shipboard outbreaks of influenza A and B can occur year-round, with exposure to strains circulating in different parts of the world. Thus, anyone planning a cruise should receive the current seasonal influenza vaccine two weeks or more before travel if the vaccine is available and no contraindications exist. For people at high risk for influenza complications, health-care providers should discuss chemoprophylaxis and how and when to initiate antiviral treatment.

LEGIONNAIRES' DISEASE

Less common on cruise ships, Legionnaires' disease is nevertheless a treatable infection that can result in severe pneumonia leading to death. Approximately 10–15 percent of all Legionnaires' disease cases reported to the CDC occur in people who have traveled during the 10 days before symptom onset. Clusters of Legionnaires' disease associated with hotel or cruise ship travel can be difficult to detect because travelers often disperse from the source of infection before symptoms begin. Data reported to the CDC during 2014–2015 included 25 confirmed cases of Legionnaires' disease associated with cruise ship exposures.

In general, Legionnaires' disease is contracted by inhaling warm, aerosolized water containing the bacteria *Legionella*. Transmission can also sometimes occur through aspiration of *Legionella*-containing water. Typically, people do not spread *Legionella* to others; a single episode of possible person-to-person transmission of Legionnaires' disease has been reported. Contaminated hot tubs are commonly implicated as a source of shipboard *Legionella* outbreaks although potable water supply systems also have been culpable. Improvements in ship design and standardization of water disinfection have reduced the risk for *Legionella* growth and colonization.

DIAGNOSIS AND REPORTING

People with suspected Legionnaires' disease require prompt antibiotic treatment. When evaluating cruise travelers for Legionnaires' disease, obtain a thorough travel history of all destinations during the 10 days before symptom onset to assist in identifying potential sources of exposure and collect urine for *Legionella* antigen testing. Most cruise ships have the capacity to perform this test, which detects *L. pneumophila* serogroup 1, the most common serogroup.

Perform culture of lower respiratory secretions on selective media to detect non–*L. pneumophila* serogroup one species and serogroups. Culture is also used for comparing clinical isolates to environmental isolates during an outbreak investigation. Notify the CDC of any travel-associated Legionnaires' disease cases by sending an email to travellegionella@cdc.gov. Quickly report all cases of Legionnaires' disease to public health officials, who can determine whether a case links to previously reported cases and work to stop potential clusters and new outbreaks.

Other Vaccine-Preventable Diseases

Although most cruise ship passengers come from countries with routine vaccination programs (e.g., Canada and the United States), many of the crew are from low- or middle-income countries where immunization rates can be low. Outbreaks of hepatitis A, measles, meningococcal disease, mumps, pertussis, rubella, and varicella have all been reported on cruise ships. The majority (82%) of these outbreaks occurred among crew members; prior to the COVID-19 pandemic, varicella was the most frequently reported VPD. Other VPDs (e.g., pertussis) occur more often among passengers.

Each cruise line sets its own policies regarding vaccinations for its crew; some have limited or no requirements. Thus, all passengers should be up-to-date with routine vaccinations before travel, as well as any required or recommended vaccinations specific to their destinations. People of childbearing age should have documented immunity to measles, rubella, and varicella (either by vaccination or titer) before cruise ship travel.

Vector-Borne Diseases

Some cruise ship ports of call include destinations where vector-borne diseases (e.g., dengue, Japanese encephalitis, malaria, yellow fever, and Zika) are known to be endemic. In addition, new diseases can surface in unexpected locations; chikungunya was reported for the first time in the Caribbean in late 2013, with subsequent spread throughout the region and numerous other North, Central, and South American countries and territories. Zika was first reported in Brazil in 2015 and subsequently spread across the Caribbean and Latin America, sparking concern because of its association with microcephaly and other congenital abnormalities in the fetus.

NONINFECTIOUS HEALTH RISKS

Stresses of cruise ship travel include varying weather and environmental conditions, unaccustomed changes to diet, and levels of physical activity. Despite modern stabilizer systems, seasickness is a common complaint, affecting up to 25 percent of travelers. Note that travel is an independent risk factor for behaviors, such as alcohol and illicit drug use and misuse and unsafe sex.[6]

[6] "Cruise Ship Travel," Centers for Disease Control and Prevention (CDC), May 1, 2023. Available online. URL: wwwnc.cdc.gov/travel/yellowbook/2024/air-land-sea/cruise-ship-travel. Accessed July 19, 2023.

Part 2 | **Viral Contagious Diseases**

Chapter 5 | **Adenovirus Infections**

WHAT ARE ADENOVIRUS INFECTIONS?

Adenoviruses are common. These viruses typically cause mild cold or flu-like illness. Adenoviruses (refer to Figure 5.1) can cause illness in people of all ages at any time of year.

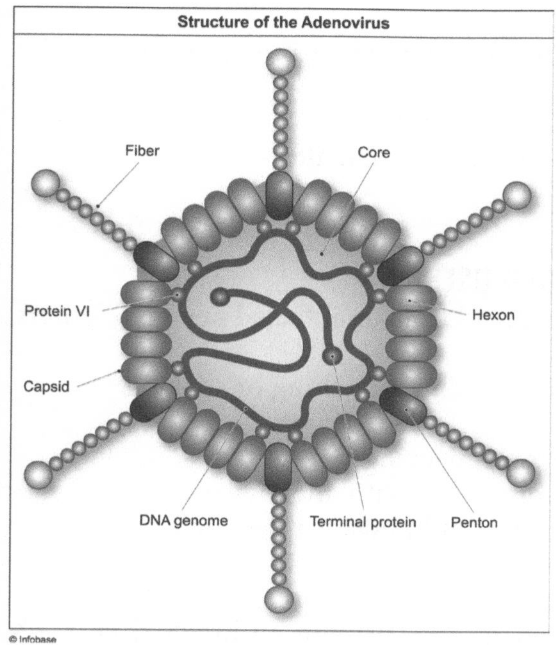

Figure 5.1. Structure of the Adenovirus

Infobase

SYMPTOMS OF ADENOVIRUSES

Adenoviruses can cause mild-to-severe illness though serious illness is less common. People with weakened immune systems, or existing respiratory or cardiac disease, are at higher risk of developing severe illness from an adenovirus infection.

Adenoviruses can cause a wide range of illnesses such as:

- common cold or flu-like symptoms
- fever
- sore throat
- acute bronchitis (inflammation of the airways of the lungs, sometimes called a "chest cold")
- pneumonia (infection of the lungs)
- pink eye (conjunctivitis)
- acute gastroenteritis (inflammation of the stomach or intestines causing diarrhea, vomiting, nausea, and stomach pain)

Less common symptoms of adenovirus infection include the following:

- bladder inflammation or infection
- neurologic disease (conditions that affect the brain and spinal cord)

TRANSMISSION OF ADENOVIRUSES

Adenoviruses are usually spread from an infected person to others through:

- close personal contact, such as touching or shaking hands
- the air by coughing and sneezing
- touching an object or surface with adenoviruses on it, then touching your mouth, nose, or eyes before washing your hands

Some adenoviruses can spread through an infected person's stool, for example, during diaper changing. Adenovirus can also spread through the water, such as swimming pools, but this is less common.

Length of Transmission

Sometimes, the virus can be shed (released from the body) for a long time after a person recovers from an adenovirus infection, especially among people who have weakened immune systems. This "virus shedding" usually occurs without any symptoms, even though the person can still spread adenovirus to other people.

TREATMENT OF ADENOVIRUSES

There are no approved antiviral medicines and no specific treatment for people with adenovirus infection. Most adenovirus infections are mild and may be managed with rest and over-the-counter (OTC) pain medicines or fever reducers to help relieve symptoms. Always read the label and use medications as directed. If you have concerns, you should speak with your health-care provider.

Adenovirus Vaccine Is for the U.S. Military Only

There is a vaccine for adenovirus types 4 and 7 that is used in military personnel who may be at higher risk for infection from these two adenovirus types. This vaccine contains live virus that can be shed in the stool and potentially cause disease in other people if transmitted. The safety and effectiveness of this vaccine has not been studied in the general population or in people with weakened immune systems, and it is not approved for use outside of the military. There is currently no adenovirus vaccine available to the general public.

PREVENTION OF ADENOVIRUSES

If you are sick, you can help protect others:

- Stay home when you are sick.
- Cough and sneeze into a tissue or your upper shirt sleeve, not your hands.
- Avoid sharing cups and eating utensils with others.
- Refrain from kissing others.
- Wash your hands often with soap and water for at least 20 seconds, especially after using the bathroom.

Frequent handwashing is especially important in childcare settings and health-care facilities.

Follow Simple Steps to Protect Yourself and Others

You can protect yourself and others from adenoviruses and other respiratory illnesses by following a few simple steps:

- Wash your hands often with soap and water for at least 20 seconds.
- Avoid touching your eyes, nose, or mouth with unwashed hands.
- Avoid close contact with people who are sick.

Maintain Proper Chlorine Levels to Prevent Outbreaks in Swimming Pools

It is important to keep adequate levels of chlorine in swimming pools to prevent outbreaks of conjunctivitis caused by adenoviruses. The Centers for Disease Control and Prevention (CDC) Healthy Swimming website (www.cdc.gov/healthywater/swimming) provides more information on how to maintain healthy and safe swimming environments.[1]

[1] "Adenoviruses," Centers for Disease Control and Prevention (CDC), November 28, 2022. Available online. URL: www.cdc.gov/adenovirus/index.html. Accessed June 22, 2023.

Chapter 6 | **Chickenpox and Shingles**

CHICKENPOX

Chickenpox is a highly contagious disease caused by the varicella-zoster virus (VZV). It can cause an itchy, blister-like rash among other symptoms. The rash first appears on the chest, back, and face and then spreads over the entire body.

Chickenpox can be serious, especially during pregnancy and in babies, adolescents, adults, and people with weakened immune systems (lowered ability to fight germs and sickness). The best way to prevent chickenpox is to get the chickenpox vaccine.

Signs and Symptoms of Chickenpox

Anyone who has not had chickenpox or gotten the chickenpox vaccine can get the disease. Chickenpox illness usually lasts about four to seven days.

The classic symptom of chickenpox is a rash that turns into itchy, fluid-filled blisters that eventually turn into scabs. The rash may first show up on the chest, back, and face and then spread over the entire body, including inside the mouth, eyelids, or genital area. It usually takes about one week for all of the blisters to become scabs. Other typical symptoms that may begin to appear one to two days before rash include:

- fever
- tiredness
- loss of appetite
- headache

Children usually miss five to six days of school or childcare due to chickenpox.

CHICKENPOX IN VACCINATED PEOPLE (BREAKTHROUGH CHICKENPOX)

Some people who have been vaccinated against chickenpox can still get the disease. However, they usually have milder symptoms with fewer or no blisters (or just red spots), a mild or no fever, and are sick for a shorter period of time than people who are not vaccinated. But some vaccinated people who get chickenpox may have a disease similar to unvaccinated people.

PEOPLE AT RISK FOR SEVERE CHICKENPOX

Some people who get chickenpox may have more severe symptoms and may be at higher risk for complications.

Transmission of Chickenpox

Chickenpox is a highly contagious disease caused by the VZV. The virus spreads easily from people with chickenpox to others who have never had the disease or have never been vaccinated. If one person has it, up to 90 percent of the people close to that person who are not immune will also become infected. The virus spreads mainly through close contact with someone who has chickenpox.

A person with chickenpox is considered contagious, beginning one to two days before rash onset until all the chickenpox lesions have crusted (scabbed). Vaccinated people who get chickenpox may develop lesions that do not crust. These people are considered contagious until no new lesions have appeared for 24 hours.

The VZV also causes shingles (refer to Figure 6.1). After chickenpox, the virus remains in the body (dormant). People get shingles when VZV reactivates in their bodies after they have already had chickenpox. People with shingles can spread VZV to people who have never had chickenpox or never received the chickenpox vaccine. This can happen through direct contact with fluid from shingles rash blisters or through breathing in virus particles that come from the blisters. If they get infected, they will develop chickenpox, not shingles.

It takes about two weeks (from 10 to 21 days) after exposure to a person with chickenpox or shingles for someone to develop chickenpox. If a vaccinated person gets the disease, they can still spread it to others. For most people, getting chickenpox once provides immunity for life. It is possible to get chickenpox more than once, but this is not common.

Complications of Chickenpox

Complications from chickenpox can occur, but they are not common in healthy people who get the disease. People who may get a serious case of chickenpox and may be at high risk for complications include:

- infants
- adolescents
- adults
- people who are pregnant
- people with bodies that have a lowered ability to fight germs and sickness (weakened immune systems) because of illness or medications, for example:
  - people with human immunodeficiency virus (HIV)/acquired immunodeficiency syndrome (AIDS) or cancer
  - patients who have had transplants
  - people on chemotherapy, immunosuppressive medications, or long-term use of steroids

Serious complications from chickenpox include:

- bacterial infections of the skin and soft tissues in children, including group A streptococcal infections
- infection of the lungs (pneumonia)
- infection or swelling of the brain (encephalitis and cerebellar ataxia)
- bleeding problems (hemorrhagic complications)
- bloodstream infections (sepsis)
- dehydration

Some people with serious complications from chickenpox can become so sick that they need to be hospitalized. Chickenpox can also cause death.

Deaths are very rare now due to the vaccine program. However, some deaths from chickenpox continue to occur in healthy, unvaccinated children and adults. In the past, many of the healthy adults who died from chickenpox contracted the disease from their unvaccinated children.

Prevention and Treatment of Chickenpox

The best way to prevent chickenpox is to get the chickenpox vaccine. Everyone—including children, adolescents, and adults—should get two doses of chickenpox vaccine if they have never had chickenpox or were never vaccinated.

Chickenpox vaccine is very safe and effective at preventing the disease. Most people who get the vaccine will not get chickenpox. If a vaccinated person does get chickenpox, the symptoms are usually milder with fewer or no blisters (they may have just red spots) and low or no fever.

The chickenpox vaccine prevents almost all cases of severe illness. Since the chickenpox vaccination program began in the United States, there has been over 97 percent decrease in chickenpox cases. Hospitalizations and deaths have become rare.

TREATMENTS AT HOME FOR PEOPLE WITH CHICKENPOX

There are several things that you can do at home to help relieve chickenpox symptoms and prevent skin infections. Calamine lotion and a cool bath with added baking soda, uncooked oatmeal, or colloidal oatmeal may help relieve some of the itching. Try to keep fingernails trimmed short and minimize scratching to prevent the virus from spreading to others and to help prevent skin infections. If you do scratch a blister by accident, wash your hands with soap and water for at least 20 seconds.

OVER-THE-COUNTER MEDICATIONS

Do not use aspirin or aspirin-containing products to relieve fever from chickenpox. The use of aspirin in children with chickenpox has been associated with Reye syndrome, a severe disease that affects the liver and brain and can cause death. Instead, use nonaspirin medications, such as acetaminophen, to relieve fever from chickenpox. The American Academy of Pediatrics (AAP) recommends avoiding treatment with ibuprofen if possible because it has been associated with life-threatening bacterial skin infections.

WHEN TO CALL A HEALTH-CARE PROVIDER

For people exposed to chickenpox or shingles, call a health-care provider if the person:

- has never had chickenpox and is not vaccinated with the chickenpox vaccine
- is pregnant
- has a lowered ability to fight germs and sickness (weakened immune system) caused by disease or medication, for example:
    - a person with HIV/AIDS or cancer
    - a person who has had a transplant
    - a person on chemotherapy, immunosuppressive medications, or long-term use of steroids

If you have symptoms, call your health-care provider. Contacting a health-care provider is especially important if the person:

- is at risk of serious complications from chickenpox because they:
    - are less than one year old
    - are older than 12 years of age
    - have a weakened immune system
    - are pregnant
- develops any of the following symptoms:
    - fever that lasts longer than four days
    - fever that rises above 102 °F (38.9 °C)
    - any areas of the rash or any part of the body becomes very red, warm, or tender or begins leaking pus (thick, discolored fluid), as these symptoms may indicate a bacterial infection
    - difficulty waking up or confused behavior
    - difficulty walking
    - stiff neck

- frequent vomiting
- difficulty breathing
- severe cough
- severe abdominal pain
- rash with bleeding or bruising (hemorrhagic rash)

TREATMENTS PRESCRIBED BY YOUR HEALTH-CARE PROVIDER FOR PEOPLE WITH CHICKENPOX

Your health-care provider can advise you on treatment options. Antiviral medications are recommended for people with chickenpox that are more likely to develop serious illness, including:

- otherwise healthy people older than 12 years of age
- people with chronic skin or lung disease
- people receiving long-term salicylate therapy or steroid therapy
- people who are pregnant
- people with a weakened immune system

There are antiviral medications licensed for the treatment of chickenpox. The medication works best if it is given as early as possible, preferably within the first 24 hours after the rash starts.[1]

SHINGLES

What Is Shingles?

Shingles, also called "herpes zoster," is a disease that triggers a painful skin rash. It is caused by the same virus as chickenpox, the VZV. After you recover from chickenpox (usually as a child), the virus continues to live in some of your nerve cells. For most adults, the virus is inactive, and it never leads to shingles (refer to Figure 6.1). But, for about one in three adults, the virus will become active again and cause shingles.

[1] "About Chickenpox," Centers for Disease Control and Prevention (CDC), October 21, 2022. Available online. URL: www.cdc.gov/chickenpox/about/index.html. Accessed June 22, 2023.

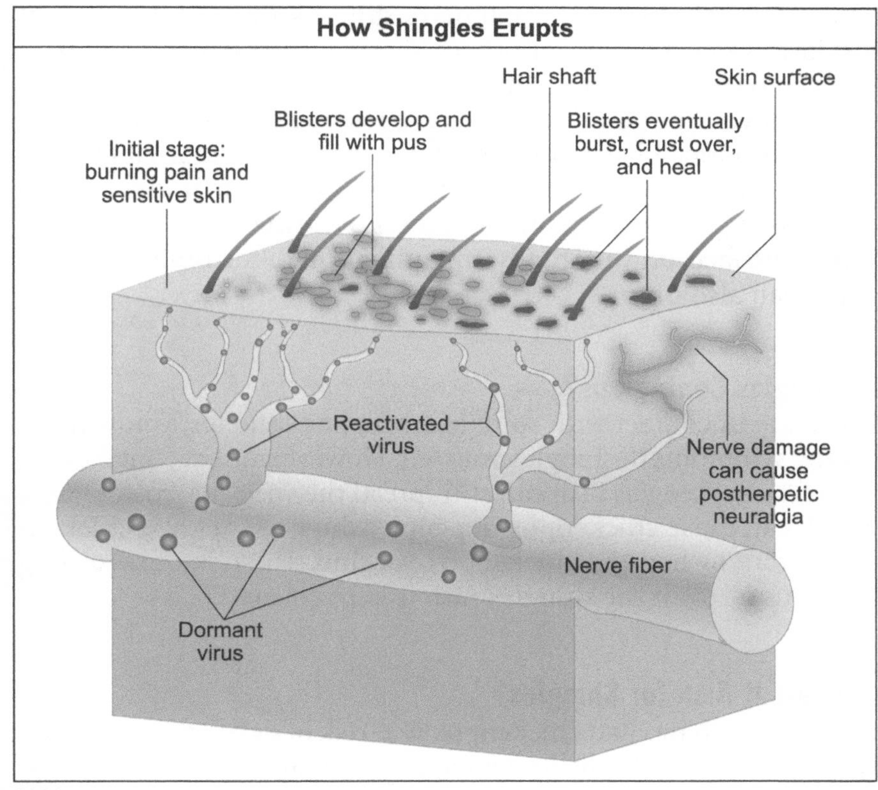

Figure 6.1. How Shingles Erupts

Infobase

What Are the Symptoms of Shingles?

Usually, shingles develops on just one side of the body or face and in a small area. The most common place for shingles to occur is in a band around one side of the waistline. Most people with shingles have one or more of the following symptoms:

- fluid-filled blisters
- burning, shooting pain
- tingling, itching, or numbness of the skin
- chills, fever, headache, or upset stomach

For some people, the symptoms of shingles are mild. They might just have some itching. For others, shingles can cause intense pain that can be felt from the gentlest touch or breeze. It is important to talk with your doctor if you notice any shingles symptoms.

If you notice blisters on your face, see your doctor right away because this is an urgent problem. Blisters near or in the eye can cause lasting eye damage and blindness. Hearing loss, a brief paralysis of the face, or, very rarely, inflammation of the brain (encephalitis) can also occur.

Is Shingles Contagious?

If you are in contact with someone who has shingles, you will not get the symptoms of shingles yourself. However, direct contact with fluid from a shingles rash can still spread the varicella-zoster virus, which can cause chickenpox in people who have not had chickenpox before or had the chickenpox vaccine. The risk of spreading the virus is low if the shingles rash is kept covered.

Are You at Risk for Shingles?

Everyone who has had chickenpox is at risk of developing shingles. Researchers do not fully understand what makes the virus become active and cause shingles. But some things make it more likely:

- **Older age**. The risk of developing shingles increases as you age. About half of all shingles cases are in adults aged 60 or older. The chance of getting shingles becomes much greater by age 70.
- **Trouble fighting infections**. Your immune system is the part of your body that responds to infections. Age can affect your immune system. So can HIV, cancer, cancer treatments, too much sun, and organ transplant drugs. Even stress or a cold can weaken your immune system for a short time. These all can put you at risk for shingles.

Most people only have shingles one time. However, it is possible to have it more than once.

How Long Does Shingles Last?

- Most cases of shingles last three to five weeks.
- The first sign is often burning or tingling pain; sometimes, it includes numbness or itching on one side of the body.
- Somewhere between one and five days after the tingling or burning feeling on the skin, a red rash will appear.
- A few days later, the rash will turn into fluid-filled blisters.
- About one week to ten days after that, the blisters dry up and crust over.
- A couple of weeks later, the scabs clear up.

LONG-TERM PAIN

After the shingles rash goes away, some people may be left with ongoing pain called "postherpetic neuralgia" (PHN). The pain is felt in the area where the rash occurred. The older you are when you get shingles, the greater your chances of developing PHN.

The PHN pain can cause depression, anxiety, sleeplessness, and weight loss. Some people with PHN find it hard to go about their daily activities, such as dressing, cooking, and eating. Talk with your doctor if you are experiencing PHN or have any of these symptoms. Usually, PHN will lessen over time.

How Are Shingles Diagnosed and Treated?

If you think you might have shingles, talk to your doctor as soon as possible. It is important to see your doctor no later than three days after the rash starts. The doctor will confirm whether you have shingles and can make a treatment plan. Most cases can be diagnosed from a visual examination. If you have a condition that weakens the immune system, your doctor may order a shingles test. Although there is no cure for shingles, early treatment with antiviral medications can help the blisters clear up faster and limit severe pain. Shingles can often be treated at home.

When Should You Get the Shingles Vaccine?

The current shingles vaccine (brand name: Shingrix) is a safe, easy, and more effective way to prevent shingles than the previous vaccine. In fact, it is over 90 percent effective at preventing shingles. Most adults aged 50 and older should get vaccinated with the shingles vaccine, which is given in two doses. You can get the shingles vaccine at your doctor's office and some pharmacies.

You should get the shingles vaccine if you:

- have already had chickenpox, the chickenpox vaccine, or shingles
- received the prior shingles vaccine called "Zostavax"
- do not remember having had chickenpox

Medicare Part D (www.medicare.gov/drug-coverage-part-d) and private health insurance plans may cover some or all of the cost. Check with Medicare or your health plan to find out if it is covered. You should not get vaccinated if you:

- currently have shingles
- are sick or have a fever
- had an allergic reaction to a previous dose of the shingles vaccine

If you are unsure about the above criteria or have other health concerns, talk with your doctor before getting the vaccine.

Tips for Coping with Shingles

If you have shingles, here are some tips that might help you feel better:

- Wear loose-fitting, natural-fiber clothing.
- Take an oatmeal bath or use calamine lotion to soothe your skin.
- Apply a cool washcloth to your blisters to ease the pain and help dry the blisters.
- Keep the area clean and try not to scratch the blisters, so they do not become infected or leave a scar.
- Do things that take your mind off your pain. For example, watch TV, read, talk with friends, listen to relaxing music, or work on a hobby, such as crafts or gardening.
- Get plenty of rest and eat well-balanced meals.

- Try simple exercises, such as stretching or walking. Check with your doctor before starting a new exercise routine.
- Avoid stress. It can make the pain worse.
- Share your feelings about your pain with family and friends. Ask for their understanding.

Also, you can limit the spreading of the virus to other people by:

- staying away from anyone who has not had chickenpox or the chickenpox vaccine or who might have a weakened immune system
- keeping the rash covered
- not touching or scratching the rash
- washing your hands often[2]

[2] National Institute on Aging (NIA), "Shingles," National Institutes of Health (NIH), October 12, 2021. Available online. URL: www.nia.nih.gov/health/shingles. Accessed June 22, 2023.

Chapter 7 | Common Colds

WHAT ARE COMMON COLDS?

Sneezing, stuffy nose, and runny nose? You might have a cold. Colds are one of the most frequent reasons for missed school and work. Every year, adults have an average of two to three colds, and children have even more. Antibiotics do not work against viruses that cause colds and will not help you feel better.

CAUSES OF COMMON COLD

More than 200 viruses can cause a cold, but rhinoviruses are the most common type. Viruses that cause colds can spread from person to person through the air and close personal contact.

RISK FACTORS OF COMMON COLD

Many factors can increase your risk of catching a cold, including the following:

- close contact with someone who has a cold
- season (Colds are more common during the fall and winter, but it is possible to get a cold any time of the year.)
- age (infants and young children have more colds per year than adults)

SYMPTOMS OF COMMON COLD

Symptoms of a cold usually peak within two to three days and can include the following:

- sneezing
- stuffy nose

- runny nose
- sore throat
- coughing
- mucus dripping down your throat (postnasal drip)
- watery eyes
- fever (although most people with colds do not have fever)

When viruses that cause colds first infect the nose and sinuses, the nose makes clear mucus. This helps wash the viruses from the nose and sinuses. After two or three days, mucus may change to a white, yellow, or green color. This is normal and does not mean you need an antibiotic. Some symptoms, especially runny or stuffy nose and cough, can last for up to 10–14 days. Those symptoms should improve over time.

WHEN TO SEEK MEDICAL CARE

See a doctor if you have:

- trouble breathing or fast breathing
- dehydration
- fever that lasts longer than four days
- symptoms that last more than 10 days without improvement
- symptoms, such as fever or cough, that improve but then return or worsen
- worsening of chronic medical conditions

This list is not all-inclusive. Please see a doctor for any symptom that is severe or concerning.

Colds can have similar symptoms to the flu. It can be difficult (or even impossible) to tell the difference between them based on symptoms alone.

TREATMENT OF COMMON COLD

Your doctor can determine if you have a cold by asking about your symptoms and examining you. Your doctor may also need to order laboratory tests.

There is no cure for a cold. It will get better on its own—without antibiotics. Antibiotics will not help you get better if you have a cold.

When antibiotics are not needed, they will not help you, and their side effects could still cause harm. Side effects can range from mild reactions, such as a rash, to more serious health problems. These problems can include severe allergic reactions, antibiotic-resistant infections, and *Clostridium difficile* infection. *Clostridium difficile* causes diarrhea that can lead to severe colon damage and death.

HOW TO FEEL BETTER

Below are some ways you can feel better while your body fights off a cold:

- Get plenty of rest.
- Drink plenty of fluids.
- Use a clean humidifier or cool mist vaporizer.
- Use saline nasal spray or drops:
  - For young children, use a rubber suction bulb to clear mucus.
- Breathe in steam from a bowl of hot water or shower.
- Use throat lozenges or cough drops. Do not give lozenges to children younger than four years of age.
- Use honey to relieve cough for adults and children at least one year of age or older.

Ask your doctor or pharmacist about over-the-counter (OTC) medicines that can help you feel better. Always use OTC medicines as directed. Remember, over-the-counter medicines may provide temporary relief of symptoms, but they will not cure your illness.[1]

[1] "Common Cold," Centers for Disease Control and Prevention (CDC), June 27, 2023. Available online. URL: www.cdc.gov/antibiotic-use/colds.html. Accessed July 18, 2023.

Chapter 8 | **Conjunctivitis**

WHAT IS CONJUNCTIVITIS?

People often call conjunctivitis "pink eye" because it can cause the white of the eye to take on a pink or red color. Symptoms of pink eye can vary but typically include redness or swelling of the white of the eye.

CAUSES OF CONJUNCTIVITIS

The most common causes of conjunctivitis (pink eye) are:

- viruses
- bacteria
- allergens

Other causes include the following:

- chemicals
- contact lens
- foreign bodies in the eye (such as a loose eyelash)
- indoor and outdoor air pollution caused, for example, by smoke, dust, fumes, or chemical vapors
- fungi
- amoeba and parasites

It can be difficult to determine the exact cause of conjunctivitis because some symptoms may be the same no matter the cause.

Viral Conjunctivitis

- infection of the eye caused by a virus
- number of different viruses, such as adenoviruses
- very contagious
- sometimes resulting in large outbreaks depending on the virus

Bacterial Conjunctivitis

- infection of the eye caused by certain bacteria
- caused by *Staphylococcus aureus, Streptococcus pneumoniae, Haemophilus influenzae, Moraxella catarrhalis*, or, less commonly, *Chlamydia trachomatis* and *Neisseria gonorrhoeae*
- spreading easily, especially with certain bacteria and in certain settings
- more common in kids than adults
- observed more frequently from December through April

Children with conjunctivitis without fever or behavioral changes can usually continue going to school.

Allergic Conjunctivitis

- the result of the body's reaction to allergens, such as pollen from trees, plants, grasses, and weeds; dust mites; molds; dander from pets; medicines; or cosmetics
- not contagious
- occurring more frequently among people with other allergic conditions, such as hay fever, asthma, and eczema
- occurring seasonally when allergens, such as pollen counts, are high
- occurring year-round due to indoor allergens, such as dust mites and animal dander

Conjunctivitis Caused by Irritants

- caused by irritation from a foreign body in the eye or contact with smoke, dust, fumes, or chemicals
- not contagious
- occurring when contact lenses are worn longer than recommended or not cleaned properly

SYMPTOMS OF CONJUNCTIVITIS

Symptoms of conjunctivitis (pink eye) can include the following:

- pink or red color in the white of the eye(s)
- swelling of the conjunctiva (the thin layer that lines the white part of the eye and the inside of the eyelid) and/or eyelids
- increased tear production
- feeling like a foreign body is in the eye(s) or an urge to rub the eye(s)
- itching, irritation, and/or burning
- discharge (pus or mucus)
- crusting of eyelids or lashes, especially in the morning
- contact lenses that feel uncomfortable and/or do not stay in place on the eye

Depending on the cause, other symptoms may occur.

Viral Conjunctivitis

- occurring with symptoms of a cold, flu, or other respiratory infection
- beginning usually in one eye and spreading to the other eye within days
- watery, rather than thick, discharge from the eye

Bacterial Conjunctivitis

- more commonly associated with discharge (pus), which can lead to eyelids sticking together
- sometimes occurring with an ear infection

Allergic Conjunctivitis

- usually occurring in both eyes
- producing intense itching, tearing, and swelling in the eyes
- occurring with symptoms of allergies, such as an itchy nose, sneezing, a scratchy throat, or asthma

Conjunctivitis Caused by Irritants

- producing watery eyes and mucus discharge

TRANSMISSION OF CONJUNCTIVITIS

How It Spreads

Several viruses and bacteria can cause conjunctivitis (pink eye), some of which are very contagious. Each of these types of germs can spread from person to person in different ways. They usually spread from an infected person to others through:

- close personal contact, such as touching or shaking hands
- the air by coughing and sneezing
- touching an object or surface with germs on it, then touching your eyes before washing your hands

When to Go Back to Work or School

If you have conjunctivitis but do not have a fever or other symptoms, you may be allowed to remain at work or school with your doctor's approval. However, if you still have symptoms and your activities at work or school include close contact with other people, you should not attend.

DIAGNOSIS OF CONJUNCTIVITIS

A doctor can often determine whether a virus, bacterium, or allergen is causing conjunctivitis (pink eye) based on patient history, symptoms, and an examination of the eye. Conjunctivitis always involves eye redness or swelling, but it also has other symptoms that can vary depending on the cause. These symptoms can help a health-care professional diagnose the cause of conjunctivitis. However, it can sometimes be difficult to make a firm diagnosis because some symptoms are the same no matter the cause.

It can also sometimes be difficult to determine the cause without doing laboratory testing. Although not routinely done, your health-care provider may collect a sample of eye discharge from the infected eye and send it to the laboratory to help them determine which form of infection you have and how best to treat it.

Viral Conjunctivitis

The cause is likely a virus if:

- conjunctivitis accompanies a common cold or respiratory tract infection
- discharge from the eye is watery rather than thick

Bacterial Conjunctivitis

The cause may be bacterial if:

- conjunctivitis occurs at the same time as an ear infection
- it occurs shortly after birth
- discharge from the eye is thick rather than watery

Allergic Conjunctivitis

The cause is likely allergic if:

- conjunctivitis occurs seasonally when pollen counts are high
- the patient's eyes itch intensely
- it occurs with other signs of allergic disease, such as hay fever, asthma, or eczema

PREVENTION OF CONJUNCTIVITIS

Preventing the Spread of Conjunctivitis

Viral and bacterial conjunctivitis (pink eye) is very contagious. They can spread easily from person to person. You can greatly reduce the risk of getting conjunctivitis or spreading it to someone else by following some simple steps for good hygiene.

If You Have Conjunctivitis

If you have conjunctivitis, you can help limit its spread to other people by following these steps:

- Wash your hands often with soap and warm water for at least 20 seconds. Wash them especially well before and after cleaning, or applying eye drops or ointment to, your infected eye. If soap and water are

not available, use an alcohol-based hand sanitizer that contains at least 60 percent alcohol to clean hands.
- Avoid touching or rubbing your eyes. This can worsen the condition or spread it to your other eye.
- With clean hands, wash any discharge from around your eye(s) several times a day using a clean, wet washcloth or fresh cotton ball. Throw away cotton balls after use and wash used washcloths with hot water and detergent and then wash your hands again with soap and warm water.
- Do not use the same eye drop dispenser/bottle for your infected and noninfected eyes.
- Wash pillowcases, sheets, washcloths, and towels often in hot water and detergent; wash your hands after handling such items.
- Stop wearing contact lenses until your eye doctor says it is okay to start wearing them again.
- Clean eyeglasses, being careful not to contaminate items (such as hand towels) that might be shared by other people.
- Clean, store, and replace your contact lenses as instructed by your eye doctor.
- Do not share personal items, such as pillows, washcloths, towels, eye drops, eye or face makeup, makeup brushes, contact lenses, contact lens storage cases, or eyeglasses.
- Do not use swimming pools.

IF YOU ARE AROUND SOMEONE WITH CONJUNCTIVITIS

If you are around someone with conjunctivitis, you can reduce your risk of infection by following these steps:

- Wash your hands often with soap and warm water for at least 20 seconds. If soap and warm water are not available, use an alcohol-based hand sanitizer that contains at least 60 percent alcohol to clean hands.
- Wash your hands after contact with an infected person or items he or she uses; for example, wash your hands

after applying eye drops or ointment to an infected person's eye(s) or after putting their bed linens in the washing machine.

- Avoid touching your eyes with unwashed hands.
- Do not share items used by an infected person; for example, do not share pillows, washcloths, towels, eye drops, eye or face makeup, makeup brushes, contact lenses, contact lens storage cases, or eyeglasses.

AVOID GETTING SICK AGAIN

In addition, if you have conjunctivitis, there are steps you can take to avoid reinfection once the infection goes away:

- Throw away and replace any eye or face makeup or makeup brushes you used while infected.
- Throw away disposable contact lenses and cases that you used while your eyes were infected.
- Throw away contact lens solutions that you used while your eyes were infected.
- Clean extended-wear lenses as directed.
- Clean eyeglasses and cases that you used while infected.

VACCINES CAN PREVENT SOME INFECTIONS ASSOCIATED WITH CONJUNCTIVITIS

There is no vaccine that prevents all types of conjunctivitis. However, there are vaccines to protect against some viral and bacterial diseases that are associated with conjunctivitis:

- rubella
- measles
- chickenpox
- Shingles
- pneumococcal
- *Haemophilus influenzae* type b (Hib)

Conjunctivitis caused by allergens or irritants is not contagious unless a secondary viral or bacterial infection develops.

TREATMENT OF CONJUNCTIVITIS

There are times when it is important to seek medical care for conjunctivitis (pink eye). However, this is not always necessary. To help relieve some of the inflammation and dryness caused by conjunctivitis, you can use cold compresses and artificial tears, which you can purchase over the counter without a prescription. You should also stop wearing contact lenses until your eye doctor says it is okay to start wearing them again. If you do not need to see a doctor, do not wear your contacts until you no longer have symptoms of pink eye.

When to Seek Medical Care

You should see a health-care provider if you have conjunctivitis along with any of the following:

- pain in the eye(s)
- sensitivity to light or blurred vision that does not improve when discharge is wiped from the eye(s)
- intense redness in the eye(s)
- symptoms that get worse or do not improve, including pink eye thought to be caused by bacteria which does not improve after 24 hours of antibiotic use
- a weakened immune system, for example, from human immunodeficiency virus (HIV) infection, cancer treatment, or other medical conditions or treatments

Newborns with symptoms of conjunctivitis should be seen by a doctor right away.

Viral Conjunctivitis

Most cases of viral conjunctivitis are mild. The infection will usually clear up in 7–14 days without treatment and without any long-term consequences. However, in some cases, viral conjunctivitis can take two to three weeks or more to clear up.

A doctor can prescribe antiviral medication to treat more serious forms of conjunctivitis. For example, conjunctivitis is caused by herpes simplex virus or varicella-zoster virus. Antibiotics will not improve viral conjunctivitis; these drugs are not effective against viruses.

Bacterial Conjunctivitis

Mild bacterial conjunctivitis may get better without antibiotic treatment and without causing any complications. It often improves in two to five days without treatment but can take two weeks to go away completely.

Your doctor may prescribe an antibiotic, usually given topically as eye drops or ointment, for bacterial conjunctivitis. Antibiotics may help shorten the length of infection, reduce complications, and reduce the spread to others. Antibiotics may be necessary in the following cases:

- with discharge (pus)
- when conjunctivitis occurs in people whose immune system is compromised
- when certain bacteria are suspected

Talk with your doctor about the best treatment options for your infection.

Allergic Conjunctivitis

Conjunctivitis caused by an allergen (such as pollen or animal dander) usually improves by removing the allergen from the person's environment. Allergy medications and certain eye drops (topical antihistamines and vasoconstrictors), including some prescription eye drops, can also provide relief from allergic conjunctivitis. In some cases, your doctor may recommend a combination of drugs to improve symptoms. Your doctor can help if you have conjunctivitis caused by an allergy.[1]

[1] "Conjunctivitis (Pink Eye)," Centers for Disease Control and Prevention (CDC), November 12, 2021. Available online. URL: www.cdc.gov/conjunctivitis/index.html. Accessed June 22, 2023.

Chapter 9 | Coronavirus Disease 2019

WHAT IS COVID-19?

Coronavirus disease 2019 (COVID-19) is a disease caused by a virus named severe acute respiratory syndrome coronavirus 2 (SARS-CoV-2). It can be very contagious and spreads quickly. Over one million people have died from COVID-19 in the United States. COVID-19 most often causes respiratory symptoms that can feel much like a cold, the flu, or pneumonia. COVID-19 may attack more than your lungs and respiratory system. Other parts of your body may also be affected by the disease. Most people with COVID-19 have mild symptoms, but some people become severely ill. Some people including those with minor or no symptoms will develop post-COVID conditions—also called "long COVID."

HOW DOES COVID-19 SPREAD?

Coronavirus disease 2019 spreads when an infected person breathes out droplets and very small particles that contain the virus. Other people can breathe in these droplets and particles, or these droplets and particles can land on their eyes, nose, or mouth. In some circumstances, these droplets may contaminate surfaces they touch. Anyone infected with COVID-19 can spread it, even if they do not have symptoms. The risk of animals spreading the virus that causes COVID-19 to people is low. The virus can spread from people to animals during close contact. People with suspected or confirmed COVID-19 should avoid contact with animals (refer to Figure 9.1).

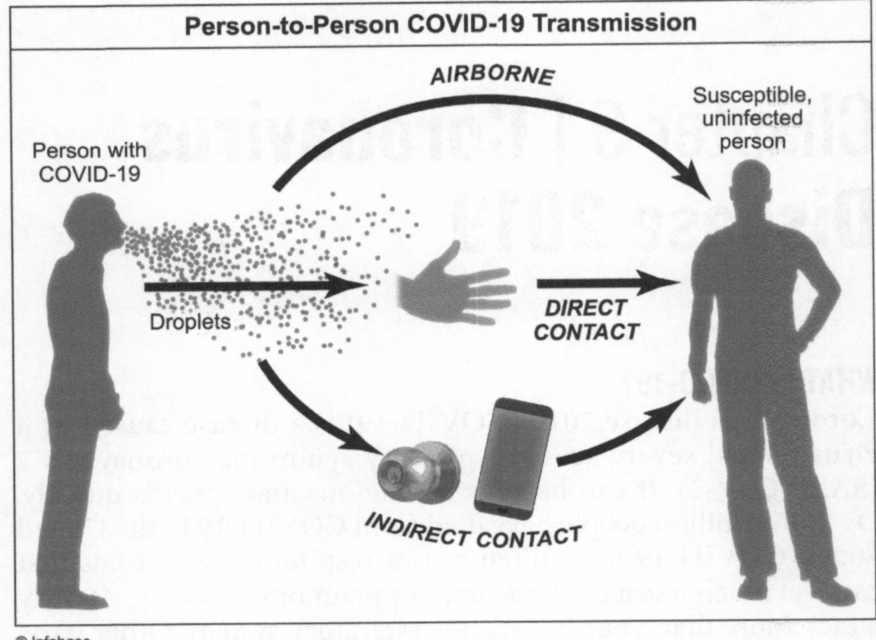

Figure 9.1. COVID-19 Transmission

Infobase

SYMPTOMS OF COVID-19

People with COVID-19 have had a wide range of symptoms reported—ranging from mild symptoms to severe illness. Symptoms may appear 2–14 days after exposure to the virus. Anyone can have mild to severe symptoms. Possible symptoms include:

- fever or chills
- cough
- shortness of breath or difficulty breathing
- fatigue
- muscle or body aches
- headache
- new loss of taste or smell
- sore throat

- congestion or runny nose
- nausea or vomiting
- diarrhea

This list does not include all possible symptoms. Symptoms may change with new COVID-19 variants and can vary depending on vaccination status. The Centers for Disease Control and Prevention (CDC) will continue to update this list as we learn more about COVID-19. Older adults and people who have underlying medical conditions such as heart or lung disease or diabetes are at higher risk for getting very sick from COVID-19.

WHEN TO SEEK EMERGENCY MEDICAL ATTENTION

Look for emergency warning signs* for COVID-19:

- trouble breathing
- persistent pain or pressure in the chest
- new confusion
- inability to wake or stay awake
- pale, gray, or blue-colored skin, lips, or nail beds, depending on skin tone

If someone is showing any of these signs, call 911 or call ahead to your local emergency facility. Notify the operator that you are seeking care for someone who has or may have COVID-19.

**This list is not all possible symptoms. Please call your medical provider for any other symptoms that are severe or concerning to you.*

WHAT ARE ANTIBODIES, AND HOW DO THEY HELP PROTECT YOU?

Antibodies are proteins your immune system makes to help fight infection and protect you from getting sick in the future. A positive antibody test result can help identify someone who has had COVID-19 in the past or has been vaccinated against COVID-19. Studies show that people who have antibodies from an infection with the virus that causes COVID-19 can improve their level of protection by getting vaccinated.

FACTORS THAT AFFECT YOUR RISK OF GETTING VERY SICK FROM COVID-19

Vaccination, past infection, or timely access to testing and treatment can help protect you from getting very sick if you get COVID-19. However, some people are more likely than others to get very sick if they get COVID-19. This includes people who are older, are immunocompromised, have certain disabilities, or have underlying health conditions. Understanding your COVID-19 risk and the risks that might affect others can help you make decisions to protect yourself and others.

FACTORS THAT RAISE YOUR RISK OF GETTING VERY SICK FROM COVID-19

Age

Older adults (especially those aged 50 and older, with risk increasing with older age) are more likely than younger people to get very sick if they get COVID-19. This means they are more likely to need hospitalization, intensive care, or a ventilator to help them breathe, or they could die. Most COVID-19 deaths occur in people older than 65.

Immunocompromised or a Weakened Immune System

Having a weakened immune system, also known as being immunocompromised, can make you more likely to get very sick if you get COVID-19. People who are immunocompromised or who are taking medicines that weaken their immune system may not be protected as well as others, even if they are up-to-date on their vaccines. For this reason, it is important to have a COVID-19 plan to protect yourself from infection and prepare for what to do if you get sick.

Underlying Health Conditions

Certain underlying health conditions you have (e.g., obesity or chronic obstructive pulmonary disorder (COPD)) may affect your risk of becoming very sick if you get COVID-19. Often, the more health conditions you have, the higher your risk. Certain conditions increase your risk more than others. For example, severe heart disease increases your risk more than high blood pressure.

FACTORS THAT CAN HELP PROTECT YOU FROM GETTING VERY SICK FROM COVID-19

Vaccination

COVID-19 vaccines are safe and effective. Staying up to date with your COVID-19 vaccines is the best way to protect yourself and others around you from getting very sick, being hospitalized, or dying from COVID-19. People who are up-to-date with their COVID-19 vaccines are far less likely to be hospitalized or die from COVID-19 than people the same age who have not been vaccinated or who are not up-to-date on their COVID-19 vaccines. However, even though vaccines reduce their risk, some people, particularly older adults with multiple underlying health conditions or people who are immunocompromised, can still get very sick from COVID-19.

Timely Treatment

If you are at increased risk of getting very sick from COVID-19, free medications are available that can reduce your chances of severe illness and death. Treatment needs to be started within a few days of infection to be effective. It can also help have a plan for what to do if you feel sick or are diagnosed with COVID-19, especially if you have barriers to testing or treatment, such as transportation challenges or lack of insurance.

Previous Infection

Having a previous infection with the virus that causes COVID-19 offers some protection from future illness. However, people who have had previous infections can still be reinfected and get severe COVID-19, especially if their previous infection was months ago or with a different variant (e.g., Delta variant). There are also risks to being repeatedly infected, including the potential of longer-term symptoms or the development of post-COVID conditions. Studies show that people with previous infections who are vaccinated are less likely to be hospitalized than those with previous infections who are not vaccinated. This means that people who have had previous infections should still get vaccinated to increase their protection against COVID-19. Getting a COVID-19 vaccination is a safer way to build protection than getting sick with COVID-19.[1]

[1] "About COVID-19," Centers for Disease Control and Prevention (CDC), July 10, 2023. Available online. URL: www.cdc.gov/coronavirus/2019-ncov/your-health/about-covid-19.html. Accessed July 25, 2023.

Chapter 10 | Ebola

WHAT IS EBOLA DISEASE?

Ebola disease is the term for a group of deadly diseases in people caused by four Ebola viruses within the genus *Ebolavirus* (refer to Figure 10.1). There are occasional Ebola disease outbreaks in people, occurring primarily on the African continent.

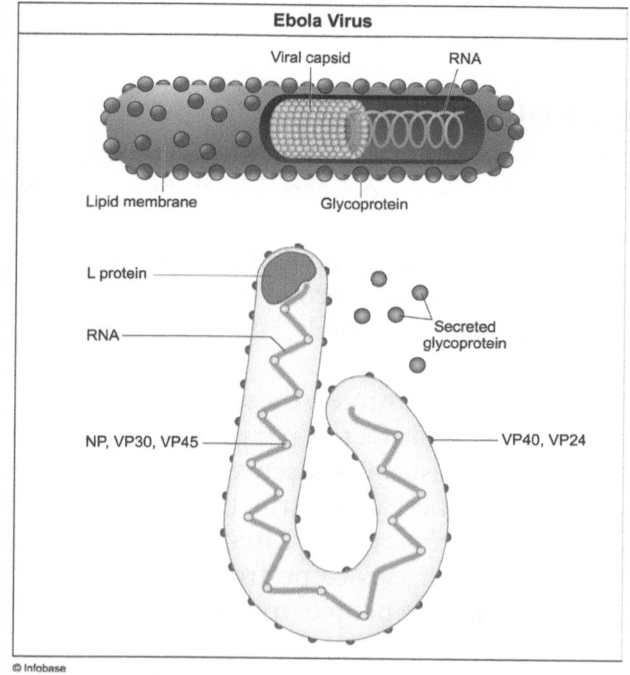

Figure 10.1. Ebola Virus

Infobase

The names of the four Ebola viruses that cause illness in people, with their associated viral species and disease name, are as follows:

- Ebola virus (species *Zaire ebolavirus*) causes Ebola virus disease.
- Sudan virus (species *Sudan ebolavirus*) causes Sudan virus disease.
- Taï Forest virus (species *Taï Forest ebolavirus*, formerly *Côte d'Ivoire ebolavirus*) causes Taï Forest virus disease.
- Bundibugyo virus (species *Bundibugyo ebolavirus*) causes Bundibugyo virus disease.

There are two additional Ebola viruses that are not known to cause disease in people. Reston virus (species *Reston ebolavirus*) is known to cause illness in nonhuman primates and pigs, but not in people. Bombali virus (species *Bombali ebolavirus*) was recently identified in bats, but it is unknown if it causes illness in either animals or people.

EMERGENCE OF EBOLA VIRUSES

Ebola viruses were first discovered in 1976 when two consecutive outbreaks of fatal hemorrhagic fever occurred in different parts of Central Africa. The first outbreak occurred in the Democratic Republic of Congo (formerly, Zaire) in a village near the Ebola River, which gave the virus its name. The second outbreak occurred in what is now South Sudan, approximately 500 miles (850 km) away.

Initially, public health officials assumed these outbreaks were a single event associated with an infected person who traveled between the two locations. Scientists later discovered that the two outbreaks were caused by two genetically distinct viruses:

Zaire ebolavirus and *Sudan ebolavirus*. After this discovery, scientists concluded that these viruses came from two different sources and spread independently to people in each of the affected areas.

Following the discovery of these Ebola viruses, scientists studied thousands of animals, insects, and plants in search of the source or reservoir host. It is believed that African fruit bats are likely involved in the spread of Ebola viruses and may even be the reservoir host. Scientists continue to search for conclusive evidence of the bat's role in the transmission of Ebola viruses. The most recent Ebola virus to be detected, the Bombali virus, was identified in samples from bats collected in Sierra Leone.

Like other viruses of its kind, it is possible that the reservoir host animal does not experience serious illness despite being infected with the virus. Ebola viruses are likely maintained in the environment by spreading from host to host or through intermediate hosts or vectors (organisms that can spread pathogens from infected animals to other living organisms). Infected animals carrying the virus can transmit it to other animals, such as apes, monkeys, duikers (antelopes), and people. Most infected animals will not get sick; however, Ebola viruses are known to cause severe illness in nonhuman primates (such as monkeys, gorillas, and chimpanzees) similar to Ebola disease in humans. Once an Ebola virus has infected a person, the virus can spread to other people through contact with the body fluids of the infected person.

Viral and epidemiologic data suggest that Ebola viruses existed long before the initial recorded outbreaks occurred. Factors such as population growth, encroachment into forested areas, and interaction with wildlife (such as animal meat consumption) may have contributed to the spread of Ebola viruses to people.

TRANSMISSION OF EBOLA VIRUSES

Scientists think people are initially infected with an Ebola virus through contact with an infected animal, such as a fruit bat or nonhuman primate. This is called a "spillover event." After that, the virus spreads from person to person, potentially affecting many people.

Ebola viruses spread through contact (such as through broken skin or mucous membranes in the eyes, nose, or mouth) with:

- blood or body fluids (urine, saliva, sweat, feces, vomit, breast milk, amniotic fluid, and semen) of a person who is sick with or has died from Ebola disease
- objects (such as clothes, bedding, needles, and medical equipment) contaminated with body fluids

from a person who is sick with or has died from Ebola disease
- infected fruit bats or nonhuman primates (such as apes and monkeys)
- semen from a man who recovered from Ebola disease (through oral, vaginal, or anal sex)

Ebola viruses can remain in certain body fluids (including semen) of a patient who has recovered from Ebola disease, even if they no longer have symptoms of severe illness. There is no evidence that Ebola viruses can spread through sex or other contact with vaginal fluids from a woman who has had Ebola disease.

When people become infected with an Ebola virus, they do not start developing signs or symptoms right away. This period between exposure to an illness and having symptoms is known as the "incubation period." A person can only spread the Ebola virus to other people after they develop signs and symptoms of Ebola disease.

Additionally, Ebola viruses are not known to be transmitted through food. However, in certain parts of the world, Ebola viruses may spread through the handling and consumption of wild animal meat or hunted wild animals infected with the Ebola virus. There is no evidence that mosquitoes or other insects can transmit Ebola viruses.

Risk

- Health workers and family members who do not use proper infection control while caring for patients with suspected or confirmed Ebola disease are at the highest risk of getting sick. Ebola viruses can spread when people come into contact with infected blood or body fluids.
- Ebola viruses pose little risk to travelers or the general public who have not cared for or been in contact with someone sick with Ebola.

Persistence of Ebola Viruses

Ebola viruses can remain in areas of the body that are immunologically privileged sites after acute infection. These are sites where viruses and pathogens, such as Ebola viruses, are shielded from the survivor's immune system, even after being cleared elsewhere in the body. These areas include the testes, interior of the eyes, placenta, and central nervous system, particularly the cerebrospinal fluid. Whether an Ebola virus is present in these body parts and for how long vary by survivor. Scientists are now studying how long Ebola viruses stay in these body fluids among Ebola disease survivors.

During an Ebola outbreak, the virus can spread quickly within health-care settings (such as clinics or hospitals). Clinicians and other health-care personnel providing care should use dedicated, preferably disposable, medical equipment. Proper cleaning and disposal of instruments such as needles and syringes are important. If instruments are not disposable, they must be sterilized before being used again.

Ebola viruses can survive on dry surfaces, such as doorknobs and countertops for several hours; in body fluids such as blood, Ebola viruses can survive up to several days at room temperature. Cleaning and disinfection should be performed using a hospital-grade disinfectant.

SIGNS AND SYMPTOMS OF EBOLA VIRUSES

Symptoms may appear anywhere from 2 to 21 days after contact with Ebola viruses, with an average of 8-10 days. The course of the illness typically progresses from "dry" symptoms initially (such as fever, aches and pains, and fatigue) and then progresses to "wet" symptoms (such as diarrhea and vomiting) as the person becomes sicker.

Primary signs and symptoms of Ebola disease often include some or several of the following:

- fever
- aches and pains, such as severe headaches and muscle and joint pain
- weakness and fatigue
- sore throat
- loss of appetite
- gastrointestinal symptoms, including abdominal pain, diarrhea, and vomiting
- unexplained hemorrhaging, bleeding, or bruising

Other symptoms may include red eyes, skin rash, and hiccups.

Many common illnesses can have the same symptoms as Ebola disease, including influenza (flu), malaria, or typhoid fever.

Ebola disease is a rare and often deadly illness. Recovery depends on good supportive clinical care and the patient's immune response. Studies show that survivors of an Ebola virus infection have antibodies (proteins made by the immune system that identify and neutralize invading viruses) that can be detected in the blood up to 10 years after recovery. Survivors are thought to have some protective immunity to the species of Ebola virus that sickened them.

DIAGNOSIS OF EBOLA VIRUSES

Diagnosing Ebola disease shortly after infection can be difficult. Early symptoms of Ebola disease such as fever, headache, and weakness are not specific to infection with Ebola viruses and often are seen in patients with other more common diseases, such as malaria and typhoid fever.

To determine whether Ebola disease is a possible diagnosis, there must be a combination of symptoms suggestive of Ebola disease and possible exposure to an Ebola virus within 21 days before the onset of symptoms. An exposure may include contact with:

- blood or body fluids from a person sick with or who died from Ebola disease
- objects contaminated with blood or body fluids of a person sick with or who died from Ebola disease
- infected fruit bats and nonhuman primates (apes or monkeys)
- semen from a man who has recovered from Ebola disease

If a person shows signs of Ebola disease and has had a possible exposure, he or she should be isolated (separated from other people), and public health authorities should be notified. Blood samples from the patient should be collected and tested to confirm infection. Ebola viruses can be detected in blood after the onset of symptoms. It may take up to three days after symptoms start for the virus to reach detectable levels.

Polymerase chain reaction (PCR) is a commonly used diagnostic method for Ebola disease because of its ability to detect low levels of the Ebola virus. PCR methods can detect the presence of a few virus particles in small amounts of blood, but the ability to detect the virus increases as the amount of virus increases during an active infection. When the virus is no longer present in great enough numbers in a patient's blood, PCR methods will no longer be effective. The detection of antibodies is another method used to confirm a person's exposure to an infection by the Ebola virus.

A positive laboratory test means that an Ebola virus infection is confirmed. Public health authorities will conduct a public health investigation, including identifying and monitoring all potentially exposed contacts.

TREATMENT OF EBOLA VIRUSES

Therapeutics

There are currently two treatments approved by the U.S. Food and Drug Administration (FDA) to treat Ebola virus disease caused by the Ebola virus, species *Zaire ebolavirus*, in adults and children. The first drug approved in October 2020, Inmazeb™, is a combination of three monoclonal antibodies. The second drug, Ebanga™, is a single monoclonal antibody and was approved in December 2020. Monoclonal antibodies (often abbreviated as mAbs) are proteins produced in a lab or other manufacturing facility that act like natural antibodies to stop a germ, such as a virus, from replicating after it has infected a person. These particular mAbs bind to a portion of the Ebola virus's surface called the "glycoprotein," which prevents the virus from entering a person's cells.

Both of these treatments, along with two others, were evaluated in a randomized controlled trial during the 2018–2020 Ebola outbreak in the Democratic Republic of the Congo. Overall survival was much higher for patients receiving either of the two treatments that are now approved by the FDA. Neither Inmazeb™ nor Ebanga™ have been evaluated for efficacy against species other than *Zaire ebolavirus*.

Supportive Care

Whether or not other treatments are available, basic interventions can significantly improve chances of survival when provided early. These are referred to as supportive care and include the following:

- providing fluids and electrolytes (body salts) orally or through infusion into the vein (intravenously)
- using medication to support blood pressure, reduce vomiting and diarrhea, and manage fever and pain
- treating other infections if they occur

PREVENTION AND VACCINE FOR EBOLA VIRUSES

In the areas where Ebola disease is most common, Ebola viruses are believed to spread at low rates among certain animal populations. Ebola viruses can spread to a person when they come in contact with an infected animal. Once infected, a person can become sick with Ebola disease and spread the virus to other people who come in contact with them.

When living in or traveling to a region where Ebola viruses are potentially present, there are several ways to protect yourself and prevent the spread of Ebola disease:

- Avoid contact with blood and body fluids (such as urine, feces, saliva, sweat, vomit, breast milk, amniotic fluid, semen, and vaginal fluids) of people who are sick.
- Avoid contact with semen from a man who has recovered from Ebola disease until testing shows that the virus is gone from his semen.
- Avoid contact with items that may have come in contact with an infected person's blood or body fluids (such as clothes, bedding, needles, and medical equipment).
- Avoid funeral or burial practices that involve touching the body of someone who is suspected or confirmed to have had Ebola disease.
- Avoid contact with bats, forest antelopes, nonhuman primates (such as monkeys and chimpanzees), and

the blood, fluids, or raw meat prepared from these or unknown animals.

These same prevention methods should be used when living in or traveling to an area affected by an Ebola outbreak. After returning from an Ebola-affected area, people should monitor their health for 21 days and seek medical care immediately if they develop symptoms of Ebola disease.

Ebola Vaccine

The FDA approved the Ebola vaccine rVSV-ZEBOV (called "Ervebo®") on December 19, 2019. This vaccine is given as a single dose vaccine and has been found to be safe and protective against the Ebola virus (species *Zaire ebolavirus*) only, which has caused the largest and most deadly Ebola outbreaks to date. This is the first FDA-approved vaccine for Ebola viruses.

On February 26, 2020, the Advisory Committee on Immunization Practices (ACIP) recommended pre-exposure prophylaxis vaccination with rVSV-ZEBOV for adults aged 18 and over in the U.S. population who are at potential occupational risk of exposure to *Zaire ebolavirus*. This recommendation includes adults who are:

- responding or planning to respond to an outbreak caused by the Ebola virus
- laboratorians or other staff working at biosafety level 4 facilities that work with live Ebola virus in the United States
- health-care personnel working at federally designated Ebola Treatment Centers in the United States

A two-dose vaccine regimen of a different vaccine that was also designed to protect against the *Zaire ebolavirus* species of Ebola was used under a research protocol in 2019 during an Ebola outbreak in the Democratic Republic of the Congo. The two doses of this vaccine use two different vaccine components (Ad26.ZEBOV and MVA-BN-Filo), and the regimen requires an initial dose and a "booster" dose 56 days later. This vaccine has not yet been approved by the FDA for routine use.

Handwashing

Ebola viruses spread through contact with the blood or body fluids of an infected person. They can enter the body through broken skin or mucous membranes in the eyes, nose, or mouth. This can easily happen by touching one's face with contaminated hands.

Hand hygiene (including alcohol-based hand rubs, soap and water, and correct glove use) is a basic component of personal and community hygiene and is an important way to prevent the spread of infections while providing healthcare. Correct hand hygiene lowers the number of germs on the hands and limits the opportunity for spread, including dangerous germs, such as Ebola viruses.

Proper hand hygiene methods are described below. Alcohol-based hand sanitizers are the preferred method for cleaning your hands in most clinical situations. When hands are visibly soiled with blood or other body fluids, wash hands with soap and water.

- Use alcohol-based hand sanitizer when hands are not visibly soiled. These products usually contain 60–95 percent ethanol or isopropanol. Alcohol-based hand sanitizer should not be used when hands are visibly soiled with dirt, blood, or other body fluids.
- Use soap and water when hands are visibly soiled with dirt, blood, or other body fluids and as an alternative to alcohol-based hand sanitizer. Antimicrobial soaps are not proven to offer benefits over washing hands with plain soap (not containing antimicrobial compounds) and water.
- Use mild (0.05%) chlorine solution in settings where hand sanitizer and soap are not available. Repeated use of 0.05 percent chlorine solution can cause skin irritation.[1]

[1] "Ebola Disease," Centers for Disease Control and Prevention (CDC), May 17, 2023. Available online. URL: www.cdc.gov/vhf/ebola/about.html. Accessed June 23, 2023.

Chapter 11 | **Fifth Disease**

WHAT IS FIFTH DISEASE?

Fifth disease is a mild rash illness caused by parvovirus B19. It is more common in children than adults. A person usually gets sick with fifth disease within 14 days after getting infected with parvovirus B19. This disease, also called "erythema infectiosum," got its name because it was fifth in a list of historical classifications of common skin rash illnesses in children.

SIGNS AND SYMPTOMS OF FIFTH DISEASE

The symptoms of fifth disease are usually mild and may include the following:

- fever
- runny nose
- headache
- rash

You Can Get a Rash on Your Face and Body

You may get a red rash on your face called a "slapped cheek" rash. This rash is the most recognized feature of fifth disease. It is more common in children than adults.

Some people may get a second rash a few days later on their chest, back, buttocks, or arms and legs. The rash may be itchy, especially on the soles of the feet. It can vary in intensity and usually goes away in 7–10 days, but it can come and go for several weeks. As it starts to go away, it may look lacy.

You May Also Have Painful or Swollen Joints

People with fifth disease can also develop pain and swelling in their joints. This is called "polyarthropathy syndrome." It is more common in adults, especially women. Some adults with fifth disease may only have painful joints, usually in the hands, feet, or knees, and no other symptoms. The joint pain usually lasts one to three weeks, but it can last for months or longer. It usually goes away without any long-term problems.

COMPLICATIONS OF FIFTH DISEASE

Fifth disease is usually mild for children and adults who are otherwise healthy. But, for some people, parvovirus B19 infection can cause serious health complications, such as chronic anemia that requires medical treatment.

You may be at risk for serious complications from fifth disease if you have a weakened immune system caused by leukemia, cancer, organ transplants, or human immunodeficiency virus (HIV) infection.

TRANSMISSION OF FIFTH DISEASE

Parvovirus B19—which causes fifth disease—spreads through respiratory secretions, such as saliva, sputum, or nasal mucus, when an infected person coughs or sneezes. You are most contagious when it seems like you have "just a fever and/or cold" and before you get the rash or joint pain and swelling. After you get the rash, you are not likely to be contagious, so it is usually safe for you or your child to go back to work or school.

People with fifth disease who have weakened immune systems may be contagious for a longer amount of time. Parvovirus B19 can also spread through blood or blood products. A pregnant woman who is infected with parvovirus B19 can pass the virus to her baby. Once you recover from fifth disease, you develop immunity that generally protects you from parvovirus B19 infection in the future.

DIAGNOSIS OF FIFTH DISEASE

Health-care providers can often diagnose fifth disease just by seeing a "slapped cheek" rash on a patient's face. They can also do a blood test to determine if you are susceptible or possibly immune to parvovirus B19 infection or if you were recently infected. This is not a routine test but can be performed in special circumstances. The blood test may be particularly helpful for pregnant women who may have been exposed to parvovirus B19 and are suspected to have fifth disease. Any pregnant woman who may have been exposed to parvovirus B19 should contact their obstetrician or health-care provider as soon as possible.

TREATMENT OF FIFTH DISEASE

Fifth disease is usually mild and will go away on its own. Children and adults who are otherwise healthy usually recover completely. Treatment usually involves relieving symptoms, such as fever, itching, joint pain, and swelling.

People who have complications from the fifth disease should see their health-care provider for medical treatment.

PREVENTION OF FIFTH DISEASE

There is no vaccine or medicine that can prevent parvovirus B19 infection. You can reduce your chance of being infected or infecting others by:

- washing your hands often, for at least 20 seconds, with soap and water
- covering your mouth and nose when you cough or sneeze
- not touching your eyes, nose, or mouth
- avoiding close contact with people who are sick
- staying home when you are sick

Once you get the rash, you are probably not contagious. So it is usually safe for you to go back to work or for your child to return to school or a childcare center. Health-care providers who are pregnant should know about potential risks to their babies and discuss this with their doctor. All health-care providers and patients should follow strict infection control practices to prevent parvovirus B19 from spreading.[1]

[1] "Parvovirus B19 and Fifth Disease," Centers for Disease Control and Prevention (CDC), November 26, 2019. Available online. URL: www.cdc.gov/parvovirusb19/fifth-disease.html. Accessed June 23, 2023.

Chapter 12 | Genital Herpes

WHAT IS GENITAL HERPES?

Genital herpes is a sexually transmitted disease (STD) caused by the herpes simplex virus type 1 (HSV-1) or type 2 (HSV-2).

HOW COMMON IS GENITAL HERPES?

Genital herpes infection is common in the United States. The Centers for Disease Control and Prevention (CDC) estimated that there were 572,000 new genital herpes infections in the United States in a single year. Nationwide, 11.9 percent of persons aged 14–49 years have HSV-2 infection (12.1% when adjusted for age). However, the prevalence of genital herpes infection is higher than that because an increasing number of genital herpes infections are caused by HSV-1. Oral HSV-1 infection is typically acquired in childhood; because the prevalence of oral HSV-1 infection has declined in recent decades, people may have become more susceptible to contracting a genital herpes infection from HSV-1.

HSV-2 infection is more common among women than among men; the percentages of those infected during 2015 and 2016 were 15.9 percent versus 8.2 percent, respectively, among 14–49-year-olds. This is possibly because genital infection is more easily transmitted from men to women than from women to men during penile–vaginal sex. HSV-2 infection is more common among non-Hispanic blacks (34.6%) than among non-Hispanic whites (8.1%). A previous analysis found that these disparities exist even among persons with similar numbers of lifetime sexual partners. Most infected persons may be unaware of their infection; in the United States, an estimated 87.4 percent of 14–49-year-olds infected with HSV-2 have never received a clinical diagnosis.

The age-adjusted percentage of persons in the United States infected with HSV-2 decreased from 18.0 percent in 1999–2000 to 12.1 percent in 2015–2016.

HOW DO PEOPLE GET GENITAL HERPES?

Infections are transmitted through contact with HSV in herpes lesions, mucosal surfaces, genital secretions, or oral secretions. HSV-1 and HSV-2 can be shed from normal-appearing oral or genital mucosa or skin. Generally, a person can only get HSV-2 infection during genital contact with someone who has a genital HSV-2 infection. However, receiving oral sex from a person with an oral HSV-1 infection can result in getting a genital HSV-1 infection. Transmission commonly occurs from contact with an infected partner who does not have visible lesions and who may not know that he or she is infected. In persons with asymptomatic HSV-2 infections, genital HSV shedding occurs on 10.2 percent of days, compared to 20.1 percent of days among those with symptomatic infections.

WHAT ARE THE SYMPTOMS OF GENITAL HERPES?

Most individuals infected with HSV are asymptomatic or have very mild symptoms that go unnoticed or are mistaken for another skin condition. When symptoms do occur, herpes lesions typically appear as one or more vesicles, or small blisters, on or around the genitals, rectum, or mouth. The average incubation period for an initial herpes infection is four days (range, 2–12) after exposure. The vesicles break and leave painful ulcers that may take two to four weeks to heal after the initial herpes infection. Experiencing these symptoms is referred to as having a first herpes "outbreak" or episode.

Clinical manifestations of genital herpes differ between the first and recurrent (i.e., subsequent) outbreaks. The first outbreak of herpes is often associated with a longer duration of herpetic lesions, increased viral shedding (making HSV transmission more likely), and systemic symptoms, including fever, body aches, swollen lymph nodes, or headache. Recurrent outbreaks of genital herpes are common, and many patients who recognize recurrences have prodromal symptoms, either localized genital pain or tingling or shooting pains in the legs, hips, or buttocks, which occur hours to days before the eruption of herpetic lesions. Symptoms of recurrent outbreaks are typically shorter in duration and less severe than the first outbreak of genital herpes. Long-term studies have indicated that the number of symptomatic recurrent outbreaks may decrease over time. Recurrences and subclinical shedding are much less frequent for genital HSV-1 infection than for genital HSV-2 infection.

WHAT ARE THE COMPLICATIONS OF GENITAL HERPES?

Genital herpes may cause painful genital ulcers that can be severe and persistent in persons with suppressed immune systems, such as persons infected with human immunodeficiency virus (HIV). Both HSV-1 and HSV-2 can also cause rare but serious complications such as aseptic meningitis (inflammation of the linings of the brain). Development of extragenital lesions (e.g., buttocks, groin, thigh, finger, or eye) may occur during the course of infection.

Some persons who contract genital herpes have concerns about how it will impact their overall health, sex life, and relationships. There can also be considerable embarrassment, shame, and stigma associated with a herpes diagnosis that can substantially interfere with a patient's relationships. Clinicians can address these concerns by encouraging patients to recognize that while herpes is not curable, it is a manageable condition. Three important steps that providers can take for their newly diagnosed patients are: giving information, providing support resources, and helping define treatment and prevention options. Patients can be counseled that risk of genital herpes transmission can be reduced, but not eliminated, by disclosure of infection to sexual partners, avoiding sex during a recurrent outbreak, use of suppressive antiviral therapy, and consistent condom use. Since a diagnosis of genital herpes may affect perceptions about existing or future sexual relationships, it is important for patients to understand how to talk to sexual partners about STDs.

There are also potential complications for a pregnant woman and her newborn child.

WHAT IS THE LINK BETWEEN GENITAL HERPES AND HIV?

Genital ulcerative disease caused by herpes makes it easier to transmit and acquire HIV infection sexually. There is an estimated twofold to fourfold increased risk of acquiring HIV if individuals with genital herpes infection are genitally exposed to HIV. Ulcers or breaks in the skin or mucous membranes (lining of the mouth, vagina, and rectum) from a herpes infection may compromise the protection normally provided by the skin and mucous membranes against infections, including HIV. In addition, having genital herpes increases the number of CD4 cells (the target cell for HIV entry) in the genital mucosa. In persons with both HIV and genital herpes, local activation of HIV replication at the site of genital herpes infection can increase the risk that HIV will be transmitted during contact with the mouth, vagina, or rectum of an HIV-uninfected sex partner.

HOW DOES GENITAL HERPES AFFECT A PREGNANT WOMAN AND HER BABY?

Neonatal herpes is one of the most serious complications of genital herpes. Health-care providers should ask all pregnant women if they have a history of genital herpes. Herpes infection can be passed from mother to child during pregnancy or childbirth, or babies may be infected shortly after birth, resulting in a potentially fatal neonatal herpes infection. Infants born to women who acquire genital herpes close to the time of delivery and are shedding viruses at delivery are at a much higher risk for developing neonatal herpes, compared with women who have recurrent genital herpes. Thus, it is important that women avoid contracting herpes during pregnancy. Women should be counseled to abstain from intercourse during the third trimester with partners known to have or suspected of having genital herpes.

While women with genital herpes may be offered antiviral medication late in pregnancy through delivery to reduce the risk of a recurrent herpes outbreak, third-trimester antiviral prophylaxis has not been shown to decrease the risk of herpes transmission to the neonate. Routine serologic HSV screening of pregnant women is not recommended. However, at the onset of labor, all women should undergo careful examination and questioning to evaluate for the presence of prodromal symptoms or herpetic lesions. If herpes symptoms are present, a cesarean delivery is recommended to prevent HSV transmission to the infant. There are detailed guidelines for how to manage asymptomatic infants born to women with active genital herpes lesions.

HOW IS GENITAL HERPES DIAGNOSED?

Herpes simplex virus nucleic acid amplification tests (NAAT) are the most sensitive and highly specific tests available for diagnosing herpes. However, in some settings, viral culture is the only test available. The sensitivity of viral culture can be low, especially among people who have recurrent or healing lesions. Because viral shedding is intermittent, it is possible for someone to have a genital herpes infection even though it was not detected by NAAT or culture.

Type-specific virologic tests can be used for diagnosing genital herpes when a person has recurrent symptoms or lesions without a confirmatory NAAT or culture result or has a partner with genital herpes. Both virologic tests and type-specific serologic tests should be available in clinical settings serving patients with, or at risk for, sexually transmitted infections (STIs).

Given performance limitations with commercially available type-specific serologic tests (especially with low index value results (less than 3)), a confirmatory test (Biokit or Western Blot) with a second method should be performed before test interpretation. If confirmatory tests are unavailable, patients should be counseled about the limitations of available testing before serologic testing. Health-care providers should also be aware that false-positive results occur. In instances of suspected recent acquisition, serologic testing within 12 weeks after acquisition may be associated with false negative test results.

HSV-1 serologic testing does not distinguish between oral and genital infection and typically should not be performed for diagnosing genital HSV-1 infection. Diagnosis of genital HSV-1 infection is confirmed by virologic tests from lesions.

The CDC does not recommend screening for HSV-1 or HSV-2 in the general population due to limitations of the type-specific serologic testing. Several scenarios where type-specific serologic HSV tests may be useful include the following:

- patients with recurrent genital symptoms or atypical symptoms and negative HSV NAAT or culture
- patients with a clinical diagnosis of genital herpes but no laboratory confirmation
- patients who report having a partner with genital herpes

Patients who are at higher risk of infection (e.g., presenting for a sexually transmitted infection evaluation, especially those with multiple sex partners) and people with HIV might need to be assessed for a history of genital herpes symptoms, followed by serology testing in those with genital symptoms.

IS THERE A CURE OR TREATMENT FOR HERPES?

There is no cure for herpes. Antiviral medications can, however, prevent or shorten outbreaks during the period of time the person takes the medication. In addition, daily suppressive therapy (i.e., daily use of antiviral medication) for herpes can reduce the likelihood of transmission to partners.

There is currently no commercially available vaccine that is protective against genital herpes infection. Candidate vaccines are in clinical trials.

HOW CAN HERPES BE PREVENTED?

Correct and consistent use of latex condoms can reduce, but not eliminate, the risk of transmitting or acquiring genital herpes because herpes virus shedding can occur in areas that are not covered by a condom.

The surest way to avoid transmission of STDs, including genital herpes, is to abstain from sexual contact or to be in a long-term mutually monogamous relationship with a partner who has been tested for STDs and is known to be uninfected.

Persons with herpes should abstain from sexual activity with partners when herpes lesions or other symptoms of herpes are present. It is important to know that even if a person does not have any symptoms, he or she can still infect sex partners. Sex partners of infected persons should be advised that they may become infected and they should use condoms to reduce the risk. Sex partners can seek testing to determine if they are infected with HSV.

Daily treatment with valacyclovir decreases the rate of HSV-2 transmission in discordant, heterosexual couples in which the source partner has a history of genital HSV-2 infection. Such couples should be encouraged to consider suppressive antiviral therapy as part of a strategy to prevent transmission, in addition to consistent condom use and avoidance of sexual activity during recurrences.

Counseling those with genital herpes, as well as their sex partners, is critical. It can help patients cope with the infection and prevent further spread into the community.[1]

[1] "Genital Herpes—CDC Detailed Fact Sheet," Centers for Disease Control and Prevention (CDC), July 22, 2021. Available online. URL: www.cdc.gov/std/herpes/stdfact-herpes-detailed.htm. Accessed June 23, 2023.

Chapter 13 | Gonorrhea

WHAT IS GONORRHEA?

Gonorrhea is a sexually transmitted disease (STD) caused by infection with the *Neisseria gonorrhoeae* bacterium. *N. gonorrhoeae* infects the mucous membranes of the reproductive tract, including the cervix, uterus, and fallopian tubes in women, and the urethra in women and men. *N. gonorrhoeae* can also infect the mucous membranes of the mouth, throat, eyes, and rectum.

HOW COMMON IS GONORRHEA?

Gonorrhea is a very common infectious disease. The Centers for Disease Control and Prevention (CDC) estimates that approximately 1.6 million new gonococcal infections occurred in the United States in 2018, and more than half occurred among young people aged 15–24. Gonorrhea is the second most commonly reported bacterial sexually transmitted infection in the United States. However, many infections are asymptomatic, so reported cases only capture a fraction of the true burden.

HOW DO PEOPLE GET GONORRHEA?

Gonorrhea is transmitted through sexual contact with the penis, vagina, mouth, or anus of an infected partner. Ejaculation does not have to occur for gonorrhea to be transmitted or acquired. Gonorrhea can also be spread perinatally from mother to baby during childbirth. People who have had gonorrhea and received treatment may be reinfected if they have sexual contact with a person infected with gonorrhea.

WHO IS AT RISK FOR GONORRHEA?

Any sexually active person can be infected with gonorrhea. In the United States, the highest reported rates of infection are among sexually active teenagers, young adults, and African Americans.

WHAT ARE THE SIGNS AND SYMPTOMS OF GONORRHEA?

Many men with gonorrhea are asymptomatic. When present, signs and symptoms of urethral infection in men include dysuria or a white, yellow, or green urethral discharge that usually appears 1–14 days after infection. In cases where urethral infection is complicated by epididymitis, men with gonorrhea may also complain of testicular or scrotal pain.

Most women with gonorrhea are asymptomatic. Even when a woman has symptoms, they are often so mild and nonspecific that they are mistaken for a bladder or vaginal infection. The initial symptoms and signs in women include dysuria, increased vaginal discharge, or vaginal bleeding between periods. Women with gonorrhea are at risk of developing serious complications from the infection, regardless of the presence or severity of symptoms.

Symptoms of rectal infection in both men and women may include discharge, anal itching, soreness, bleeding, or painful bowel movements. Rectal infection may also be asymptomatic. Pharyngeal infection may cause a sore throat but usually is asymptomatic.

WHAT ARE THE COMPLICATIONS OF GONORRHEA?

Untreated gonorrhea can cause serious and permanent health problems in both women and men. In women, gonorrhea can spread into the uterus or fallopian tubes and cause pelvic inflammatory disease (PID). The symptoms may be quite mild or can be very severe and can include abdominal pain and fever. PID can lead to internal abscesses and chronic pelvic pain. PID can also damage the fallopian tubes enough to cause infertility or increase the risk of ectopic pregnancy.

In men, gonorrhea may be complicated by epididymitis. In rare cases, this may lead to infertility. If left untreated, gonorrhea can also spread to the blood and cause disseminated gonococcal infection (DGI). DGI is usually characterized by arthritis, tenosynovitis, and/or dermatitis. This condition can be life-threatening.

WHAT ABOUT GONORRHEA AND HUMAN IMMUNODEFICIENCY VIRUS?

Untreated gonorrhea can increase a person's risk of acquiring or transmitting the human immunodeficiency virus (HIV), the virus that causes acquired immunodeficiency syndrome (AIDS).

HOW DOES GONORRHEA AFFECT A PREGNANT WOMAN AND HER BABY?

If a pregnant woman has gonorrhea, she may give the infection to her baby as the baby passes through the birth canal during delivery. This can cause blindness, joint infection, or a life-threatening blood infection in the baby.

Treatment of gonorrhea as soon as it is detected in pregnant women will reduce the risk of these complications. Pregnant women should consult a health-care provider for appropriate examination, testing, and treatment, as necessary.

WHO SHOULD BE TESTED FOR GONORRHEA?

Any sexually active person can be infected with gonorrhea. Anyone with genital symptoms such as discharge, burning during urination, unusual sores, or rash should stop having sex and see a health-care provider immediately. Also, anyone with an oral, anal, or vaginal sex partner who has been recently diagnosed with an STD should see a health-care provider for evaluation.

Some people should be tested (screened) for gonorrhea even if they do not have symptoms or know of a sex partner who has gonorrhea. Anyone who is sexually active should discuss his or her risk factors with a health-care provider and ask whether he or she should be tested for gonorrhea or other STDs.

The CDC recommends yearly gonorrhea screening for all sexually active women younger than 25 years of age, as well as older women with risk factors such as new or multiple sex partners or a sex partner who has a sexually transmitted infection. People who have gonorrhea should also be tested for other STDs.

HOW IS GONORRHEA DIAGNOSED?

Urogenital gonorrhea can be diagnosed by testing urine, urethral specimens (for men), or endocervical or vaginal specimens (for women) using nucleic acid amplification testing (NAAT). It can also be diagnosed using gonorrhea culture, which requires endocervical or urethral swab specimens. The rectal and oral diagnostic tests for gonorrhea (as well as chlamydia) approved by the U.S. Food and Drug Administration (FDA) have been validated for clinical use.

WHAT IS THE TREATMENT FOR GONORRHEA?

Gonorrhea can be cured with the right treatment. The CDC now recommends a single 500 mg intramuscular dose of ceftriaxone for the treatment of gonorrhea. Alternative regimens are available when ceftriaxone cannot be used to treat urogenital or rectal gonorrhea. Although medication will stop the infection, it will not repair any permanent damage done by the disease. Antimicrobial resistance in gonorrhea is of increasing concern, and successful treatment of gonorrhea is becoming more difficult. A test of cure—follow-up testing to be sure the infection was treated successfully—is not needed for genital and rectal infections; however, if a person's symptoms continue for more than a few days after receiving treatment, he or she should return to a health-care provider to be reevaluated. A test of cure is needed 7–14 days after treatment for people who are treated for pharyngeal (infection of the throat) gonorrhea.

Because reinfection is common, men and women with gonorrhea should be retested three months after treatment of the initial infection, regardless of whether they believe that their sex partners were successfully treated.

WHAT ABOUT PARTNERS?

If a person has been diagnosed and treated for gonorrhea, he or she should tell all recent anal, vaginal, or oral sex partners, so they can see a health provider and be treated. This will reduce the risk that the sex partners will develop serious complications from gonorrhea and will also reduce the person's risk of becoming reinfected. A person with gonorrhea and all of his or her sex partners must avoid having sex until they have completed their treatment for gonorrhea and until they no longer have symptoms.

HOW CAN GONORRHEA BE PREVENTED?

Latex condoms, when used consistently and correctly, can reduce the risk of transmission of gonorrhea. The surest way to avoid transmission of gonorrhea or other STDs is to abstain from vaginal, anal, and oral sex or to be in a long-term mutually monogamous relationship with a partner who has been tested and is known to be uninfected.[1]

[1] "Gonorrhea—CDC Detailed Fact Sheet," Centers for Disease Control and Prevention (CDC), April 11, 2023. Available online. URL: www.cdc.gov/std/gonorrhea/stdfact-gonorrhea-detailed.htm. Accessed June 23, 2023.

Chapter 14 | Hand-Foot-and-Mouth Disease

Hand-foot-and-mouth disease (HFMD) is common in children under five years old, but anyone can get it. The illness is usually not serious, but it is very contagious. It can spread quickly at schools and day care centers.

HOW DOES HAND-FOOT-AND-MOUTH DISEASE SPREAD?

Hand-foot-and-mouth disease spreads easily through:

- person-to-person contact
- droplets made when a person who is sick with HFMD sneezes, coughs, or talks
- contact with contaminated surfaces and objects

Is Hand-Foot-and-Mouth Disease Contagious?

Yes. HFMD is caused by viruses. A person infected with one of these viruses is contagious, which means that they can pass the virus to other people. If someone is sick with HFMD, the virus can be found in their:

- nose and throat secretions, such as saliva, drool, or nasal mucus
- fluid from blisters
- feces (poop)

People with HFMD are usually most contagious during the first week that they are sick. However, people can still sometimes spread the virus to others for days or weeks after symptoms go away or even if they have no symptoms at all.

How Do You Get Hand-Foot-and-Mouth Disease?

- contact with droplets that contain the virus made when a person sick with HFMD coughs, sneezes, or talks
- touching an infected person or making other close contact with them, such as kissing, hugging, or sharing cups or eating utensils
- touching an infected person's poop, such as changing diapers, and then touching your eyes, nose, or mouth
- touching objects and surfaces that have the virus on them, such as doorknobs or toys, and then touching your eyes, nose, or mouth

Although rare, you can also get the virus by swallowing recreational water, such as in swimming pools. This can happen if the water is not properly treated with chlorine and becomes contaminated with the poop from a person who has HFMD.

IS HAND-FOOT-AND-MOUTH DISEASE COMMON?

Yes. HFMD is common and in the United States occurs mostly in the summer and fall, but you can get it any time of year.

WHAT VIRUSES CAUSE HAND-FOOT-AND-MOUTH DISEASE?

Hand-foot-and-mouth disease is caused by viruses that belong to the enterovirus family:

- Coxsackievirus A16 is typically the most common cause of HFMD in the United States. Other coxsackieviruses can also cause the illness.
- Coxsackievirus A6 can also cause HFMD, and the symptoms may be more severe.
- Enterovirus 71 (EV-A71) has been associated with cases and outbreaks in East and Southeast Asia. Although rare, EV-A71 has been associated with more severe diseases such as encephalitis (swelling of the brain).

SYMPTOMS OF HAND-FOOT-AND-MOUTH DISEASE

Symptoms of HFMD usually include fever, mouth sores, and skin rash. The rash is commonly found on the hands and feet.

HFMD disease is common in infants and children younger than five years old. Most children have mild symptoms for 7–10 days.

Fever and Flu-Like Symptoms

Children often get a fever and other flu-like symptoms three to five days after they catch the virus. These can include the following:

- fever
- eating or drinking less
- sore throat
- feeling unwell

Mouth Sores

Your child can get painful mouth sores. These sores usually start as small red spots, often on the tongue and insides of the mouth, that blister and can become painful. Signs that swallowing might be painful for your child are as follows:

- not eating or drinking
- drooling more than usual
- only wanting to drink cold fluids

Skin Rash

Your child can get a skin rash on the palms of the hands and soles of the feet. It can also show up on the buttocks, legs, and arms.

The rash is usually not itchy and looks like flat or slightly raised red spots, sometimes with blisters that have an area of redness at their base. Fluid in the blister can contain the virus that causes HFMD. Keep blisters clean and avoid touching them.

When to See a Health-Care Provider

- Your child is not able to drink normally, and you are worried they might be getting dehydrated.
- Your child's fever lasts longer than three days.
- Symptoms do not improve after 10 days.
- Your child has a weakened immune system (the body's ability to fight germs and sickness).

- Symptoms are severe.
- Your child is very young, especially younger than six months.

Health-care providers can usually tell if someone has HFMD by examining the patient and the rash appearance while considering the patient's age and other symptoms.

Sometimes, health-care providers might collect samples from the patient's throat or feces (poop) and send them to a laboratory to test for the virus. However, these tests are rarely done.

COMPLICATIONS OF HAND-FOOT-AND-MOUTH DISEASE

Hand-foot-and-mouth disease is usually not serious. Nearly all people get better in 7–10 days with no or minimal medical treatment. Complications from HFMD are rare.

Dehydration

Some people, especially young children, can get dehydrated if they are not able to swallow enough liquids because of painful mouth sores. Parents can prevent dehydration by making sure their child drinks enough liquids.

Fingernail and Toenail Loss

Although very rare, people may lose a fingernail or toenail after having HFMD. Most reports of fingernail and toenail loss have been in children. In these reported cases, the person usually loses the nail within a few weeks after being sick. The nail usually grows back on its own. However, there is no evidence that HFMD is the cause of nail loss.

Viral (Aseptic) Meningitis

Although very rare, a small number of people with HFMD get viral meningitis. It causes fever, headache, stiff neck, or back pain and may require the infected person to be hospitalized for a few days.

Encephalitis or Paralysis

Although extremely rare, a small number of people with HFMD get encephalitis (swelling of the brain) or paralysis (inability to move parts of the body).

HOW TO TREAT HAND-FOOT-AND-MOUTH DISEASE

Most people with HFMD get better on their own in 7–10 days. There is no specific medical treatment for HFMD.

Treat Symptoms and Prevent Dehydration

You can take steps to relieve symptoms and prevent dehydration while you or your child are sick. Take over-the-counter (OTC) medications to relieve fever and pain caused by mouth sores. These medications can include acetaminophen or ibuprofen. Never give aspirin to children.

Give them enough liquids. Mouth sores can make it painful to swallow, so your child may not want to drink much. Make sure they drink enough to stay hydrated.

PREVENT HAND-FOOT-AND-MOUTH DISEASE

Hand-foot-and-mouth disease is very contagious. You can help prevent catching or spreading HFMD by following some simple steps.

Wash Your Hands

Wash your hands often with soap and water for at least 20 seconds. If soap and water are not available, use an alcohol-based hand sanitizer. Always wash your hands:

- after changing diapers
- after using the toilet
- after blowing your nose, coughing, or sneezing
- before and after caring for someone who is sick

Help children wash their hands. Teach them how to wash their hands and make sure they wash them often. Help them keep blisters clean and avoid touching them.

Avoid Close Contact with People Who Are Sick

Avoid touching someone who has HFMD, such as hugging or kissing them.

CAN MY CHILD RETURN TO SCHOOL IF THEY ARE SICK?

Because HFMD is normally mild, children can continue to go to childcare and schools as long as they:

- have no fever
- have no uncontrolled drooling with mouth sores
- feel well enough to participate in classroom activities

Talk with your child's health-care provider if you are still not sure when it is okay for them to return. In some cases, the local health department may require children with HFMD to stay home to control an outbreak.

Avoid Touching Your Eyes, Nose, and Mouth

You can get infected with HFMD if you have the virus on your hands and then touch your eyes, nose, or mouth. To reduce your chance of getting sick, do not touch your eyes, nose, and mouth with unwashed hands.

Clean and Disinfect

Clean and disinfect frequently touched surfaces and shared items, such as toys and doorknobs.[1]

[1] "Hand, Foot, and Mouth Disease (HFMD)," Centers for Disease Control and Prevention (CDC), May 11, 2023. Available online. URL: www.cdc.gov/hand-foot-mouth/index.html. Accessed June 26, 2023.

Chapter 15 | Hepatitis

WHAT IS HEPATITIS?

Hepatitis means inflammation of the liver. When the liver is inflamed or damaged, its function can be affected. Heavy alcohol use, toxins, some medications, and certain medical conditions can cause hepatitis, but it is often caused by a virus. In the United States, the most common hepatitis viruses are hepatitis A virus (HAV), hepatitis B virus (HBV), and hepatitis C virus (HCV).

WHAT IS THE DIFFERENCE BETWEEN HEPATITIS A, HEPATITIS B, AND HEPATITIS C?

Hepatitis A, hepatitis B, and hepatitis C are liver infections caused by three different viruses. Although each can cause similar symptoms, they are spread in different ways and can affect the liver differently. Hepatitis A is usually a short-term infection and does not become chronic. Hepatitis B and hepatitis C can also begin as short-term, acute infections, but in some people, the virus remains in the body, resulting in chronic disease and long-term liver problems. There are vaccines to prevent hepatitis A and hepatitis B; however, there is no vaccine for hepatitis C.

HEPATITIS A

Hepatitis A is a highly contagious, short-term liver infection caused by HAV. Since 2016, person-to-person outbreaks of hepatitis A have been occurring across the United States, mainly among people who use injection drugs or are experiencing homelessness. Since the hepatitis A vaccine was first recommended in 1996, cases of hepatitis A in the United States declined dramatically. Unfortunately, in recent years, the number of people infected has been increasing because there have been multiple outbreaks of hepatitis A in the United States resulting from person-to-person contact, especially among people who use drugs, people experiencing homelessness, and men who have sex with men (MSM).

Transmission

- **Person-to-person contact.** Hepatitis A can be spread from close, personal contact with an infected person, such as through certain types of sexual contact (such as oral-anal sex), caring for someone who is ill, or using drugs with others. Hepatitis A is very contagious, and people can even spread the virus before they feel sick.
- **Eating contaminated food or drink.** Contamination of food with the HAV can happen at any point: growing, harvesting, processing, handling, and even after cooking. Contamination of food and water happens more often in countries where hepatitis A is common. Although uncommon, foodborne outbreaks have occurred in the United States from people eating contaminated fresh and frozen imported food products.

Symptoms of Hepatitis A

Not everyone with hepatitis A has symptoms. Adults are more likely to have symptoms than children. If symptoms develop, they usually appear two to seven weeks after infection. Symptoms usually last less than two months although some people can be ill for as long as six months. If symptoms develop, they can include the following:

- yellow skin or eyes
- not wanting to eat
- upset stomach
- throwing up
- stomach pain
- fever
- dark urine or light-colored stools
- diarrhea
- joint pain
- feeling tired

Diagnosis and Treatment of Hepatitis A

A doctor can determine if you have hepatitis A by discussing your symptoms and ordering a blood test that can tell whether you have been recently infected with the virus that causes hepatitis A.

Prevention of Hepatitis A

The best way to prevent hepatitis A is through vaccination with the hepatitis A vaccine. To get the full benefit of the hepatitis A vaccine, more than one shot is needed. The number and timing of these shots depend on the type of vaccine you are given. Practicing good hand hygiene—including thoroughly washing hands after using the bathroom, changing diapers, and before preparing or eating food—plays an important role in preventing the spread of hepatitis A.

HEPATITIS B

Hepatitis B is a vaccine-preventable liver infection caused by the HBV. Hepatitis B is spread when blood, semen, or other body fluids from a person infected with the virus enter the body of someone who is not infected. This can happen through sexual contact; sharing needles, syringes, or other drug-injection equipment; or during pregnancy or delivery. Not all people newly infected with HBV have symptoms, but for those that do, symptoms can include fatigue, poor appetite, stomach pain, nausea, and jaundice. For many people, hepatitis B is a short-term illness. For others, it can become a long-term, chronic infection that can lead to serious, even life-threatening health issues such as liver disease or liver cancer. Age plays a role in whether hepatitis B will become chronic. The younger a person is when infected with the HBV, the greater the chance of developing chronic infection. About 9 in 10 infants who become infected go on to develop life-long, chronic infections. The risk goes down as a child gets older. About one in three children who get infected before age six will develop chronic hepatitis B. By contrast, almost all children aged six and older and adults infected with the HBV recover completely and do not develop chronic infection.

Symptoms of Hepatitis B

Not all people with acute HBV infection have symptoms. Symptoms can range from asymptomatic or mild disease to, rarely, fulminant hepatitis. The presence of signs and symptoms varies by age. Infants, children under five years of age, and immunosuppressed adults with acute HBV infection are typically asymptomatic. People less than 30 years old are less likely to be symptomatic compared with persons aged 30 years and older. When present, signs and symptoms of acute HBV infections can include:

- fever
- fatigue
- loss of appetite
- nausea
- vomiting
- abdominal pain
- dark urine
- clay-colored stool
- joint pain
- jaundice

Most people with chronic HBV infection are asymptomatic and have no evidence of liver disease or injury. However, some people develop chronic hepatitis (elevation of aspartate transaminase (AST)/alanine transaminase (ALT), cirrhosis, or hepatocellular carcinoma (i.e., primary liver cancer).

Transmission

HBV is transmitted from a person who has an HBV infection to a person who is not infected through activities that involve percutaneous (i.e., puncture through the skin) or mucosal contact with infectious blood or body fluids (e.g., semen and saliva), including:

- a mother to her baby during pregnancy or delivery
- sexual contact with an infected partner
- injection drug use that involves sharing needles, syringes, or drug-preparation equipment
- contact with blood from or open sores
- exposures to needle sticks or sharp instruments

- sharing certain items that can break the skin or mucous membranes (e.g., razors, toothbrushes, and glucose monitoring equipment), potentially resulting in exposure to blood
- poor infection control practices in health-care settings (e.g., dialysis units, diabetes clinics).

HBV can survive outside the body and remains infectious for at least seven days.

Screening and Testing of Hepatitis B

During screening, clinicians will test for hepatitis B surface antigen (HBsAg), antibody to hepatitis B surface antigen (anti-HBs), and total antibody to hepatitis B core antigen (total anti-HBc). This is known as a "triple panel."

Clinicians will periodically test susceptible people, regardless of age, who have ongoing risk for exposure, while these risks persist. To ensure increased access to testing, anyone who requests HBV testing should receive it, regardless of disclosure of risk, because many people might be reluctant to disclose stigmatizing risks. Susceptible people include those who have never been infected with HBV (i.e., total anti-HBc negative) and either did not complete a hepatitis B vaccine series as recommended by the Advisory Committee on Immunization Practices (ACIP) or who are known to be vaccine nonresponders.

Clinicians should test all pregnant people for HBsAg during each pregnancy, preferably in the first trimester, regardless of vaccination status or history of testing. Clinicians should test pregnant people with a history of appropriately timed triple panel screening and without subsequent risk for exposure to HBV (i.e., no new HBV exposures since triple panel screening) need HBsAg.

Treatment of Hepatitis B

Generally, the provider will treat people with acute infection using supportive care depending on their symptoms. There are several antiviral medications available for people with chronic infections. It is important to link these patients to care with regular monitoring to prevent liver damage and/or hepatocellular carcinoma.

The risk for chronic infection varies according to the age at infection and is greatest among young children. Approximately 90 percent of infected infants and 30 percent of children infected between the ages of 1 and 5 will remain chronically infected with HBV. By contrast, approximately 95 percent of infected adults recover completely from HBV infection and do not become chronically infected.

Vaccination

The ACIP recommends hepatitis B vaccination among all adults aged 19–59 years and adults aged 60 and over with risk factors for hepatitis B or without identified risk factors but seeking protection.

There are three single-antigen vaccines, one three-antigen vaccine, and three combination vaccines currently licensed in the United States:

- single-antigen hepatitis B vaccines:
    - Engerix-B
    - Recombivax HB
    - Heplisav-B
- three-antigen hepatitis B vaccines:
    - PreHevbrio (13)
- combination vaccines:
    - **Pediarix**. Combined hepatitis B, diphtheria, tetanus, acellular pertussis (DTaP), and inactivated poliovirus (IPV) vaccine
    - **Twinrix**. Combined hepatitis A and hepatitis B vaccine
    - **Vaxelis**. Combined DTaP, IPV, *Haemophilus influenzae* type b, and hepatitis B vaccine

The vaccination schedule most often used for children and adults is three intramuscular injections, the second and third doses administered at one and six months, respectively, after the first dose. Alternate schedules have been approved for certain vaccines and/or populations. A new formulation, Heplisav-B (HepB-CpG), is approved for two doses, one month apart.

HEPATITIS C

Hepatitis C is a liver infection caused by the HCV. Hepatitis C is spread through contact with blood from an infected person. Today, most people become infected with the HCV by sharing needles or other equipment used to prepare and inject drugs. For some people, hepatitis C is a short-term illness, but for more than half of people who become infected with the HCV, it becomes a long-term, chronic infection. Chronic hepatitis C can result in serious, even life-threatening health problems such as cirrhosis and liver cancer. People with chronic hepatitis C can often have no symptoms and do not feel sick. When symptoms appear, they often are a sign of advanced liver disease. There is no vaccine for hepatitis C. The best way to prevent hepatitis C is by avoiding behaviors that can spread the disease, especially injecting drugs. Getting tested for hepatitis C is important because treatments can cure most people with hepatitis C in 8–12 weeks.

Transmission and Symptoms of Hepatitis C

HCV is transmitted primarily through parenteral exposures to infectious blood or body fluids that contain blood. Possible exposures include the following:

- injection-drug use (currently the most common mode of HCV transmission in the United States)
- birth to an HCV-infected mother

Although less frequent, HCV can also be spread through:

- sex with an HCV-infected person (an inefficient means of transmission although MSM infected with human immunodeficiency virus (HIV) have increased risk of sexual transmission)
- sharing personal items contaminated with infectious blood, such as razors or toothbrushes
- other health-care procedures that involve invasive procedures, such as injections (usually recognized in the context of outbreaks)
- unregulated tattooing

- receipt of donated blood, blood products, and organs (rare in the United States since blood screening became available in 1992)
- needlestick injuries in health-care settings

People with newly acquired HCV infection usually are asymptomatic or have mild symptoms that are unlikely to prompt a visit to a health-care professional. When symptoms do occur, they can include the following:

- fever
- fatigue
- dark urine
- clay-colored stool
- abdominal pain
- loss of appetite
- nausea
- vomiting
- joint pain
- jaundice

In those people who do develop symptoms, the average period from exposure to symptom onset is 2–12 weeks (range: 2–26 weeks). Some people with chronic HCV infection develop medical conditions due to hepatitis C that are not limited to the liver. Such conditions can include the following:

- diabetes mellitus
- glomerulonephritis
- essential mixed cryoglobulinemia
- porphyria cutanea tarda
- non-Hodgkin lymphoma

Testing and Diagnosis of Hepatitis C

The CDC now recommends universal hepatitis C screening for all U.S. adults and all pregnant women during every pregnancy, except in settings where the prevalence of HCV infection is less than 0.1 percent. Routine periodic testing is recommended for people with ongoing risk factors, while risk factors persist, including those who currently inject drugs and share needles, syringes, or other drug preparation equipment, along with people who have certain medical conditions (e.g., people who ever received maintenance hemodialysis). Testing of people at risk should occur regardless of setting prevalence.

Several blood tests can detect HCV infection, including:

- screening tests for antibodies to HCV (anti-HCV)
- enzyme immunoassay (EIA)
- enhanced chemiluminescence immunoassay (CLIA)
- chemiluminescence microparticle immunoassay (CMIA)
- microparticle immunoassay (MEIA)
- electrochemiluminescence immunoassay (ECLIA)
- immunochromatographic assay (rapid test)
- qualitative nucleic acid tests to detect the presence of HCV ribonucleic acid (RNA)
- quantitative nucleic acid tests to detect levels of HCV RNA

Management and Treatment of Hepatitis C

The CDC recommends that people who are diagnosed with hepatitis C be provided medical evaluation (by either a primary-care clinician or specialist (e.g., in hepatology, gastroenterology, or infectious disease)) for chronic liver disease, including treatment and monitoring;

- hepatitis A and hepatitis B vaccination
- screening and brief intervention for alcohol consumption
- HIV risk assessment and testing

With the exception of pregnant women and children under three years of age, people with acute hepatitis C (i.e., those with measurable HCV RNA) should be treated for their infection. Over 90 percent of people infected with HCV can be cured of their infection, regardless of HCV genotype, with 8–12 weeks of oral therapy.

HEPATITIS D

Hepatitis D, also known as "delta hepatitis," is a liver infection caused by the hepatitis D virus (HDV). Hepatitis D only occurs in people who are also infected with the HBV. Hepatitis D is spread when blood or other body fluids from a person infected with the virus enter the body of someone who is not infected. Hepatitis D can be an acute, short-term infection or become a long-term, chronic infection. Hepatitis D can cause severe symptoms and serious illness that can lead to life-long liver damage and even death. People can become infected with both hepatitis B and HDV at the same time (known as "coinfection") or get hepatitis D after first being infected with the HBV (known as "superinfection"). There is no vaccine to prevent hepatitis D. However, prevention of hepatitis B with hepatitis B vaccine also protects against future hepatitis D infection.

Transmission and Exposure

HDV is mainly transmitted through activities that involve percutaneous (i.e., puncture through the skin) and to a lesser extent through mucosal contact with infectious blood or body fluids (e.g., semen and saliva), including:

- sex with an infected partner
- injection-drug use that involves sharing needles, syringes, or drug-preparation equipment
- birth to an infected mother (rare)
- contact with blood from or the open sores of an infected person
- needle sticks or exposures to sharp instruments
- sharing items (e.g., razors and toothbrushes) with an infected person

HDV is not spread through food or water, sharing eating utensils, breastfeeding, hugging, kissing, hand holding, coughing, or sneezing.

Signs and Symptoms of Hepatitis D

HDV causes infection and clinical illness only in HBV-infected people. The signs and symptoms of acute HDV infection are indistinguishable from those of other types of acute viral hepatitis infections. These include:

- fever
- fatigue
- loss of appetite
- nausea
- vomiting
- abdominal pain
- dark urine
- clay-colored bowel movements
- joint pain
- jaundice

These signs and symptoms typically appear three to seven weeks after initial infection. Acute hepatitis occurs in HBV/HDV-coinfected people, and their symptoms may follow a biphasic course. Symptoms of HBV/HDV coinfection can range from mild to severe (fulminant hepatitis), but for most people, coinfection is self-limited: less than 5 percent of coinfected people go on to develop chronic infections. Regardless, acute liver failure is more common among people with HBV/HDV coinfection than among those infected with HBV alone.

Diagnosis and Treatment of Hepatitis D

Because cases of hepatitis D are not clinically distinguishable from other types of acute viral hepatitis, diagnosis can be confirmed only by testing for the presence of antibodies against HDV and/or HDV RNA. HDV infection should be considered in any person with a positive HBsAg who has severe symptoms of hepatitis or acute exacerbations.

No treatment is available for HDV infection specifically. Pegylated interferon alpha has shown some efficacy, but the sustained virologic response rate (a measure of viral clearance) is low (25%). New therapies are being evaluated. In cases of fulminant hepatitis and end-stage liver disease, liver transplantation may be considered.

Prevention

Although no vaccine is available for hepatitis D, vaccination with the hepatitis B vaccine can protect people from HDV infection.

HEPATITIS E

Hepatitis E is a liver infection caused by the hepatitis E virus (HEV). HEV is found in the stool of an infected person. It is spread when someone unknowingly ingests the virus—even in microscopic amounts. In developing countries, people most often get hepatitis E from drinking water contaminated by feces from people who are infected with the virus. In the United States and other developed countries where hepatitis E is not common, people have gotten sick with hepatitis E after eating raw or undercooked pork, venison, wild boar meat, or shellfish. In the past, most cases in developed countries involved people who have recently traveled to countries where hepatitis E is common.

Symptoms of hepatitis E can include fatigue, poor appetite, stomach pain, nausea, and jaundice. However, many people with hepatitis E, especially young children, have no symptoms. Except for the rare occurrence of chronic hepatitis E in people with compromised immune systems, most people recover fully from the disease without any complications. No vaccine for hepatitis E is currently available in the United States.

Transmission and Exposure

HEV is usually spread by the fecal–oral route. In developing countries, where HEV genotypes 1 and 2 predominate, the most common source of HEV infection is contaminated drinking water. In developed countries, sporadic cases of HEV genotype 3 have occurred following consumption of uncooked/undercooked pork or deer meat. Consumption of shellfish was a risk factor in a recently described outbreak that occurred among cruise ship passengers. HEV genotype 4, detected in China, Taiwan, and Japan, has also been associated with foodborne transmission.

Hepatitis E can infect certain mammals, and consumption of uncooked/undercooked meat or organs from infected animals can lead to foodborne transmission to humans. HEV RNA (genotypes 3 and 4) has been extracted from pork, boar, and deer meat.

Symptoms of Hepatitis E

When they occur, the signs and symptoms of hepatitis E are similar to those of other types of acute viral hepatitis and liver injury. They include the following:

- fever
- fatigue
- loss of appetite
- nausea
- vomiting
- abdominal pain
- jaundice
- dark urine
- clay-colored stool
- joint pain

The ratio of symptomatic to asymptomatic infection ranges from 1:2 to 1:13. Many people with hepatitis E do not have symptoms of acute infection. Pregnant women are more likely to experience severe illness, including fulminant hepatitis and death. When symptoms occur, they usually develop 15–60 days (mean: 40 days) after exposure. Most people with hepatitis E recover completely. During hepatitis E outbreaks, the overall case-fatality rate is about 1 percent.

However, for pregnant women, hepatitis E can be a serious illness, with mortality reaching 10–30 percent among pregnant women in their third trimester. Hepatitis E can also pose serious health threats to people with preexisting chronic liver disease and organ-transplant recipients on immunosuppressive therapy, resulting in decompensated liver disease and death.

Diagnosis and Treatment of Hepatitis E

HEV infection should be considered in any person with symptoms of viral hepatitis who tests negative for hepatitis A, hepatitis B, hepatitis C, other hepatotropic viruses, and all other causes of acute liver injury. Any symptomatic person who has traveled either to or from a hepatitis E-endemic area or outbreak-afflicted region should also be evaluated for HEV infection. A detailed history regarding travel, sources of drinking water, uncooked food, and contact with jaundiced persons should be obtained from these patients to aid in diagnosis. Because domestically acquired cases of hepatitis E are occurring in the United States, HEV infection also should be considered in any person with unexplained symptoms of liver injury, regardless of travel history.

Because cases of hepatitis E are not clinically distinguishable from other types of acute viral hepatitis, diagnosis can be confirmed only by testing for the presence of antibodies against HEV or HEV RNA. Both serologic and nucleic acid tests are commercially available, but they have not been approved by the U.S. Food and Drug Administration (FDA) for use in the United States. These tests are used for research purposes, but some commercial laboratories use commercially available assays from other countries.

Hepatitis E usually resolves on its own without treatment. There is no specific antiviral therapy for acute hepatitis E. Physicians will offer supportive therapy. Patients are typically advised to rest, get adequate nutrition and fluids, avoid alcohol, and check with their physician before taking any medications that can damage the liver, especially acetaminophen. Hospitalization is sometimes required in severe cases and should be considered for pregnant women.

Prevention

Prevention of hepatitis E relies primarily on good sanitation and the availability of clean drinking water. Travelers to developing countries can reduce their risk of infection by not drinking unpurified water. Boiling and chlorination of water will inactivate HEV.

Hepatitis

Avoiding raw pork and venison can reduce the risk of HEV genotype 3 transmission. Immune globulin is not effective in preventing hepatitis E. No FDA-approved vaccine for hepatitis E is currently available in the United States; however, in 2012, a recombinant vaccine was approved for use in China.[1]

[1] "Hepatitis A Questions and Answers for the Public," Centers for Disease Control and Prevention (CDC), July 28, 2020. Available online. URL: www.cdc.gov/hepatitis/hav/afaq.htm. Accessed July 17, 2023.

Chapter 16 | **Human Immunodeficiency Virus and Acquired Immunodeficiency Syndrome**

WHAT IS HUMAN IMMUNODEFICIENCY VIRUS?

Human immunodeficiency virus (HIV) is a virus that attacks cells that help the body fight infection, making a person more vulnerable to other infections and diseases. It is spread by contact with certain bodily fluids of a person with HIV, most commonly during unprotected sex (sex without a condom or HIV medicine to prevent or treat HIV), or through sharing injection drug equipment. If left untreated, HIV can lead to the disease-acquired immunodeficiency syndrome (AIDS). The human body cannot get rid of HIV, and no effective HIV cure exists. So, once you have HIV, you have it for life.

Luckily, however, effective treatment with HIV medicine (called "antiretroviral therapy" (ART)) is available. If taken as prescribed, HIV medicine can reduce the amount of HIV in the blood (also called the "viral load") to a very low level. This is called "viral suppression." If a person's viral load is so low that a standard lab cannot detect it, this is called having an undetectable viral load. People with HIV who take HIV medicine as prescribed and get and keep an undetectable viral load can live long and healthy lives and will not transmit HIV to their HIV-negative partners through sex.

In addition, there are effective methods to prevent getting HIV through sex or drug use, including PrEP, medicine people at risk for HIV take to prevent getting HIV from sex or injection drug use, and post-exposure prophylaxis (PEP), HIV medicine taken within 72 hours after a possible exposure to prevent the virus from taking hold.

WHAT IS ACQUIRED IMMUNODEFICIENCY SYNDROME?

Acquired immunodeficiency syndrome is the late stage of HIV infection that occurs when the body's immune system is badly damaged because of the virus. In the United States, most people with HIV do not develop AIDS because taking HIV medicine as prescribed stops the progression of the disease. A person with HIV is considered to have progressed to AIDS when:

- the number of their CD4 cells falls below 200 cells/mm^3 (In someone with a healthy immune system, CD4 counts are between 500 and 1,600 cells/mm^3.)
- they develop one or more opportunistic infections regardless of their CD4 count.

Without HIV medicine, people with AIDS typically survive about three years. Once someone has a dangerous opportunistic illness, life expectancy without treatment falls to about one year. HIV medicine can still help people at this stage of HIV infection, and it can even be lifesaving. But people who start HIV medicine soon after they get HIV experience more benefits—that is why HIV testing is so important.

HOW DO YOU KNOW IF YOU HAVE HUMAN IMMUNODEFICIENCY VIRUS?

The only way to know for sure if you have HIV is to get tested. Testing is relatively simple. You can ask your health-care provider for an HIV test. Many medical clinics, substance abuse programs, community health centers, and hospitals offer them too. To find an HIV testing location near you, use the HIV Services Locator (https://locator.hiv.gov). HIV self-testing is also an option.

Self-testing allows people to take an HIV test and find out their result in their own home or other private location. You can buy a self-test kit at a pharmacy or online. Some health departments or community-based organizations also provide self-test kits for a reduced cost or for free. You can only get HIV by coming into direct contact with certain body fluids from a person with HIV who has a detectable viral load. These fluids are:

- blood
- semen (cum) and pre-seminal fluid (pre-cum)
- rectal fluids
- vaginal fluids
- breast milk

For transmission to occur, the HIV in these fluids must get into the bloodstream of an HIV-negative person through a mucous membrane (found in the rectum, vagina, mouth, or tip of the penis), through open cuts or sores, or by direct injection (from a needle or syringe). People with HIV who take HIV medicine as prescribed and get and keep an undetectable viral load can live long and healthy lives and will not transmit HIV to their HIV-negative partners through sex.

HOW IS HUMAN IMMUNODEFICIENCY VIRUS SPREAD FROM PERSON TO PERSON?

Human immunodeficiency virus can only be spread through specific activities. In the United States, the most common ways are as follows:

- having vaginal or anal sex with someone who has HIV without using a condom the right way every time or taking medicines to prevent or treat HIV (Anal sex is riskier than vaginal sex for HIV transmission.)
- sharing injection drug equipment, such as needles, syringes, or other drug injection equipment ("works") with someone who has HIV because these items may have blood in them and blood can carry HIV (People who inject hormones, silicone, or steroids can also get or transmit HIV by sharing needles, syringes, or other injection equipment.)

Less common ways are as follows:

- **An HIV-positive person transmitting HIV to their baby during pregnancy, birth, or breastfeeding.** However, the use of HIV medicines and other strategies have helped lower the risk of perinatal transmission of HIV to less than 1 percent in the United States.
- **Being exposed to HIV through a needlestick or sharps injury**. This is a risk mainly for health-care workers. The risk is very low.

HIV is spread only in extremely rare cases in the following ways:

- **Having oral sex**. Oral sex carries little to no risk of getting or transmitting HIV. Theoretically, it is possible if an HIV-positive man ejaculates in his partner's mouth during oral sex. Factors that may increase the risk of transmitting HIV through oral sex are oral ulcers, bleeding gums, genital sores, and the presence of other sexually transmitted diseases (STDs), which may or may not be visible. However, the risk is still extremely low and much lower than with anal or vaginal sex.
- **Receiving blood transfusions, blood products, or organ/tissue transplants that are contaminated with HIV**. The risk is extremely small these days because of rigorous testing of the U.S. blood supply and donated organs and tissues. (And you cannot get HIV from donating blood. Blood collection procedures are highly regular and very safe.)
- **Being bitten by a person with HIV**. Each of the very small number of documented cases has involved severe trauma with extensive tissue damage and the presence of blood. This rare transmission can occur through contact between broken skin, wounds, or mucous membranes and blood or body fluids from a person who has HIV. There is no risk of transmission if the skin is not broken. There are no documented cases of HIV being transmitted through spitting as HIV is not transmitted through saliva.

- **Deep, open-mouth kissing.** HIV may spread through this way if both partners have sores or bleeding gums and blood from the HIV-positive partner gets into the bloodstream of the HIV-negative partner. HIV is not spread through saliva.
- **Eating food that has been pre-chewed by a person with HIV.** The only known cases are among infants. HIV transmission can occur when the blood from an HIV-positive caregiver's mouth mixes with food while chewing and an infant eats it. However, you cannot get HIV by consuming food handled by someone with HIV.

HOW IS HUMAN IMMUNODEFICIENCY VIRUS NOT SPREAD?

Human immunodeficiency virus is not spread by:

- air or water
- mosquitoes, ticks, or other insects
- saliva, tears, sweat, feces, or urine that is not mixed with the blood of a person with HIV
- shaking hands; hugging; sharing toilets; sharing dishes, silverware, or drinking glasses; or engaging in closed-mouth or "social" kissing with a person with HIV
- drinking fountains
- other sexual activities that do not involve the exchange of body fluids (e.g., touching)
- donating blood

HIV cannot be passed through healthy, unbroken skin.

IS THE RISK OF HUMAN IMMUNODEFICIENCY VIRUS DIFFERENT FOR DIFFERENT GROUPS?

Human immunodeficiency virus can affect anyone regardless of sexual orientation, race, ethnicity, gender, age, or where they live. However, certain groups of people in the United States are more likely to get HIV than others because of particular factors, including the communities in which they live, what subpopulations they belong to, and their risk behaviors.

- **Communities**. When you live in a community where many people have HIV, the chance of being exposed to the virus by having sex or sharing needles or other injection equipment with someone who has HIV is higher. You can use the HIV, STD, hepatitis, and tuberculosis Atlas Plus of the Centers for Disease Control and Prevention (CDC; www.cdc.gov/NCHHSTP/Atlas) to see the percentage of people with HIV ("prevalence") in different U.S. counties and states, as well as other data. Within any community, the prevalence of HIV can vary among different subpopulations.
- **Subpopulations**. In the United States, gay, bisexual, and other men who have sex with men are the population most affected by HIV. According to the CDC, of the 30,635 new HIV diagnoses in the United States in 2020, 68 percent (20,758) were among gay and bisexual men. By race/ethnicity, Blacks/African Americans and Hispanics/Latinos are disproportionately affected by HIV compared to other racial and ethnic groups. Also, transgender women who have sex with men are among the groups at highest risk for HIV infection. People who inject drugs remain at significant risk for getting HIV as well.
- **Risk behaviors**. In the United States, HIV is spread mainly through having anal or vaginal sex or sharing needles or syringes with an HIV-positive partner. Anal sex is the highest-risk behavior. Fortunately, there are more HIV prevention tools available today than ever before. These include using condoms correctly, every time you have sex; PrEP, medicine people at risk for HIV take to prevent getting HIV from sex or injection drug use; and treatment as prevention, a method in which people with HIV take HIV medicine as prescribed to achieve and maintain an undetectable viral load, a level of HIV in the blood so low that it cannot be detected in a standard blood test. People

with HIV who take HIV medicine (called "ART") as prescribed and get and keep an undetectable viral load can live long and healthy lives and will not transmit HIV to their HIV-negative partners through sex.

WHAT ARE THE SYMPTOMS OF HUMAN IMMUNODEFICIENCY VIRUS?

There are several symptoms of HIV. Not everyone will have the same symptoms. It depends on the person and what stage of the disease they are in. Below are the three stages of HIV and some of the symptoms people may experience.

Stage 1: Acute Human Immunodeficiency Virus Infection

Within two to four weeks after infection with HIV, about two-thirds of people will have a flu-like illness. This is the body's natural response to HIV infection.

Flu-like symptoms can include the following:

- fever
- chills
- rash
- night sweats
- muscle aches
- sore throat
- fatigue
- swollen lymph nodes
- mouth ulcers

These symptoms can last anywhere from a few days to several weeks. But some people do not have any symptoms at all during this early stage of HIV. Do not assume you have HIV just because you have any of these symptoms—they can be similar to those caused by other illnesses. But, if you think you may have been exposed to HIV, get an HIV test.

Here is what to do:

- **Find an HIV testing site near you.** You can get an HIV test at your primary care provider's office, your local health department, a health clinic, or many other

places. Use the HIV Services Locator (https://locator.hiv.gov) to find an HIV testing site near you.
- **Request an HIV test for a recent infection.** Most HIV tests detect antibodies (proteins your body makes as a reaction to HIV), not HIV itself. But it can take a few weeks after you have HIV for your body to produce these antibodies. There are other types of tests that can detect HIV infection sooner. Tell your doctor or clinic if you think you were recently exposed to HIV and ask if their tests can detect early infection.
- **Know your status.** After you get tested, be sure to learn your test results. If you are HIV-positive, see a health-care provider as soon as possible, so you can start treatment with HIV medicine. And be aware: When you are in the early stage of infection, you are at very high risk of transmitting HIV to others. It is important to take steps to reduce your risk of transmission. If you are HIV-negative, there are prevention tools such as PrEP that can help you stay negative.

Stage 2: Clinical Latency

In this stage, the virus still multiplies but at very low levels. People in this stage may not feel sick or have any symptoms. This stage is also called "chronic HIV infection." Without HIV treatment, people can stay in this stage for 10 or 15 years, but some move through this stage faster. If you take HIV medicine exactly as prescribed and get and keep an undetectable viral load, you can live and long and healthy life and will not transmit HIV to your HIV-negative partners through sex. But, if your viral load is detectable, you can transmit HIV during this stage, even when you have no symptoms. It is important to see your health-care provider regularly to get your viral load checked.

Stage 3: Acquired Immunodeficiency Syndrome

If you have HIV and you are not on HIV treatment, eventually, the virus will weaken your body's immune system, and you will progress to AIDS. This is the late stage of HIV infection.

Symptoms of AIDS can include the following:

- rapid weight loss
- recurring fever or profuse night sweats
- extreme and unexplained tiredness
- prolonged swelling of the lymph glands in the armpits, groin, or neck
- diarrhea that lasts for more than a week
- sores of the mouth, anus, or genitals
- pneumonia
- red, brown, pink, or purplish blotches on or under the skin or inside the mouth, nose, or eyelids
- memory loss, depression, and other neurologic disorders

Each of these symptoms can also be related to other illnesses. The only way to know for sure if you have HIV is to get tested. If you are HIV-positive, a health-care provider will diagnose if your HIV has progressed to stage 3 (AIDS) based on certain medical criteria.

Many of the severe symptoms and illnesses of HIV disease come from the opportunistic infections that occur because your body's immune system has been damaged. See your health-care provider if you are experiencing any of these symptoms.

But be aware: Thanks to effective treatment, most people in the United States with HIV do not progress to AIDS. If you have HIV and remain in care, take HIV medicine as prescribed, and get and keep an undetectable viral load, you will stay healthy and will not progress to AIDS.[1]

HUMAN IMMUNODEFICIENCY VIRUS TESTS FOR SCREENING AND DIAGNOSIS

Human immunodeficiency virus tests are very accurate, but no test can detect the virus immediately after infection. How soon a test can detect HIV depends on the type of test being used. The

[1] HIV.gov, "What Are HIV and AIDS?" U.S. Department of Health and Human Services (HHS), January 13, 2023. Available online. URL: www.hiv.gov/hiv-basics/overview/about-hiv-and-aids/what-are-hiv-and-aids. Accessed June 26, 2023.

following are the three types of HIV tests: antibody tests, antigen/antibody tests, and nucleic acid tests (NAT).

- **Antibody tests.** These tests look for antibodies to HIV in a person's blood or oral fluid. Antibody tests can take 23–90 days to detect HIV after exposure. Most rapid tests and the only FDA-approved HIV self-test are antibody tests. In general, antibody tests that use blood from a vein can detect HIV sooner after infection than tests done with blood from a finger stick or with oral fluid.
- **Antigen/antibody tests.** These tests look for both HIV antibodies and antigens. Antibodies are produced by a person's immune system when they are exposed to viruses, such as HIV. Antigens are foreign substances that cause a person's immune system to activate. If a person has HIV, an antigen called "p24" is produced before antibodies develop.
  Antigen/antibody tests are recommended for testing done in labs and are common in the United States.
  An antigen/antibody test performed by a lab on blood from a vein can usually detect HIV 18–45 days after exposure. There is also a rapid antigen/antibody test available that is done with a finger stick. Antigen/antibody tests done with blood from a finger stick can take 18–90 days after exposure.
- **Nucleic acid tests (NATs).** NATs look for the actual virus in the blood. This test should be considered for people who have had a recent exposure or a possible exposure with early symptoms of HIV and have tested negative with an antibody or antigen/antibody test. A NAT can usually detect HIV 10–33 days after exposure.

An initial HIV test usually will either be an antigen/antibody test or an antibody test. If the initial HIV test is a rapid or self-test and it is positive, the person should go to a health-care provider to get follow-up testing. If the initial HIV test is a lab test and it is positive, the lab will usually conduct follow-up testing on the same blood sample as the initial test. Although HIV tests are generally accurate, follow-up tests allow the health-care provider to confirm the result.[2]

WHAT ARE THE TREATMENTS FOR HUMAN IMMUNODEFICIENCY VIRUS?

There is no cure for HIV infection, but it can be treated with medicines. This is called "ART." ART can make HIV infection a manageable chronic condition. It also reduces the risk of spreading the virus to others.

Most people with HIV live long and healthy lives if they get ART as soon as possible and stay on it. It is also important to take care of yourself. Making sure that you have the support you need, living a healthy lifestyle, and getting regular medical care can help you enjoy a better quality of life.

CAN HUMAN IMMUNODEFICIENCY VIRUS INFECTION BE PREVENTED?

You can reduce the risk of getting or spreading HIV by:

- getting tested for HIV
- choosing less risky sexual behaviors (This includes limiting the number of sexual partners you have and using latex condoms every time you have sex. If you or your partner is allergic to latex, you can use polyurethane condoms.)
- getting tested and treated for STDs
- not injecting drugs
- talking to your health-care provider about medicines to prevent HIV:
    - **Pre-exposure prophylaxis (PrEP).** PrEP is for people who do not already have HIV but are at very high risk of getting it. PrEP is a daily medicine that can reduce this risk.

[2] "HIV Testing," Centers for Disease Control and Prevention (CDC), June 9, 2022. Available online. URL: www.cdc.gov/hiv/testing/index.html#:~:text=An%20antigen%2Fantibody%20test%20performed,to%2090%20days%20after%20exposure. Accessed June 26, 2023.

- **Post-exposure prophylaxis (PEP)**. PEP is for people who have possibly been exposed to HIV. It is only for emergency situations. PEP must be started within 72 hours after a possible exposure to HIV.[3]

[3] MedlinePlus, "HIV Symptoms," National Institutes of Health (NIH), February 14, 2023. Available online. URL: https://medlineplus.gov/hiv.html. Accessed June 26, 2023.

Chapter 17 | **Human Papillomavirus Infection**

Human papillomavirus (HPV) is the most common sexually transmitted infection (STI) in the United States. HPV vaccines can prevent some of the health effects HPV causes.

WHAT IS HUMAN PAPILLOMAVIRUS?

There were about 43 million HPV infections in 2018, many among people in their late teens and early 20s. There are many different types of HPV. Some types can cause health problems, including genital warts and cancers. But there are vaccines that can stop these health problems from happening. HPV is a different virus than human immunodeficiency virus (HIV) and herpes simplex virus (HSV).

HOW IS HUMAN PAPILLOMAVIRUS SPREAD?

You can get HPV by having vaginal, anal, or oral sex with someone who has the virus. It is most commonly spread during vaginal or anal sex. It also spreads through close skin-to-skin touching during sex. A person with HPV can pass the infection to someone even when they have no signs or symptoms. If you are sexually active, you can get HPV, even if you have had sex with only one person. You can also develop symptoms years after having sex with someone who has the infection. This makes it hard to know when you first got it.

DOES HUMAN PAPILLOMAVIRUS CAUSE HEALTH PROBLEMS?

In most cases (9 out of 10), HPV goes away on its own within two years without health problems. But, when HPV does not go away, it can cause health problems such as genital warts and cancer. Genital warts usually appear as a small bump or group of bumps in the genital area. They can be small or large, raised or flat, or shaped like a cauliflower. A health-care provider can usually diagnose warts by looking at the genital area.

DOES HUMAN PAPILLOMAVIRUS CAUSE CANCER?

Human papillomavirus can cause cervical and other cancers, including cancer of the vulva, vagina, penis, or anus. It can also cause cancer in the back of the throat (called "oropharyngeal cancer"). This can include the base of the tongue and tonsils. Cancer often takes years, even decades, to develop after a person gets HPV. Genital warts and cancers result from different types of HPV. There is no way to know who will develop cancer or other health problems from HPV. People with weak immune systems (including those with HIV) may be less able to fight off HPV. They may also be more likely to develop health problems from HPV.

HOW CAN YOU AVOID HUMAN PAPILLOMAVIRUS AND THE HEALTH PROBLEMS IT CAN CAUSE?

You can do several things to lower your chances of getting HPV.

Get Vaccinated

The HPV vaccine is safe and effective. It can protect against diseases (including cancers) caused by HPV when given in the recommended age groups.

Get Screened for Cervical Cancer

Routine screening for women aged 21–65 can prevent cervical cancer. If you are sexually active, do the following:

- Use condoms the right way every time you have sex. This can lower your chances of getting HPV. But

HPV can infect areas the condom does not cover. So condoms may not fully protect against getting HPV.
- Be in a mutually monogamous relationship—or have sex only with someone who only has sex with you.

WHO SHOULD GET THE HUMAN PAPILLOMAVIRUS VACCINE?

The Centers for Disease Control and Prevention (CDC) recommends HPV vaccination for:
- all preteens (including boys and girls) at age 11 or 12 (or can start at age 9).
- everyone through age 26 if not vaccinated already.

Vaccination is not recommended for everyone older than age 26. However, some adults aged 27–45 who are not already vaccinated may decide to get the HPV vaccine after speaking with their health-care provider about their risk for new HPV infections and the possible benefits of vaccination. HPV vaccination in this age range provides less benefit. Most sexually active adults have already been exposed to HPV although not necessarily all of the HPV types targeted by vaccination. At any age, having a new sex partner is a risk factor for getting a new HPV infection. People who are already in a long-term, mutually monogamous relationship are not likely to get a new HPV infection.

HOW DO YOU KNOW IF YOU HAVE HUMAN PAPILLOMAVIRUS?

There is no test to find out a person's "HPV status." Also, there is no approved HPV test to find HPV in the mouth or throat. There are HPV tests that can screen for cervical cancer. Health-care providers only use these tests for screening women aged 30 and older. HPV tests are not recommended to screen men, adolescents, or women under the age of 30. Most people with HPV do not know they have the infection. They never develop symptoms or health problems from it. Some people find out they have HPV when they get genital warts. Women may find out they have HPV when they get an abnormal Papanicolaou (Pap) test result (during cervical cancer screening). Others may only find out once they have developed more serious problems from HPV, such as cancers.

HOW COMMON ARE HUMAN PAPILLOMAVIRUS AND HEALTH PROBLEMS THAT DEVELOP FROM IT?

- **HPV (the virus).** The CDC estimates that there were 43 million HPV infections in 2018. In that same year, there were 13 million new infections. HPV is so common that almost every sexually active person will get HPV at some point if they do not get vaccinated. Health problems related to HPV include genital warts and cervical cancer.
- **Genital warts.** Prior to HPV vaccines, genital warts caused by HPV affected roughly 340,000–360,000 people yearly.* About one in 100 sexually active adults in the United States has genital warts at any given time.
- **Cervical cancer.** Every year, nearly 12,000 women living in the United States will have cervical cancer. More than 4,000 women die from cervical cancer—even with screening and treatment.

There are other conditions and cancers caused by HPV that occur in people living in the United States. Every year, about 19,400 women and 12,100 men experience cancers caused by HPV.

******These figures only look at the number of people who sought care for genital warts. This could be less than the actual number of people who get genital warts.*

CAN HUMAN PAPILLOMAVIRUS AFFECT YOUR PREGNANCY?

Pregnant people with HPV can get genital warts or develop abnormal cell changes on the cervix. Routine cervical cancer screening can help find abnormal cell changes. You should get routine cervical cancer screening even when you are pregnant.

IS THERE TREATMENT FOR HUMAN PAPILLOMAVIRUS OR HEALTH PROBLEMS THAT DEVELOP FROM IT?

There is no treatment for the virus itself. However, there are treatments for the health problems that HPV can cause:

- Genital warts can go away with treatment from your health-care provider or with prescription medicine. If left untreated, genital warts may go away, stay the same, or grow in size or number.

- Cervical precancer treatment is available. Women who get routine Pap tests and follow-up as needed can find problems before cancer develops. Prevention is always better than treatment.
- Other HPV-related cancers are also more treatable when found and treated early.[1]

[1] "Genital HPV Infection—Basic Fact Sheet," Centers for Disease Control and Prevention (CDC), April 12, 2022. Available online. URL: www.cdc.gov/std/hpv/stdfact-hpv.htm. Accessed June 26, 2023.

Chapter 18 | **Infectious Mononucleosis**

WHAT IS INFECTIOUS MONONUCLEOSIS?

Infectious mononucleosis, also called "mono," is a contagious disease. Epstein-Barr virus (EBV) is the most common cause of infectious mononucleosis, but other viruses can also cause this disease. It is common among teenagers and young adults, especially college students. At least one out of four teenagers and young adults who get infected with EBV will develop infectious mononucleosis.

SYMPTOMS OF INFECTIOUS MONONUCLEOSIS

Typical symptoms of infectious mononucleosis usually appear four to six weeks after you get infected with EBV. Symptoms may develop slowly and may not all occur at the same time. These symptoms include the following:

- extreme fatigue
- fever
- sore throat
- head and body aches
- swollen lymph nodes in the neck and armpits
- swollen liver or spleen or both
- rash

An enlarged spleen and a swollen liver are less common symptoms. For some people, their liver or spleen or both may remain enlarged even after their fatigue ends. Most people get better in two to four weeks; however, some people may feel fatigued for several more weeks. Occasionally, the symptoms of infectious mononucleosis can last for six months or longer.

DIAGNOSING INFECTIOUS MONONUCLEOSIS

Health-care providers typically diagnose infectious mononucleosis based on symptoms. Laboratory tests are not usually needed to diagnose infectious mononucleosis. However, specific laboratory tests may be needed to identify the cause of illness in people who do not have a typical case of infectious mononucleosis. The blood work of patients who have infectious mononucleosis due to EBV infection may show:

- more white blood cells (lymphocytes) than normal
- unusual-looking white blood cells (atypical lymphocytes)
- fewer than normal neutrophils or platelets
- abnormal liver function

TRANSMISSION OF INFECTIOUS MONONUCLEOSIS

Epstein-Barr virus is the most common cause of infectious mononucleosis, but other viruses can cause this disease. Typically, these viruses spread through bodily fluids, especially saliva. However, these viruses can also spread through blood and semen during sexual contact, blood transfusions, and organ transplantations.

PREVENTION AND TREATMENT OF INFECTIOUS MONONUCLEOSIS

There is no vaccine to protect against infectious mononucleosis. You can help protect yourself by not kissing or sharing drinks, food, or personal items, such as toothbrushes, with people who have infectious mononucleosis. You can help relieve symptoms of infectious mononucleosis by:

- drinking fluids to stay hydrated
- getting plenty of rest
- taking over-the-counter (OTC) medications for pain and fever

If you have infectious mononucleosis, you should not take penicillin antibiotics such as ampicillin or amoxicillin. Based on the severity of the symptoms, a health-care provider may recommend treatment of specific organ systems affected by infectious mononucleosis.

Infectious Mononucleosis

Because your spleen may become enlarged as a result of infectious mononucleosis, you should avoid contact sports until you fully recover. Participating in contact sports can be strenuous and may cause the spleen to rupture. Other infections that can cause infectious mononucleosis are as follows:

- cytomegalovirus (CMV)
- toxoplasmosis
- human immunodeficiency virus (HIV)
- rubella
- hepatitis A, B, or C
- adenovirus[1]

[1] "Epstein-Barr Virus and Infectious Mononucleosis," Centers for Disease Control and Prevention (CDC), September 28, 2020. Available online. URL: www.cdc.gov/epstein-barr/index.html. Accessed June 23, 2023.

Chapter 19 | Influenza

Chapter Contents

Section 19.1 | Avian Flu

Although avian (bird) influenza (flu) A viruses usually do not infect people, there have been some rare cases of human infection with these viruses. Illnesses in humans from bird flu virus infections have ranged in severity from no symptoms or mild illness to severe disease that resulted in death. Asian lineage H7N9 and highly pathogenic avian influenza Asian lineage H5N1 viruses have been responsible for most human illness from bird flu viruses worldwide to date, including the most serious illnesses and illnesses with the highest mortality.

Infected birds shed the bird flu virus through their saliva, mucous, and feces. Human infections with bird flu viruses can happen when the virus gets into a person's eyes, nose, or mouth or is inhaled. This can happen when the virus is in the air (in droplets or possibly dust) and a person breathes it in or possibly when a person touches something that has the virus on it and then touches their mouth, eyes, or nose. Human infections with bird flu viruses have occurred most often after unprotected contact with infected birds or surfaces contaminated with bird flu viruses (refer to Figure 19.1). However, some infections have been identified where direct contact with infected birds or their environment was not known to have occurred.

The spread of bird flu viruses from one infected person to a close contact is very rare, and when it has happened, it has only spread to a few people. However, because of the possibility that bird flu viruses could change and gain the ability to spread easily between people, monitoring for human infection and person-to-person spread is extremely important for public health.

SIGNS AND SYMPTOMS OF AVIAN INFLUENZA A VIRUS INFECTIONS IN HUMANS

The reported signs and symptoms of bird flu virus infections in humans have ranged from no symptoms or mild illness (such as eye redness (conjunctivitis) or mild flu-like upper respiratory symptoms) to severe (such as pneumonia requiring hospitalization) and included fever (temperature of 100 °F (37.8 °C) or greater) or feeling feverish*, cough, sore throat, runny or stuffy nose, muscle or body aches, headaches, fatigue, and shortness of breath or difficulty breathing. Less common signs and symptoms include diarrhea, nausea, vomiting, or seizures.

**Fever may not always be present.*

PREVENTION OF AVIAN INFLUENZA A VIRUS INFECTIONS

- As a general precaution, whenever possible, people should avoid direct contact with wild birds and observe them only from a distance.
- Wild birds can be infected with avian (bird) influenza (flu) A viruses even if they do not look sick.
- Avoid unprotected contact with domestic birds (poultry) that look sick or have died.
- Do not touch surfaces that may be contaminated with saliva, mucous, or feces from wild or domestic birds.

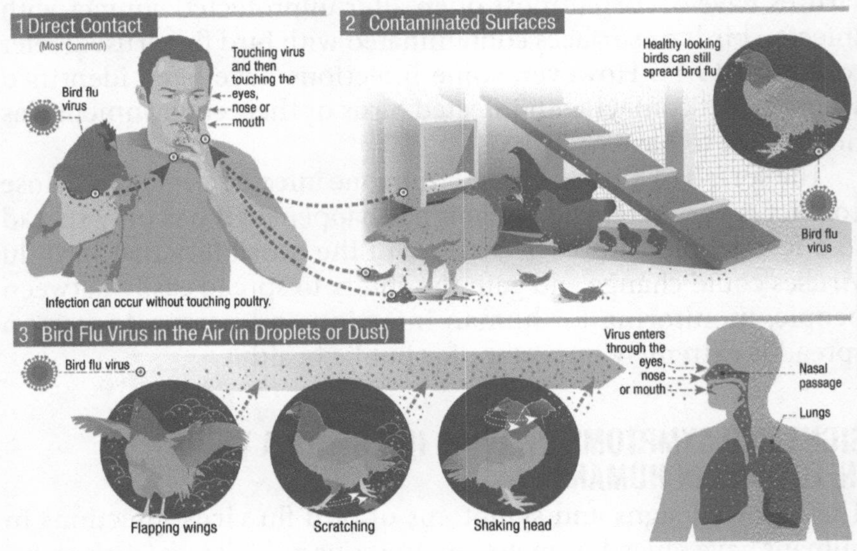

Figure 19.1. Avian Flu Transmission

Centers for Disease Control and Prevention (CDC)

DETECTING BIRD FLU AVIAN INFLUENZA A VIRUS INFECTION IN HUMANS

Bird flu virus infection in people cannot be diagnosed by clinical signs and symptoms alone; laboratory testing is needed. Bird flu virus infection is usually diagnosed by collecting a swab from the upper respiratory tract (nose or throat) of the sick person. Testing is more accurate when the swab is collected during the first few days of illness.

For critically ill patients, collection and testing of lower respiratory tract specimens may also lead to the diagnosis of bird flu virus infection. However, for some patients who are no longer very sick or who have fully recovered, it may be difficult to detect bird flu virus in a specimen.

The Centers for Disease Control and Prevention (CDC) has posted guidance for clinicians and public health professionals in the United States on appropriate testing, specimen collection, and processing of samples from patients who might be infected with avian influenza A viruses.[1]

Section 19.2 | H1N1 Flu

WHAT IS H1N1?

H1N1 (sometimes called "swine flu") is an influenza virus causing illness in people. This new virus was first detected in people in the United States in April 2009. This virus is spreading from person to person worldwide, probably in much the same way that regular seasonal influenza viruses spread. On June 11, 2009, the World Health Organization (WHO) declared that a pandemic of H1N1 flu was underway.

[1] "Bird Flu Virus Infections in Humans," Centers for Disease Control and Prevention (CDC), May 4, 2022. Available online. URL: www.cdc.gov/flu/avianflu/avian-in-humans.htm. Accessed June 27, 2023.

WHY IS THE H1N1 VIRUS SOMETIMES CALLED "SWINE FLU"?

This virus was originally referred to as "swine flu" because laboratory testing showed that many of the genes in the virus were very similar to influenza viruses that normally occur in pigs (swine) in North America. But further study has shown that the H1N1 is very different from what normally circulates in North American pigs. It has two genes from flu viruses that normally circulate in pigs in Europe and Asia and bird (avian) genes and human genes. Scientists call this a "quadruple reassortant" virus.

H1N1 FLU IN HUMANS

Are There Human Infections with the H1N1 Virus in the United States?

Yes. While H1N1 activity declined after October 2009, human illness with H1N1 is ongoing in the United States. In fact, the H1N1 virus is the predominant influenza virus in circulation so far during the 2009-2010 flu season. The United States experienced its first wave of H1N1 activity in the spring of 2009, followed by a second wave in the fall, with the number of people infected peaking at the end of October. There are still uncertainties surrounding the rest of this flu season, including the possibility that seasonal influenza viruses will spread during the winter as they usually do while H1N1 viruses continue to cause illness. In past pandemics, flu activity has occurred in waves, and it is possible that the United States could experience another wave either later in the 2010 winter or later. In the past, when new viruses have emerged to cause flu pandemics, the new virus has continued to spread among people. Experts believe it is likely that the new H1N1 virus will continue to circulate among people for some time, perhaps as a typical winter flu. In fact, an H1N1 virus has been selected as the H1N1 vaccine component for the Southern Hemisphere's upcoming seasonal flu vaccine.

The Centers for Disease Control and Prevention (CDC) routinely works with states to collect, compile, and analyze information about influenza and has done the same for the H1N1 virus since the beginning of the outbreak.

Is the H1N1 Virus Contagious?

The H1N1 virus is contagious and spreads from human to human.

HOW DOES THE H1N1 VIRUS SPREAD?

Spread of the H1N1 virus is thought to occur in the same way that seasonal flu spreads. Flu viruses are spread mainly from person to person through coughing, sneezing, or talking by people with influenza. Sometimes, people may become infected by touching something—such as a surface or object—with flu viruses on it and then touching their mouth or nose.

CAN YOU GET H1N1 MORE THAN ONCE?

Getting infected with any influenza virus, including H1N1, should cause your body to develop immune resistance to that virus, so it is not likely that a person would be infected with the identical influenza virus more than once. (However, people with weakened immune systems might not develop full immunity after infection and might be more likely to get infected with the same influenza virus more than once.) However, it is also possible that a person could have a positive test result for flu infection more than once in an influenza season. This can occur for the following two reasons:

- A person may be infected with different influenza viruses (e.g., the first time with H1N1 and the second time with a regular seasonal flu virus). Most rapid tests cannot distinguish which influenza virus is responsible for the illness.
- Influenza tests can occasionally give false positive and false negative results, so it is possible that one of the test results was incorrect. This is more likely to happen when the diagnosis is made with rapid flu tests.

WHAT ARE THE SIGNS AND SYMPTOMS OF THE H1N1 FLU VIRUS IN PEOPLE?

The symptoms of the H1N1 flu virus in people include fever, cough, sore throat, runny or stuffy nose, body aches, headache, chills, and fatigue. Some people may have vomiting and diarrhea. People may be infected with the flu, including H1N1, and have respiratory symptoms without a fever. Severe illnesses and deaths have occurred as a result of illness associated with this virus.

HOW SEVERE IS THE ILLNESS THAT IS ASSOCIATED WITH H1N1 FLU VIRUS?

Illness with the H1N1 virus has ranged from mild to severe. While most people who have been sick have recovered without needing medical treatment, hospitalizations and deaths from infection with this virus have occurred.

In seasonal flu, certain people are at "high risk" of serious complications. This includes people aged 65 and older, children younger than five years old, pregnant women, and people of any age with certain chronic medical conditions. More than 70 percent of adults who have been hospitalized with the H1N1 virus have had one or more medical conditions previously recognized as placing people at "higher risk" of serious seasonal flu-related complications. This includes pregnancy, diabetes, heart disease, asthma, and kidney disease. In one study, 57 percent of children who had been hospitalized as a result of H1N1 have had one or more "higher risk" medical conditions.

Young children are also at high risk of serious complications from H1N1, just as they are from seasonal flu. And while people 65 and older are less likely to be infected with H1N1 flu, if they get sick, they are also at "high risk" of developing serious complications from their illness. The CDC laboratory studies have shown that no children and very few adults younger than 60 years old have existing antibodies to the H1N1 flu virus; however, about one-third of adults older than 60 may have antibodies against this virus. It is unknown how much, if any, protection may be afforded against H1N1 flu by any existing antibody.

WHO IS AT HIGHER RISK FROM SERIOUS H1N1-RELATED COMPLICATIONS?

Most people who get the flu (either seasonal or H1N1) will have mild illness, will not need medical care or antiviral drugs, and will recover in less than two weeks. Some people, however, are more likely to get flu complications that result in being hospitalized and occasionally result in death. Pneumonia, bronchitis, sinus infections, and ear infections are examples of flu-related complications. The flu can also make chronic health problems worse. For example, people with asthma may experience asthma attacks while they have the flu, and people with chronic congestive heart failure may have worsening of this condition that is triggered by the flu. The following list includes the groups of people more likely to get flu-related complications if they get sick from influenza. People at high risk for developing flu-related complications:

- children younger than five, but especially children younger than two years old
- adults aged 65 and older
- pregnant women

People who have medical conditions including:

- asthma
- neurological and neurodevelopmental conditions (including disorders of the brain, spinal cord, peripheral nerve, and muscle such as cerebral palsy (CP), epilepsy (seizure disorders), stroke, intellectual disability (mental retardation), moderate to severe developmental delay, muscular dystrophy (MD), or spinal cord injury (SCI)).
- chronic lung disease (such as chronic obstructive pulmonary disease (COPD) and cystic fibrosis (CF))
- heart disease (such as congenital heart disease (CHD), congestive heart failure (CHF), and coronary artery disease (CAD))
- blood disorders (such as sickle cell disease (SCD))
- endocrine disorders (such as diabetes mellitus)
- kidney disorders
- liver disorders
- metabolic disorders (such as inherited metabolic disorders and mitochondrial disorders)
- weakened immune system due to disease or medication (such as people with human immunodeficiency virus

(HIV) or acquired immunodeficiency syndrome (AIDS) or cancer or those on chronic steroids)
- people younger than 19 years of age who are receiving long-term aspirin therapy

In addition, some studies have shown that obese persons (body mass index greater than or equal to 30) and particularly morbidly obese persons (body mass index greater than or equal to 40) are at higher risk, perhaps because they have one of the higher risk conditions above but do not realize it.

HOW DOES H1N1 FLU COMPARE TO SEASONAL FLU IN TERMS OF ITS SEVERITY AND INFECTION RATES?

Flu seasons vary in terms of timing, duration, and severity. Seasonal influenza can cause mild to severe illness and at times can lead to death. Each year, in the United States, on average 36,000 people die from flu-related complications, and more than 200,000 people are hospitalized from flu-related causes. Of those hospitalized, 20,000 are children younger than five years old. More than 90 percent of deaths and about 60 percent of hospitalizations occur in people older than 65.

The CDC estimates of the numbers of H1N1 cases, hospitalizations, and deaths are that people younger than 65 years of age are more severely affected by H1N1 flu relative to people 65 and older compared with seasonal flu. The CDC estimates that with H1N1, approximately 90 percent of hospitalizations and 88 percent of estimated deaths from April through December 12, 2009, occurred in people younger than 65 years old. However, because severe illness and deaths have occurred among people 65 and older and because supplies of the H1N1 vaccine have increased dramatically, the CDC is now encouraging all people six months and older, including people older than 65, to get vaccinated against H1N1.

HOW LONG CAN AN INFECTED PERSON SPREAD THE H1N1 VIRUS TO OTHERS?

People infected with seasonal and H1N1 flu shed viruses and may be able to infect others from one day before getting sick to five to seven days after. This can be longer in some people, especially children and people with weakened immune systems, and in people infected with H1N1 viruses.

PREVENTION AND TREATMENT

What Can You Do to Protect Yourself from Getting Sick?

This season, there is a seasonal flu vaccine to protect against seasonal flu viruses and an H1N1 vaccine to protect against the H1N1 influenza virus. A flu vaccine is by far the most important step in protecting against flu infection.

There are also everyday actions that can help prevent the spread of germs that cause respiratory illnesses, such as the flu.

Take these everyday steps to protect your health:

- Cover your nose and mouth with a tissue when you cough or sneeze. Throw the tissue in the trash after you use it.
- Wash your hands often with soap and water. If soap and water are not available, use an alcohol-based hand rub.
- Avoid touching your eyes, nose, or mouth. Germs spread this way.
- Try to avoid close contact with sick people.
- If you are sick with flu-like illness, the CDC recommends that you stay home for at least 24 hours after your fever is gone except to get medical care or for other necessities. (Your fever should be gone without the use of a fever-reducing medicine.) Keep away from others as much as possible to keep from making others sick.

Other important actions that you can take are as follows:

- Follow public health advice regarding school closures, avoiding crowds, and other social distancing measures.
- Be prepared in case you get sick and need to stay home for a week or so; a supply of over-the-counter (OTC) medicines, alcohol-based hand rubs (for when soap and water are not available), tissues, and other related items could help you avoid the need to make trips out in public while you are sick and contagious.

What Is the Best Way to Keep from Spreading the Virus through Coughing or Sneezing?

If you are sick with flu-like illness, the CDC recommends that you stay home for at least 24 hours after your fever is gone except to get medical care or for other necessities. (Your fever should be gone without the use of a fever-reducing medicine.)

Keep away from others as much as possible. Cover your mouth and nose with a tissue when coughing or sneezing. Put your used tissue in the waste basket. Then clean your hands and do so every time you cough or sneeze.

If You Have a Family Member at Home Who Is Sick with H1N1 Flu, Should You Go to Work?

Employees who are well but who have an ill family member at home with H1N1 flu can go to work as usual. These employees should monitor their health every day and take everyday precautions including covering their coughs and sneezes and washing their hands often with soap and water, especially after they cough or sneeze. If soap and water are not available, they should use an alcohol-based hand rub. If they become ill, they should notify their supervisor and stay home. Employees who have an underlying medical condition or who are pregnant should call their health-care provider for advice because they might need to receive influenza antiviral drugs.

What Is the Best Technique for Washing Your Hands to Avoid Getting the Flu?

Washing your hands will often help protect you from germs. The CDC recommends that when you wash your hands—with soap and warm water— you wash for 15–20 seconds. When soap and water are not available, alcohol-based disposable hand wipes or gel sanitizers may be used. You can find them in most supermarkets and drugstores. If using gel, rub your hands until the gel is dry. The gel does not need water to work; the alcohol in it kills the germs on your hands.

What Should You Do If You Get Sick?

For information about what to do if you get sick with flu-like symptoms this season, see What To Do If You Get Sick: H1N1 and Seasonal Flu (www.cdc.gov/h1n1flu/sick.htm). A downloadable flyer (www.cdc.gov/flu/freeresources/2009-10/pdf/what_to_do_if_you_get_sick.pdf) containing this information is also available.

What Should You Do If You Have a Fever?

Fever can be one of the symptoms of a flu-like illness for many people. A fever is an oral temperature of at least 100 °F (37.8 °C). Signs of a fever include chills, a flushed appearance, feeling very warm, or sweating.

Fever-reducing medicines typically contain acetaminophen (such as Tylenol) or ibuprofen (such as Motrin). These medicines can both help bring fever down and relieve pain. Aspirin (acetylsalicylic acid) should not be given to children or teenagers (anyone aged 18 and younger) who have flu; this can cause a rare but serious illness called "Reye syndrome."

To help avoid spreading the flu, if you have a fever, stay at home for at least 24 hours after you no longer have a fever or signs of a fever. However, if you are taking fever-reducing medicines, you cannot tell if your fever is truly gone. Therefore, when you start to feel better, increase the interval between doses of fever-reducing medicines and continue to monitor your temperature to make sure your fever does not return.

What Are "Emergency Warning Signs" That Should Signal Anyone to Seek Medical Care Urgently?

IN CHILDREN

- fast breathing or trouble breathing
- bluish skin color
- not drinking enough fluids
- not waking up or not interacting
- being so irritable that the child does not want to be held
- flu-like symptoms that improve but then return with fever and worse cough
- fever with a rash

IN ADULTS

- difficulty breathing or shortness of breath
- pain or pressure in the chest or abdomen
- sudden dizziness
- confusion
- severe or persistent vomiting
- flu-like symptoms that improve but then return with fever and worse cough

ARE THERE MEDICINES TO TREAT H1N1 INFECTION?

Yes. There are drugs your doctor may prescribe for treating both seasonal and H1N1 called "antiviral drugs." These drugs can make you better faster and may also prevent serious complications. It is very important that antiviral drugs be used early to treat flu in people who are very sick (e.g., people who are in the hospital) and people who are sick with flu and have a greater chance of getting serious flu complications. Other people may also be treated with antiviral drugs by their doctor this season. Most healthy people with flu, however, do not need to be treated with antiviral drugs.

CENTERS FOR DISEASE CONTROL AND PREVENTION ADVISES AGAINST "SWINE FLU PARTIES"

"Swine flu parties" are gatherings during which people have close contact with a person who has H1N1 flu in order to become infected with the virus. The intent of these parties is for a person to become infected with what for many people has been a mild disease, in the hope of having natural immunity to the H1N1 flu virus that might circulate later and cause more severe disease.

The CDC does not recommend "swine flu parties" as a way to protect against H1N1 flu in the future. While the disease seen in the current H1N1 flu outbreak has been mild for many people, it has been severe and even fatal for others. There is no way to predict with certainty what the outcome will be for an individual or, equally important, for others to whom the intentionally infected person may spread the virus. Vaccination against H1N1 with the H1N1 vaccine is the best way to protect against this virus. Supplies of the H1N1 vaccine are ample, and the CDC is now recommending that everyone get vaccinated.

The CDC recommends that people with H1N1 flu avoid contact with others as much as possible. If you are sick with flu-like illness, the CDC recommends that you stay home for at least 24 hours after your fever is gone except to get medical care or for other necessities. (Your fever should be gone without the use of a fever-reducing medicine.) Stay away from others as much as possible to keep from making others sick.

CONTAMINATION AND CLEANING

How Long Can Influenza Virus Remain Viable on Objects (Such as Books and Doorknobs)?

Studies have shown that the influenza virus can survive on environmental surfaces and can infect a person for two to eight hours after being deposited on the surface.

What Kills Influenza Virus?

Influenza virus is destroyed by heat (167–212 °F (75–100 °C)). In addition, several chemical germicides, including chlorine, hydrogen peroxide, detergents (soap), iodophors (iodine-based antiseptics), and alcohols, are effective against human influenza viruses if used in proper concentration for a sufficient length of time.

What If Soap and Water Are Not Available and Alcohol-Based Products Are Not Allowed in Your Facility?

If soap and water are not available and alcohol-based products are not allowed, other hand sanitizers that do not contain alcohol may be useful.

What Are the Most Likely Sources of Contamination?

Germs can be spread when a person touches something that is contaminated with germs and then touches his or her eyes, nose, or mouth. Droplets from a cough or sneeze of an infected person move through the air. Germs can be spread when a person touches respiratory droplets from another person on a surface such as a desk, for example, and then touches their own eyes, mouth, or nose before washing their hands.

How Should Waste Disposal Be Handled to Prevent the Spread of Influenza Virus?

To prevent the spread of the influenza virus, it is recommended that tissues and other disposable items used by an infected person be thrown in the trash. Additionally, persons should wash their hands with soap and water after touching used tissues and similar waste.

What Household Cleaning Should Be Done to Prevent the Spread of Influenza Virus?

To prevent the spread of the influenza virus, it is important to keep surfaces (especially bedside tables, surfaces in the bathroom, kitchen counters, and toys for children) clean by wiping them down with a household disinfectant according to directions on the product label.

How Should Linens, Eating Utensils, and Dishes of Persons Infected with the Influenza Virus Be Handled?

Linens, eating utensils, and dishes belonging to those who are sick do not need to be cleaned separately, but importantly, these items should not be shared without washing thoroughly first.

Linens (such as bedsheets and towels) should be washed by using household laundry soap and tumbled dry in a hot setting. Individuals should avoid "hugging" laundry prior to washing it to prevent contaminating themselves. Individuals should wash their hands with soap and water or alcohol-based hand rub immediately after handling dirty laundry.

Eating utensils should be washed either in a dishwasher or by hand with water and soap.

OTHER EXPOSURES TO H1N1 FLU

Can You Get Infected with the H1N1 Virus from Eating or Preparing Pork?

No. H1N1 viruses are not spread by food. You cannot get infected with 2009 HIN1 from eating pork or pork products. Eating properly handled and cooked pork products is safe.

Is There a Risk from Drinking Water?

Tap water that has been treated by conventional disinfection processes does not likely pose a risk for transmission of influenza viruses. Current drinking water treatment regulations provide a high degree of protection from viruses. No research has been completed on the susceptibility of the H1N1 flu virus to conventional drinking water treatment processes. However, recent studies have demonstrated that free chlorine levels typically used in drinking water treatment are adequate to inactivate highly pathogenic H5N1 avian influenza. It is likely that other influenza viruses, such as H1N1, would also be similarly inactivated by chlorination. To date, there have been no documented human cases of influenza caused by exposure to influenza-contaminated drinking water.

Can the H1N1 Flu Virus Be Spread through Water in Swimming Pools, Spas, Water Parks, Interactive Fountains, and Other Treated Recreational Water Venues?

Influenza viruses infect the human upper respiratory tract. There has never been a documented case of influenza virus infection associated with water exposure. Recreational water that has been treated at CDC-recommended disinfectant levels does not likely pose a risk for transmission of influenza viruses. No research has been completed on the susceptibility of the H1N1 influenza virus to chlorine and other disinfectants used in swimming pools, spas, water parks, interactive fountains, and other treated recreational venues. However, recent studies have demonstrated that free chlorine levels recommended by the CDC (1–3 ppm or mg/L for pools and 2–5 ppm for spas) are adequate to disinfect the avian influenza A (H5N1) virus. It is likely that other influenza viruses, such as the H1N1 virus, would also be similarly disinfected by chlorine.

Can the H1N1 Influenza Virus Be Spread at Recreational Water Venues Outside the Water?

Yes, recreational water venues are no different than any other group setting. The spread of this H1N1 flu is thought to be happening in the same way that seasonal flu spreads. Flu viruses are spread mainly from person to person through coughing or sneezing of people with influenza. Sometimes, people may become infected by touching something with flu viruses on it and then touching their mouth or nose.

H1N1 IN PETS

What Animals Can Be Infected with the H1N1 Virus?

In addition to humans, live swine and turkeys, a small number of ferrets (which are highly susceptible to influenza A viruses), domestic cats, and dogs have been infected with the H1N1 virus. In addition, H1N1 virus infection was reported in a cheetah in the United States. The CDC is working closely with domestic and international public and animal health partners to continually monitor reports of H1N1 in animals and will provide additional information to the public as it becomes available.

How Do Pets Become Infected with H1N1?

All available information suggests that the ferrets and domestic cats infected with H1N1 infections acquired the virus through close contact with ill humans.

Can You Get H1N1 Influenza from Your Pet?

Available evidence suggests that transmission has been from ill humans to their companion animals. No evidence is available to suggest that animals are infecting humans with the H1N1 virus.

What Do You Do If You Are Sick with Flu-Like Symptoms and You Have Pets?

If you are sick with influenza-like-illness, take the same precautions with your pets that you would to keep your family and friends healthy:

- Cover your coughs and sneezes.
- Wash your hands frequently.
- Minimize contact with your pets until 24 hours after your fever is gone without the use of fever-reducing medication

What Should You Do If You Suspect Your Pet Has the H1N1 Influenza Virus?

If members of your household have flu-like symptoms and your pet exhibits respiratory illness, contact your veterinarian.

Is There a Vaccine Available for Your Pet?

Currently, there is no licensed and approved H1N1 vaccine for pets. (There is a canine influenza vaccine, which protects dogs from the H3N8 canine flu virus, but it will not protect pets against the H1N1 virus, and the H3N8 vaccine should not be used in any species other than dogs.)

How Serious Is This Disease in Pets?

Pet ferrets with naturally occurring H1N1 infection have exhibited illnesses similar in severity to that seen in ferrets exposed to seasonal influenza viruses and to the H1N1 virus in laboratory settings. Clinical signs exhibited have included sneezing, inactivity, and weight loss. Of the reported cases, most of the pets have recovered fully with supportive care although some have died.[2]

---

[2] "2009 H1N1 Flu ('Swine Flu') and You," Centers for Disease Control and Prevention (CDC), February 10, 2010. Available online. URL: www.cdc.gov/h1n1flu/qa.htm. Accessed June 27, 2023.

Section 19.3 | Pandemic Flu

WHAT IS AN INFLUENZA PANDEMIC?

An influenza pandemic is a global outbreak of a new influenza A virus that is very different from current and recently circulating human seasonal influenza A viruses. Pandemics happen when new (novel) influenza A viruses emerge that are able to infect people easily and spread from person to person in an efficient and sustained way.

WHERE DO PANDEMIC INFLUENZA VIRUSES COME FROM?

Different animals—including birds and pigs—are hosts to influenza A viruses that do not normally infect people. Influenza A viruses are constantly changing, making it possible on very rare occasions for nonhuman influenza viruses to change in such a way that they can infect people easily and spread efficiently from person to person.

HOW DO INFLUENZA A VIRUSES CHANGE TO CAUSE A PANDEMIC?

Influenza A viruses are divided into subtypes based on two proteins on the surface of the virus: the hemagglutinin (H) and the neuraminidase (N). There are 18 different hemagglutinin subtypes and 11 different neuraminidase subtypes (H1 through H18 and N1 through N11). Theoretically, any combination of the 18 hemagglutinins and 11 neuraminidase proteins is possible, but not all have been found in animals, and even fewer have been found to infect humans.

Influenza viruses can change in two different ways, one of which is called "antigenic shift" and can result in the emergence of a new influenza virus. Antigenic shift represents an abrupt, major change in an influenza A virus. This can result from direct infection of humans with a nonhuman influenza A virus, such as a virus circulating among birds or pigs. Antigenic shift can also happen when a nonhuman influenza A virus (e.g., an avian influenza virus) exchanges genetic information with other influenza A viruses in a process called "genetic reassortment," and the resultant new virus is able to infect people. For example, an exchange of genes between a human influenza A virus and an avian influenza A virus can create a new influenza A virus with a hemagglutinin protein or both a hemagglutinin protein and a neuraminidase protein from an avian influenza A virus. If this new virus causes illness in infected people and can spread easily from person to person, an influenza pandemic can occur.

WHAT HAPPENS WHEN A PANDEMIC INFLUENZA VIRUS EMERGES?

When a pandemic influenza virus emerges, the virus can spread quickly because most people will not be immune and a vaccine might not be widely available to offer immediate protection. During the H1N1 pandemic, for example, a new H1N1 virus was first identified in April 2009. By June 2009, that novel H1N1 virus had spread worldwide, and the World Health Organization (WHO) declared a pandemic. Spread of a pandemic influenza virus may occur in multiple disease "waves" that are separated by several months. As a pandemic influenza virus spreads, large numbers of people may need medical care worldwide. Schools, childcare centers, workplaces, and other places for mass gatherings may experience more absenteeism. Public health and health-care systems can become overloaded, with elevated rates of hospitalizations and deaths. Other critical infrastructure, such as law enforcement, emergency medical services, and the transportation industry may also be affected.

WILL SEASONAL FLU VACCINES PROTECT AGAINST PANDEMIC FLU?

It is unlikely that seasonal flu vaccines would protect against a pandemic influenza virus. Seasonal flu vaccines that are used annually protect against currently circulating human influenza A and B viruses. They are not designed to protect against new influenza A viruses. A pandemic influenza virus would be very different from circulating seasonal influenza A viruses, and thus, seasonal vaccines would not be expected to offer protection.

ARE THERE VACCINES TO PROTECT AGAINST PANDEMIC FLU?

The federal government has created a stockpile of some vaccines against select influenza A viruses with pandemic potential that could be used in the event of a pandemic, including vaccines against certain avian influenza A (e.g., H5N1 and H7N9) viruses. If a similar virus were to begin a pandemic, some vaccines would already be available.

The Department of Health and Human Services (HHS) is the lead agency for public health preparedness and medical response to an influenza pandemic. Within the HHS, the Biomedical Advanced Research and Development Authority (BARDA) Influenza Division is charged with the advanced development and procurement of medical and nonpharmaceutical countermeasures for pandemic influenza preparedness and response.

HOW LONG WOULD IT TAKE TO DEVELOP A NEW PANDEMIC VACCINE?

If a new pandemic influenza virus (not included in the pre-pandemic vaccine stockpile) were to emerge, it is likely that a vaccine would have to be developed against that virus in order for a sufficient supply of vaccine to become available for everyone who wishes to be vaccinated. How long it would take to produce a pandemic flu vaccine would depend on many factors, including how long it would take to create a candidate vaccine virus (CVV) and what vaccine manufacturing process would be used. For the seasonal influenza vaccine, it usually takes at least six months to produce large quantities of flu vaccine. During the H1N1 pandemic, it took about the same amount of time.

The Centers for Disease Control and Prevention (CDC) began developing a CVV to make a monovalent (one component) H1N1pdm09 vaccine in mid-April. The first doses of vaccine were administered in early October, and large quantities of vaccine became available in late November. Efforts are underway now to shorten the time it takes to produce influenza vaccines, but because of the current amount of time needed to make flu vaccines, early supplies of pandemic vaccines might not be enough to meet demand, especially if most people need two doses of vaccine for protective immunity.

HOW MANY DOSES OF PANDEMIC VACCINE WOULD EACH PERSON NEED?

People with no immunity against a new influenza virus may need two doses to be fully protected against that virus. The first dose primes the immune system, and the second dose creates a protective response. During the H1N1 influenza pandemic, CDC recommended that two doses of the vaccine be given to children aged six months through nine years in order to increase the immune response.

WHAT TREATMENTS ARE AVAILABLE FOR PANDEMIC FLU?

During a flu pandemic, antiviral drugs would be an important tool to treat and prevent the spread of influenza illness. Antiviral drugs are medicines (pills, liquid, or an inhaled powder) that fight against the influenza viruses infecting the respiratory tract. Antiviral drugs are recommended to treat seasonal influenza in people who are very sick or who are at high risk of serious flu complications. These same drugs may be useful for treating pandemic influenza, depending upon whether the pandemic influenza virus is susceptible or resistant to available antiviral drugs. Antiviral drugs are prescription drugs (they are not sold over the counter) and are different from prescription antibiotics that treat bacterial infections.

ARE THERE OTHER WAYS TO SLOW A PANDEMIC?

Nonpharmaceutical interventions (NPIs) are actions, apart from getting vaccinated and taking medicine, which people and communities can take to help slow the spread of respiratory illnesses, such as pandemic flu. Again, these actions do not include medicines, vaccines, or other pharmaceutical interventions. Given that it may take months to produce a pandemic flu vaccine (not included in the pre-pandemic vaccine stockpile) and that antiviral drugs may be reserved for treatment, NPIs will likely be the only prevention tools available during the early stages of a pandemic and, thus, critically important to help slow the spread of infection.

HOW WOULD NONPHARMACEUTICAL INTERVENTIONS BE USED DURING A PANDEMIC?

The NPIs, also known as "community mitigation strategies," may be more efficient when used early in a flu pandemic and in a layered fashion. Public health officials will recommend that people practice everyday preventive actions at all times. These actions include staying home when sick, covering coughs and sneezes with a tissue, washing hands often, and cleaning frequently touched surfaces and objects. During severe, very severe, or extreme flu pandemics, public health officials may recommend additional actions, such as using face masks when sick and in close contact with other people, temporarily dismissing childcare facilities and schools, and increasing the space between people and decreasing the frequency of contact among people (i.e., social distancing).

PLANNING FOR NONPHARMACEUTICAL INTERVENTIONS DURING A FLU PANDEMIC

The CDC has developed an updated set of guidelines, called the "Community Mitigation Guidelines to Prevent Pandemic Influenza–United States, 2017"; supplemental plain-language guides for specific community groups; and online communication and education materials that outline strategies for planning and preparing for a flu pandemic and for using NPIs. Additionally, the CDC has developed an NPI 101 training for public health professionals to help them learn more about NPIs and share information with their communities on how to use NPIs.

NOVEL INFLUENZA A VIRUSES OF EXTRA CONCERN FOR PANDEMIC THREAT

Novel influenza (flu) virus is an influenza A virus that has caused human infection and that is different from current human seasonal influenza A viruses. Any novel influenza A virus, such as those of avian or swine origin, has the potential to cause an influenza pandemic. Some novel flu A viruses are believed to pose a greater pandemic threat and are more concerning to public health officials than others because they have already caused serious human illness and death and also have been able to spread in a limited manner from person to person. Novel influenza A viruses are of extra concern because of the potential impact they could have on public health if they gained the ability to spread from person to person easily and thus trigger an influenza pandemic. Examples of novel influenza A viruses of extra concern because of their potential to cause a severe pandemic include avian influenza A (H5N1) and avian influenza A (H7N9) viruses. These two different avian influenza A viruses have caused sporadic human infections and some limited person-to-person spread and resulted in critical illness and death in people.

Influenza viruses that normally circulate in pigs also have infected people; these viruses include influenza A (H1N1v, H1N2v, and H3N2v). When influenza viruses that normally circulate in swine are found in people, they are called "variant" viruses; the "v" after the virus name indicates a variant virus. Limited, unsustained spread from person to person also has been detected with these viruses, but in general, these variant viruses have been associated with less severe illness and fewer deaths than avian influenza viruses. In general, human infections with H5N1, H7N9, H1N1v, H1N2v, and H3N2v viruses have occurred rarely, but if these viruses were to change in such a way that they were able to infect humans easily and spread from person to person in a sustained manner, a flu pandemic could result.[3]

[3] "Influenza (Flu)—Questions and Answers," Centers for Disease Control and Prevention (CDC), May 15, 2017. Available online. URL: www.cdc.gov/flu/pandemic-resources/basics/faq.html. Accessed June 27, 2023.

Section 19.4 | Seasonal Flu

WHAT IS FLU?

Flu is a respiratory illness that spreads from person to person. It can cause mild to severe illness. Serious outcomes of flu can result in hospitalization or death.

Some people, such as older people, young children, pregnant women, and people with certain health conditions, are at high risk of serious flu complications.

CAUSES OF FLU

Flu is caused by a virus that is spread from person to person. It causes seasonal epidemics each year and is also called "seasonal flu."

SYMPTOMS OF FLU

Flu symptoms can occur suddenly. You might have the flu if you have some or all of these symptoms:

- fever (not everyone with flu will have a fever)
- cough
- body aches
- sore throat
- runny or stuffy nose
- headache
- chills
- fatigue
- sometimes diarrhea and vomiting

COMPLICATIONS OF FLU

Most people who get the flu will recover in a few days to less than two weeks. But some people will develop complications (such as pneumonia) as a result of flu, some of which can be life-threatening and result in death.

Moderate complications of flu include the following:

- sinus infections
- ear infections

Possible serious complications triggered by flu can include the following:

- lung infection (pneumonia)
- inflammation of the heart, brain, or muscle
- organ failure (e.g., respiratory and kidney failure)
- sepsis, which can be deadly

Flu can also make chronic medical problems worse. The following are a few examples:

- If you have asthma, flu may trigger asthma attacks.
- If you have chronic heart disease, flu may make your condition worse.

WHEN TO SEEK MEDICAL CARE

These are the emergency warning signs of flu sickness.

In Children

- fast breathing or trouble breathing
- bluish lips or face
- ribs pulling in with each breath
- chest pain
- severe muscle pain (child refuses to walk)
- dehydration (no urine for eight hours, dry mouth, no tears when crying)
- not alert or interacting when awake
- seizures
- fever above 104 °F (40 °C)
- any fever in children younger than 12 weeks old
- fever or cough that improves but then returns or worsens
- worsening of chronic medical conditions

In Adults

- difficulty breathing or shortness of breath
- persistent pain or pressure in the chest or abdomen
- persistent dizziness, confusion, or inability to arouse

- seizures
- not urinating
- severe muscle pain
- severe weakness or unsteadiness
- fever or cough that improves but then returns or worsens
- worsening of chronic medical conditions

High-Risk Group

If you have symptoms of flu and are in a high-risk group or are very sick or worried about your illness, contact your doctor.

High-risk groups include the following:

- young children
- children with neurologic conditions
- pregnant women
- adults aged 65 and older
- anyone with the following conditions:
  - asthma
  - heart disease
  - stroke
  - diabetes
  - human immunodeficiency virus (HIV)/acquired immunodeficiency syndrome (AIDS)
  - cancer

TREATMENT OF FLU

Your doctor might prescribe antiviral drugs for the flu. These drugs can make you better faster and may also prevent serious complications.

If you are in a high-risk group and develop flu symptoms, you need to contact your doctor when you first notice flu symptoms. Remind them about your high-risk status for flu.

Antiviral drugs need to be taken within two days of your first flu symptoms.

Antibiotics Will Not Help

When you have flu, antibiotics will not help you feel better. Antibiotics will not help you, and their side effects could cause harm.

Side effects of antibiotics can range from minor issues, such as a rash, to very serious health problems, such as:

- antibiotic-resistant infections, which are difficult to treat and cure
- *Clostridium difficile* infection, which causes severe diarrhea that can lead to severe colon damage and death.

If you use over-the-counter (OTC) medicines, take them as directed. Remember, OTC medicines may provide temporary relief of symptoms, but they will not cure your illness.

Over-the-Counter Medicine and Children

Be careful about giving OTC medicines to children. Not all OTC medicines are recommended for children of certain ages.

PAIN RELIEVERS

- **Children younger than six months**. Only give acetaminophen.
- **Children aged six months or older**. Acetaminophen or ibuprofen can be given.

COUGH AND COLD MEDICINES

- **Children younger than four years old**. Do not use these unless specifically directed by a doctor. The use of OTC cough and cold medicines in young children can result in serious and potentially life-threatening side effects.
- **Children aged four years or older**. Discuss with your child's doctor if OTC cough and cold medicines are safe to give to your child for temporary symptom relief.

Be sure to ask your doctor or pharmacist about the right dosage of OTC medicines for your child's age and size. Also, tell your child's doctor and pharmacist about all prescription and OTC medicines they are taking.

Never give aspirin to children younger than 19 years old. Aspirin can cause Reye syndrome, a rare but very serious illness that harms the liver and brain.

PREVENTION OF FLU

The best way to prevent flu is by getting vaccinated with the flu vaccine each year.

Other ways to avoid the flu are as follows:

- Try to avoid contact with sick people.
- If you are sick, limit contact with others as much as possible to keep from infecting them.
- Cover your nose and mouth with a tissue when you cough or sneeze. After using a tissue, do the following:
    - Throw it in the trash.
    - Wash your hands.
- Wash your hands often with soap and water. If soap and water are not available, use an alcohol-based hand rub.
- Avoid touching your eyes, nose, and mouth. Germs spread this way.
- Clean and disinfect surfaces and objects that may be contaminated with germs such as flu.

WHEN CAN YOU RETURN TO WORK OR SCHOOL?

The Centers for Disease Control and Prevention (CDC) recommends that you stay at home for at least 24 hours after your fever is gone except to get medical care or other necessities.

Your fever should be gone without the use of fever-reducing medicines.[4]

[4] "Flu (Influenza)," Centers for Disease Control and Prevention (CDC), October 6, 2021. Available online. URL: www.cdc.gov/antibiotic-use/flu.html. Accessed June 27, 2023.

Chapter 20 | Measles

Measles is a highly contagious virus that can lead to complications. Learn about its history, answers to common questions, and, if you are a parent, how you can protect your child.

SIGNS AND SYMPTOMS OF MEASLES

Measles symptoms appear 7–14 days after contact with the virus and typically include high fever, cough, runny nose, and watery eyes. The measles rash appears three to five days after the first symptoms.

7–14 Days after a Measles Infection: First Symptoms

Measles is not just a little rash. Measles can be dangerous, especially for babies and young children. Measles typically begins with:

- high fever (which may spike to more than 104 °F (40 °C))
- cough
- runny nose (coryza)
- red, watery eyes (conjunctivitis)

2–3 Days after Symptoms Begin: Koplik Spots

Tiny white spots (Koplik spots) may appear inside the mouth two to three days after symptoms begin.

3–5 Days after Symptoms Begin: Measles Rash

Three to five days after symptoms begin, a rash breaks out. It usually begins as flat red spots that appear on the face at the hairline and spread downward to the neck, trunk, arms, legs, and feet.

- Small raised bumps may also appear on top of the flat red spots.
- The spots may become joined together as they spread from the head to the rest of the body.
- When the rash appears, a person's fever may spike to more than 104 °F (40 °C).

TRANSMISSION OF MEASLES

Measles is highly contagious. Call your health-care provider immediately if you think you or your child have been exposed.

How Measles Spreads

Measles is a highly contagious virus that lives in the nose and throat mucus of an infected person. It can spread to others through coughing and sneezing.

If other people breathe the contaminated air or touch the infected surface and then touch their eyes, noses, or mouths, they can become infected. Animals do not get or spread measles.

Measles is one of the most contagious diseases. Measles is so contagious that if one person has it, up to 90 percent of the people close to that person who are not immune will also become infected.

Infected people can spread measles to others from four days before through four days after the rash appears. The measles virus can live for up to two hours in an airspace after an infected person leaves an area.

COMPLICATIONS OF MEASLES

Measles can be serious. Children younger than five years of age and adults older than 20 years of age are more likely to suffer from complications. Common complications are ear infections and diarrhea. Serious complications include pneumonia and encephalitis.

People and Groups at Risk of Measles Complications

Measles can be serious in all age groups. However, there are several groups that are more likely to suffer from measles complications:

- children younger than five years of age
- adults older than 20 years of age
- pregnant women
- people with compromised immune systems, such as from leukemia or human immunodeficiency virus (HIV) infection

Common Complications

- Ear infections occur in about 1 out of every 10 children with measles.
- Diarrhea is reported in less than 1 out of 10 people with measles.

Severe Complications in Children and Adults

Some people may suffer from severe complications, such as pneumonia (infection of the lungs) and encephalitis (swelling of the brain). They may need to be hospitalized and could die.

- **Hospitalization.** About one in five unvaccinated people in the United States who get measles is hospitalized.
- **Pneumonia.** As many as 1 out of every 20 children with measles gets pneumonia, the most common cause of death from measles in young children.
- **Encephalitis.** About 1 child out of every 1,000 who get measles will develop encephalitis (swelling of the brain) that can lead to convulsions and can leave the child deaf or with intellectual disability.
- **Death.** Nearly 1–3 of every 1,000 children who become infected with measles will die from respiratory and neurologic complications.

- **Complications during pregnancy**. Measles may cause pregnant women who have not had the measles, mumps, and rubella (MMR) vaccine to give birth prematurely or have a low-birth-weight baby.

Long-Term Complications

Subacute sclerosing panencephalitis (SSPE) is a very rare, but fatal disease of the central nervous system that results from a measles virus infection acquired earlier in life.

- SSPE generally develops 7–10 years after a person has measles, even though the person seems to have fully recovered from the illness.
- Since measles was eliminated in 2000, SSPE is rarely reported in the United States.
- Among people who contracted measles during the resurgence in the United States in 1989–1991, 7–11 out of every 100,000 were estimated to be at risk for developing SSPE.
- The risk of developing SSPE may be higher for a person who gets measles before they are two years of age.

VACCINE FOR MEASLES

Prevent Measles with the Measles, Mumps, and Rubella Vaccine

Measles can be prevented with the MMR vaccine. The vaccine protects against three diseases: measles, mumps, and rubella.

Schedule for the Measles, Mumps, and Rubella Vaccine If You Are Not Traveling

Table 20.1 shows the schedule for the MMR vaccine if you are not traveling.

CHECK IF YOUR CHILD IS DUE FOR THE MEASLES, MUMPS, AND RUBELLA VACCINE

If you have children, see if they are due for the MMR vaccine:

- Check your child's vaccination record.

- Contact their health-care provider.
- Visit the immunization scheduler for newborn to six-year-old children.

Table 20.1. Schedule for the MMR Vaccine

	First Dose	Second Dose
Children*	Age: 12–15 months	Age: 4–6 years
Teenagers and adults with no evidence of immunity**	As soon as possible	N/A

* The *Centers for Disease Control and Prevention (CDC) recommends this schedule for children aged 12 months and older. Infants aged 6–11 months and children aged 12 months and older traveling outside the United States should follow another schedule.*
***Acceptable evidence of immunity against measles includes at least one of the following: written documentation of adequate vaccination, laboratory evidence of immunity, laboratory confirmation of measles, or birth in the United States before 1957.*

MEASLES, MUMPS, AND RUBELLA VACCINE IS SAFE AND EFFECTIVE

Two doses of the MMR vaccine are about 97 percent effective at preventing measles; one dose is about 93 percent effective.

MEASLES CAN ALSO BE PREVENTED WITH THE MEASLES, MUMPS, AND RUBELLA VACCINE

Children may also get the MMRV vaccine, which protects against measles, mumps, rubella, and varicella (chickenpox). This vaccine is only licensed for use in children who are 12 months through 12 years of age.

PAYING FOR THE MEASLES VACCINE

- **If you have insurance.** Most health insurance plans cover the cost of vaccines. But you may want to check with your health insurance provider before your visit.
- **If you do not have insurance or your insurance does not cover vaccines for your child.** If you have a child

and do not have insurance or if your insurance does not cover vaccines for your child, the Vaccines for Children Program (VFC) may be able to help. This program helps families of eligible children who might not otherwise have access to vaccines. To find out if your child is eligible, visit the VFC website (www.cdc.gov/vaccines/programs/vfc/parents/qa-detailed.html) or ask your child's health-care provider. You can also contact your state VFC coordinator.

MEASLES IS A SERIOUS DISEASE THAT CAN LEAD TO COMPLICATIONS AND DEATH

Measles is a very contagious disease caused by a virus. It spreads through the air when an infected person coughs or sneezes. In fact, the measles virus can stay in the air for up to two hours after an infected person was there. So you can get infected by simply being in a room where an infected person once was. It is so contagious that if one person has it, up to 90 percent of the people close to him or her will also become infected if they are not protected.

Measles starts with a fever. Soon after, it causes a cough, runny nose, and red eyes. Then a rash of tiny, red spots breaks out. It starts at the head and spreads to the rest of the body. Vaccination prevents measles-related complications and death. Before the measles vaccination program started in 1963:

- an estimated 3–4 million people got measles each year in the United States
- of these, approximately 500,000 cases were reported each year to the CDC
- of these, 400–500 died; 48,000 were hospitalized; and 1,000 developed encephalitis (brain swelling) from measles

Since then, widespread use of the measles vaccine has led to a greater than 99 percent reduction in measles cases compared with the pre-vaccine era.[1]

[1] "About Measles," Centers for Disease Control and Prevention (CDC), July 28, 2020. Available online. URL: www.cdc.gov/measles/about/index.html. Accessed July 17, 2023.

Chapter 21 | Mumps

WHAT IS MUMPS?

Mumps is a contagious disease that is caused by a virus. It typically starts with a few days of fever. Then most people will have swelling of their salivary glands (often referred to as parotitis when the parotid gland, located in front and below the ear, swells).

SIGNS AND SYMPTOMS OF MUMPS

Mumps is best known for the puffy cheeks and tender, swollen jaw that it causes. This is a result of swollen salivary glands under the ears on one or both sides, often referred to as parotitis. Other symptoms that might begin a few days before parotitis include the following:

- fever
- headache
- muscle aches
- tiredness
- loss of appetite

Symptoms typically appear 16–18 days after infection, but this period can range from 12 to 25 days after infection. Some people who get mumps have very mild symptoms (such as a cold) or no symptoms at all and may not know they have the disease. In rare cases, mumps can cause more severe complications. Most people with mumps recover completely within two weeks.

TRANSMISSION OF MUMPS

Mumps is a contagious disease caused by a virus. It spreads through direct contact with saliva or respiratory droplets from the mouth, nose, or throat. An infected person can spread the virus by:

- coughing, sneezing, or talking
- sharing items that may have saliva on them, such as water bottles or cups
- participating in close-contact activities with others, such as playing sports, dancing, or kissing

An infected person can spread mumps from a few days before their salivary glands begin to swell up to five days after the swelling begins. A person with mumps should limit their contact with others during this time. For example, stay home from school and do not attend social events.

Mumps Virus Is Still Around

Mumps occurs in the United States, and the measles, mumps, and rubella (MMR) vaccine is the best way to prevent the disease.

- Check your child's immunization record or contact the doctor to see whether your child has already received the MMR vaccine.
- Get your child vaccinated on time; visit the immunization scheduler. (www2a.cdc.gov/nip/kidstuff/newscheduler_le) for newborn to six-year-old children.
- Remember that some preteens, teens, and adults also need the MMR vaccine; review the preteens and teen schedule (www.cdc.gov/vaccines/schedules/easy-to-read/adolescent-easyread.html) and the adult schedule (www.cdc.gov/vaccines/schedules/hcp/imz/adult.html).
- Get an additional vaccine dose if your health department recommends it to a group you are part of during an outbreak.
- Recognize the signs and symptoms of mumps.
- Let your doctor know right away if you think you or someone in your family may have mumps.

Mumps Outbreaks

Even though the vaccine has drastically reduced mumps cases, outbreaks still occur. Outbreaks have most commonly occurred among groups of people who have prolonged, close contact, such as sharing water bottles or cups, kissing, practicing sports together, or living in close quarters, with a person who has mumps. Some vaccinated people may still get mumps if they are exposed to the virus. However, disease symptoms are milder in vaccinated people. Make sure you are protected against mumps with the MMR vaccine.

COMPLICATIONS OF MUMPS

Mumps can occasionally cause complications, especially in adults. Complications can include the following:

- inflammation of the testicles (orchitis), which may lead to a decrease in testicular size (testicular atrophy)
- inflammation of the ovaries (oophoritis) and/or breast tissue (mastitis)
- inflammation in the pancreas (pancreatitis)
- inflammation of the brain (encephalitis)
- inflammation of the tissue covering the brain and spinal cord (meningitis)
- deafness

Inflammation of the testicles could lead to temporary sterility or decreased fertility in men, but no studies have assessed if it results in permanent infertility.[1]

[1] "Mumps," Centers for Disease Control and Prevention (CDC), March 8, 2021. Available online. URL: www.cdc.gov/mumps/index.html. Accessed June 28, 2023.

Chapter 22 | Nonpolio Enterovirus

Nonpolio enteroviruses cause about 10–15 million infections and tens of thousands of hospitalizations each year in the United States. Most people who get infected with these viruses do not get sick, or they only have mild illnesses, such as the common cold. But some people can have serious complications, especially infants and people with weakened immune systems.

SYMPTOMS OF NONPOLIO ENTEROVIRUS

Most people who get infected with nonpolio enteroviruses do not get sick, or they only have mild illnesses, such as the common cold. Infants, children, and teenagers are more likely than adults to get infected and become sick because they do not yet have immunity (protection) from previous exposures to the viruses. Adults can get infected too, but they are less likely to have symptoms, or their symptoms may be milder. Symptoms of mild illness may include the following:

- fever
- runny nose, sneezing, and/or cough
- skin rash
- mouth blisters
- body and muscle aches

Some nonpolio enterovirus infections can cause:

- viral conjunctivitis
- hand-foot-and-mouth disease
- viral meningitis (infection of the covering of the spinal cord and/or brain)

- viral encephalitis (infection of the brain)
- myocarditis (infection of the heart)
- pericarditis (infection of the sac around the heart)
- acute flaccid paralysis (a sudden onset of weakness in one or more arms or legs)
- inflammatory muscle disease (slow, progressive muscle weakness)

Infants and people with weakened immune systems have a greater chance of having these complications.

People who develop myocarditis may have heart failure and require long-term care. Some people who develop encephalitis or paralysis may not fully recover. Newborns infected with a nonpolio enterovirus may develop sepsis (the body's overwhelming response to infection that can lead to tissue damage, organ failure, and death). However, this is very rare. Nonpolio enterovirus infections may play a role in the development of type 1 diabetes in children.

TRANSMISSION OF NONPOLIO ENTEROVIRUS

Nonpolio enteroviruses can be found in an infected person's:

- feces (stool)
- eye, nose, and mouth secretions (such as saliva, nasal mucus, or sputum)
- blister fluid

You can get exposed to the virus by:

- having close contact, such as touching or shaking hands, with an infected person
- touching objects or surfaces that have the virus on them and then touching your eyes, nose, or mouth before washing your hands
- changing the diapers of an infected person and then touching your eyes, nose, or mouth before washing your hands
- drinking water that has the virus in it

Once infected, you can shed (pass from your body into the environment) the virus for several weeks, even if you do not have symptoms. Pregnant women who get infected with a nonpolio enterovirus shortly before delivery can pass the virus to their babies. Mothers who are breastfeeding should talk with their doctor if they are sick or think they may have an infection.

TREATMENT OF NONPOLIO ENTEROVIRUS

There is no specific treatment for nonpolio enterovirus infection. People with mild illness caused by nonpolio enterovirus infection typically only need to treat their symptoms. This includes drinking enough water to stay hydrated and taking over-the-counter (OTC) cold medications as needed. Most people recover completely. However, some illnesses caused by nonpolio enteroviruses can be severe enough to require hospitalization. If you are concerned about your symptoms, you should contact your health-care provider.

PREVENTION OF NONPOLIO ENTEROVIRUS

Many people who get infected with nonpolio enteroviruses do not have symptoms but can still spread the virus to other people. This makes it difficult to prevent them from spreading. The best way to help protect yourself and others from nonpolio enterovirus infections is to:

- wash your hands often with soap and water for 20 seconds, especially after using the toilet or changing diapers
- avoid close contact, such as touching and shaking hands, with people who are sick
- clean and disinfect frequently touched surfaces

There is no vaccine to protect you from nonpolio enterovirus infection.[1]

[1] "Non-Polio Enterovirus," Centers for Disease Control and Prevention (CDC), August 8, 2020. Available online. URL: www.cdc.gov/non-polio-enterovirus/index.html. Accessed June 28, 2023.

Chapter 23 | Norovirus Infection

Norovirus is the leading cause of vomiting, diarrhea, and foodborne illness in the United States. People of all ages can get infected and sick with norovirus, which spreads very easily and quickly.

You can get norovirus illness many times in your life because there are many different types of noroviruses. Infection with one type of norovirus may not protect you against other types. It is possible to develop protection against specific types. But it is not known exactly how long protection lasts. This may explain why so many people of all ages get infected during norovirus outbreaks. Your likelihood of getting a norovirus infection is also determined in part by your genes.

HOW NOROVIRUS SPREADS

Norovirus is very contagious and spreads very easily and quickly in different ways. You can get norovirus by accidentally getting tiny particles of feces (poop) or vomit in your mouth from a person infected with norovirus. If you get norovirus illness, you can shed billions of norovirus particles that you cannot see without a microscope. It only takes a few norovirus particles to make you and other people sick.

You can get norovirus by:

- having direct contact with someone with norovirus, such as by caring for them, sharing food or eating utensils with them, or eating food handled by them
- eating food or drinking liquids that are contaminated with norovirus

- touching surfaces or objects contaminated with norovirus and then putting your unwashed fingers in your mouth

You are most contagious:

- when you have symptoms of norovirus illness, especially vomiting
- during the first few days after you feel better

However, studies have shown that you can still spread norovirus for two weeks or more after you feel better.

Norovirus spreads through contaminated food.

This can happen when:

- a person with norovirus touches food with their bare hands
- food is placed on a counter or surface that has poop or vomit particles on it
- tiny drops of vomit from a person with norovirus spray through the air and land on the food
- food is grown with contaminated water, such as oysters, or fruit and vegetables are watered with contaminated water in the field

Norovirus spreads through contaminated water.

Recreational or drinking water can get contaminated with norovirus:

- at the source, such as when a septic tank leaks into a well
- when a person with norovirus vomits or poops in the water
- when water is not treated properly, such as with not enough chlorine

Norovirus spreads through sick people and contaminated surfaces. This can happen when:

- a person with norovirus touches surfaces with their bare hands
- food, water, or objects that are contaminated with norovirus are placed on surfaces

- tiny drops of vomit from a person with norovirus spray through the air, landing on surfaces or entering another person's mouth
- a person with norovirus has diarrhea that splatters onto surfaces

SYMPTOMS OF NOROVIRUS

Do you think you have the "stomach flu" or a "stomach bug"? It is probably norovirus, a common virus that is not related to the flu. Norovirus is the most common cause of vomiting, diarrhea, and foodborne illness.

The most common symptoms of norovirus are:

- diarrhea
- vomiting
- nausea
- stomach pain

Other symptoms include the following:

- fever
- headache
- body aches

Norovirus causes inflammation of the stomach or intestines. This is called "acute gastroenteritis."

A person usually develops symptoms 12–48 hours after being exposed to norovirus. Most people with norovirus illness get better within one to three days, but they can still spread the virus for a few days after.

If you have norovirus illness, you can feel extremely ill and vomit or have diarrhea many times a day. This can lead to dehydration, especially in young children, older adults, and people with other illnesses. Children who are dehydrated may cry with few or no tears and be unusually sleepy or fussy.

Symptoms of dehydration include the following:

- decrease in urination
- dry mouth and throat
- feeling dizzy when standing up

HOW TO TREAT NOROVIRUS

There is no specific medicine to treat people with norovirus illness.

Drink Plenty of Liquids

If you have norovirus illness, you should drink plenty of liquids to replace fluid lost from vomiting and diarrhea. This will help prevent dehydration. Sports drinks and other drinks without caffeine or alcohol can help with mild dehydration. However, these drinks may not replace important nutrients and minerals. Oral rehydration fluids that you can get over the counter are most helpful for mild dehydration.

Dehydration can lead to serious problems. Severe dehydration may require hospitalization for treatment with fluids given through your vein (intravenous (IV) fluids). Watch for signs of dehydration in children who have norovirus illness. Children who are dehydrated may cry with few or no tears and be unusually sleepy or fussy.

If you think you or someone you are caring for is severely dehydrated, call your doctor. Antibiotic drugs will not help treat norovirus infections because they fight bacteria, not viruses.

HOW TO PREVENT NOROVIRUS

Wash Your Hands Well

Wash your hands often with soap and water for at least 20 seconds, especially:

- after using the toilet or changing diapers
- before eating, preparing, or handling food
- before giving yourself or someone else medicine

It is important to continue washing your hands often even after you feel better. Norovirus can be found in your vomit or feces (poop) even before you start feeling sick. The virus can also stay in your poop for two weeks or more after you feel better, and you can still spread norovirus during that time.

Hand sanitizer does not work well against norovirus. You can use hand sanitizers in addition to handwashing, but hand sanitizer is not a substitute for handwashing, which is best.

Handle and Prepare Food Safely

Before preparing and eating your food:

- wash fruits and vegetables well
- cook oysters and other shellfish thoroughly to an internal temperature of at least 145 °F (62.8 °C)
- routinely clean and sanitize kitchen utensils, counters, and surfaces

Be aware that:

- noroviruses are relatively resistant to heat and can survive temperatures as high as 145 °F (62.8 °C)
- quick steaming processes may not heat foods enough to kill noroviruses
- food that might be contaminated with norovirus should be thrown out

Do Not Prepare and Handle Food or Care for Others When You Are Sick

You should not prepare food for others or provide health care while you are sick and for at least two days (48 hours) after symptoms stop. This also applies to sick workers in restaurants, schools, day cares, long-term care facilities, and other places where they may expose people to norovirus.

Clean and Disinfect Surfaces

After someone vomits or has diarrhea, always clean well and disinfect the entire area immediately.

MAKE HOUSEHOLD BLEACH SOLUTION

To disinfect, you should use a chlorine bleach solution with a concentration of 1,000–5,000 ppm (5–25 tablespoons of household bleach (5–8%) per gallon of water) or use a disinfecting product against norovirus registered with the U.S. Environmental Protection Agency (EPA). You should:

- wear rubber or disposable gloves and wipe the entire area with paper towels and throw them in a plastic trash bag

- disinfect the area as directed on the product label
- leave the bleach disinfectant on the affected area for at least five minutes
- clean the entire area again with soap and hot water
- wash laundry, take out the trash, and wash your hands

Wash Laundry Well

Immediately remove and wash clothes or linens that may have vomit or poop on them.

You should:

- wear rubber or disposable gloves
- handle items carefully without shaking them
- wash the items with detergent and hot water at the maximum available cycle length and then machine dry them at the highest heat setting
- wash your hands afterward with soap and water

What You Need to Know

- Norovirus is very contagious, but you can take steps to stop it from spreading.
- Wash hands well with soap and water.
- Clean and disinfect surfaces with bleach.
- Wash laundry in hot water.[1]

[1] "Norovirus," Centers for Disease Control and Prevention (CDC), May 10, 2023. Available online. URL: www.cdc.gov/norovirus/about/index.html. Accessed June 28, 2023.

Chapter 24 | Polio

WHAT IS POLIO?

Polio, or poliomyelitis, is a disabling and life-threatening disease caused by the poliovirus. The virus spreads from person to person and can infect a person's spinal cord, causing paralysis (inability to move parts of the body).

SYMPTOMS OF POLIO

Most people who get infected with poliovirus will not have any visible symptoms. About one out of four people with poliovirus infection will have flu-like symptoms that can include the following:

- sore throat
- fever
- tiredness
- nausea
- headache
- stomach pain

These symptoms usually last two to five days and then go away on their own. A smaller proportion of people with poliovirus infection will develop other, more serious symptoms that affect the brain and spinal cord:

- meningitis (infection of the covering of the spinal cord and/or brain)occurs in about 1–5 out of 100 people with poliovirus infection, depending on the virus type
- paralysis (inability to move parts of the body) or weakness in the arms, legs, or both occurs in about 1 out of 200 people to 1 in 2,000 people, depending on the virus type

Paralysis is the most severe symptom associated with poliovirus because it can lead to permanent disability and death. Between 2 and 10 out of 100 people who have paralysis from poliovirus infection die because the virus affects the muscles that help them breathe.

Even children who seem to fully recover can develop new muscle pain, weakness, or paralysis as adults, 15–40 years later. This is called "post-polio syndrome" (PPS).

Note that "poliomyelitis" (or "polio" for short) is defined as a paralytic disease. So only people with the paralytic infection are considered to have the disease.

Post-Polio Syndrome

Polio has been around since ancient times. An ancient Egyptian tomb painting showed a man with a withered leg unable to bear weight without the use of a walking stick. This means that most muscle fibers are replaced with scarring (muscle-wasting) that is permanent.

If someone had polio as a child or young adult but had kept or recovered some or all movement of weakened arms or legs, even to the point of being athletic afterward, they can become weaker in late adulthood. That is post-polio syndrome, a condition that can affect polio survivors decades after they recover from their initial poliovirus infection. Some PPS patients become wheelchair-bound when they had not been before.

TRANSMISSION OF POLIO

- Poliovirus is very contagious and spreads through person-to-person contact.
- It lives in an infected person's throat and intestines.
- It can contaminate food and water in unsanitary conditions.

Poliovirus only infects people. It enters the body through the mouth. It spreads through:

- contact with the feces (poop) of an infected person

- droplets from a sneeze or cough of an infected person (less common)

You can get infected with poliovirus if:

- you have picked up minute pieces of feces on your hands and you touch your mouth
- you put in your mouth objects, such as toys, that are contaminated with feces

An infected person can spread the virus to others immediately before and up to two weeks after symptoms appear.

- The virus can live in an infected person's intestines for many weeks. It can contaminate food and water in unsanitary conditions.
- People who do not have symptoms can still pass the virus to others and make them sick.

DIAGNOSIS OF POLIO

Health-care providers who suspect a patient has polio should hospitalize the patient right away; do a physical exam; take a detailed medical history, including vaccination history and history of any recent travel; collect samples (stool, throat swab, blood, urine, and spinal fluid); and obtain a magnetic resonance imaging (MRI) to look at pictures of the spinal cord. Poliovirus is most likely to be detected in stool specimens.

TREATMENT OF POLIO

There is no cure for paralytic polio and no specific treatment. Physical or occupational therapy can help with arm or leg weakness caused by polio and might improve long-term outcomes, especially if implemented early in the course of illness. Health-care providers should consider consulting neurology and infectious disease experts to discuss possible treatments and recommend certain interventions on a case-by-case basis.

If you think you or someone in your family has symptoms of polio, please call your health-care provider right away or go to an emergency room.

PREVENTION OF POLIO

The following are the two types of vaccines that can prevent polio:

- **Inactivated poliovirus vaccine (IPV)**. IPV is given as an injection in the leg or arm, depending on the patient's age. Only IPV has been used in the United States since 2000.
- **Oral poliovirus vaccine (OPV)**. OPV is still used throughout much of the world.

Polio vaccine protects children by preparing their bodies to fight the poliovirus. Almost all children (more than 99%) who get all the recommended doses of the inactivated polio vaccine will be protected from polio.

It is also very important to practice good hand hygiene and wash hands often with soap and water. Note that alcohol-based hand sanitizers do not kill poliovirus.[1]

[1] "Polio (Poliomyelitis)," Centers for Disease Control and Prevention (CDC), October 6, 2021. Available online. URL: www.cdc.gov/polio/index.htm. Accessed June 28, 2023.

Chapter 25 | Respiratory Syncytial Virus Infection

WHAT IS RESPIRATORY SYNCYTIAL VIRUS?

Respiratory syncytial virus (RSV) is a common respiratory virus that usually causes mild, cold-like symptoms. Most people recover in a week or two, but RSV can be serious, especially for infants and older adults. RSV is the most common cause of bronchiolitis (inflammation of the small airways in the lung) and pneumonia (infection of the lungs) in children younger than one year of age in the United States.

SYMPTOMS OF RESPIRATORY SYNCYTIAL VIRUS

People infected with RSV usually show symptoms within four to six days after getting infected. Symptoms of RSV infection usually include the following:

- runny nose
- decrease in appetite
- coughing
- sneezing
- fever
- wheezing

These symptoms usually appear in stages and not all at once. In very young infants with RSV, the only symptoms may be irritability, decreased activity, and breathing difficulties. Almost all children will have had an RSV infection by their second birthday.

CARE OF RESPIRATORY SYNCYTIAL VIRUS

Most RSV infections go away on their own in a week or two. There is no specific treatment for RSV infection though researchers are working to develop vaccines and antivirals (medicines that fight viruses).

Take Steps to Relieve Symptoms

- Manage fever and pain with over-the-counter (OTC) fever reducers and pain relievers, such as acetaminophen or ibuprofen. (Never give aspirin to children.)
- Drink enough fluids. It is important for people with RSV infection to drink enough fluids to prevent dehydration (loss of body fluids).
- Talk to your health-care provider before giving your child nonprescription cold medicines. Some medicines contain ingredients that are not good for children.

Respiratory Syncytial Virus Can Cause More Serious Health Problems

RSV can also cause more severe infections such as bronchiolitis, an inflammation of the small airways in the lung, and pneumonia, an infection of the lungs. It is the most common cause of bronchiolitis and pneumonia in children younger than one year of age.

Healthy adults and infants infected with RSV do not usually need to be hospitalized. But some people with RSV infection, especially older adults and infants younger than six months of age, may need to be hospitalized if they are having trouble breathing or are dehydrated. In the most severe cases, a person may require additional oxygen or intravenous (IV) fluids (if they cannot eat or drink enough), or intubation (have a breathing tube inserted through the mouth and down to the airway) with mechanical ventilation (a machine to help a person breathe). In most of these cases, hospitalization only lasts a few days.

TRANSMISSION OF RESPIRATORY SYNCYTIAL VIRUS

Respiratory syncytial virus can spread when:

- an infected person coughs or sneezes
- you get virus droplets from a cough or sneeze in your eyes, nose, or mouth
- you have direct contact with the virus, such as kissing the face of a child with RSV
- you touch a surface that has the virus on it, such as a doorknob, and then touch your face before washing your hands

People infected with RSV are usually contagious for three to eight days and may become contagious a day or two before they start showing signs of illness. However, some infants and people with weakened immune systems can continue to spread the virus even after they stop showing symptoms, for as long as four weeks. Children are often exposed to and infected with RSV outside the home, such as in school or childcare centers. They can then transmit the virus to other members of the family.

Respiratory syncytial virus can survive for many hours on hard surfaces, such as tables and crib rails. It typically lives on soft surfaces, such as tissues and hands, for shorter amounts of time.

People are typically infected with RSV for the first time as an infant or toddler and nearly all children are infected before their second birthday. However, repeat infections may occur throughout life, and people of any age can be infected. Infections in healthy children and adults are generally less severe than among infants and older adults with certain medical conditions. People at highest risk for severe disease include the following:

- premature infants
- young children with congenital (from birth) heart or chronic lung disease
- young children with compromised (weakened) immune systems due to a medical condition or medical treatment

- children with neuromuscular disorders
- adults with compromised immune systems
- older adults, especially those with underlying heart or lung disease

In most regions of the United States and other areas with similar climates, RSV season generally starts during fall and peaks in the winter. The timing and severity of RSV season in a given community can vary from year to year.

PREVENTION OF RESPIRATORY SYNCYTIAL VIRUS

There are steps you can take to help prevent the spread of RSV. Specifically, if you have cold-like symptoms you should:

- cover your coughs and sneezes with a tissue or your upper shirt sleeve, not your hands
- wash your hands often with soap and water for at least 20 seconds
- avoid close contact, such as kissing, shaking hands, and sharing cups and eating utensils, with others
- clean frequently touched surfaces such as doorknobs and mobile devices

Respiratory Syncytial Virus Vaccine

RSV vaccine helps protect adults aged 60 and older from RSV disease. Older adults are at greater risk than young adults for serious complications from RSV because immune systems weaken with age. In addition, certain underlying medical conditions may increase the risk of getting very sick from RSV, and older adults with these conditions may especially benefit from getting the RSV vaccine. If you are aged 60 or older, talk to your health-care provider to see if RSV vaccination is right for you.

Prevention for Children at High Risk for Severe Respiratory Syncytial Virus

A drug called "palivizumab" is available to prevent severe RSV illness in certain infants and children who are at high risk for severe disease. This could include, for example, infants born prematurely or with congenital (present from birth) heart disease or chronic lung disease. The drug can help prevent serious RSV disease, but it cannot help cure or treat children already suffering from serious RSV disease, and it cannot prevent infection with RSV. If your child is at high risk for severe RSV disease, talk to your health-care provider to see if palivizumab can be used as a preventive measure.

Ideally, people with cold-like symptoms should not interact with children at high risk for severe RSV disease, including premature infants, children younger than two years of age with chronic lung or heart conditions, children with weakened immune systems, or children with neuromuscular disorders. If this is not possible, they should carefully follow the prevention steps mentioned above and wash their hands before interacting with such children. They should also refrain from kissing high-risk children while they have cold-like symptoms.

Parents of children at high risk for developing severe RSV disease should help their child, when possible, do the following:

- Avoid close contact with sick people.
- Wash their hands often with soap and water for at least 20 seconds.
- Avoid touching their face with unwashed hands.
- Limit the time they spend in childcare centers or other potentially contagious settings during periods of high RSV activity. This may help prevent infection and spread of the virus during the RSV season.[1]

[1] "Respiratory Syncytial Virus Infection (RSV)," Centers for Disease Control and Prevention (CDC), October 28, 2022. Available online. URL: www.cdc.gov/rsv/index.html. Accessed June 28, 2023.

Chapter 26 | Rotavirus

Rotavirus commonly causes severe, watery diarrhea and vomiting in infants and young children. Children may become dehydrated and need to be hospitalized and can even die.

SYMPTOMS OF ROTAVIRUS

The most common symptoms of rotavirus are severe watery diarrhea, vomiting, fever, and/or abdominal pain. Symptoms usually start about two days after a person is exposed to rotavirus. Vomiting and watery diarrhea can last three to eight days. Additional symptoms may include loss of appetite and dehydration (loss of body fluids), which can be especially dangerous for infants and young children.

Symptoms of dehydration include the following:

- decreased urination
- dry mouth and throat
- feeling dizzy when standing up
- crying with few or no tears and
- unusual sleepiness or fussiness

TRANSMISSION OF ROTAVIRUS

You can get infected with rotavirus if you get rotavirus particles in your mouth. This can happen if you:

- put your unwashed hands that are contaminated with poop into your mouth
- touch contaminated objects or surfaces and then put your fingers in your mouth
- eat contaminated food

People who are infected with rotavirus shed the virus in their stool (poop). This is how the virus gets into the environment and can infect other people. People shed rotavirus the most and are more likely to infect others, both when they have symptoms and during the first three days after they recover. People with rotavirus can also infect others before they have symptoms.

Rotavirus spreads easily among infants and young children. They can spread rotavirus to family members and other people with whom they have close contact. Children are most likely to get rotavirus in the winter and spring (January through June).

Good hygiene, such as handwashing and cleanliness, are important but are not enough to control the spread of the disease. Rotavirus vaccination is the best way to protect your child from rotavirus disease.

TREATMENT FOR ROTAVIRUS

There is no specific medicine to treat rotavirus infection, but your doctor may recommend medicine to treat the symptoms. Antibiotics will not help because they fight bacteria, not viruses.

Since rotavirus disease can cause severe vomiting and diarrhea, it can lead to dehydration (loss of body fluids). The best way to protect against dehydration is to drink plenty of liquids. You can get oral rehydration solutions over the counter in U.S. food and drug stores; these are most helpful for mild dehydration. Severe dehydration may require hospitalization for treatment with intravenous (IV) fluids that patients receive directly through their veins. If you or someone you are caring for is severely dehydrated, contact your doctor. Infants and young children, older adults, and people with other illnesses are most at risk of dehydration.

Symptoms of dehydration include the following:

- decreased urination
- dry mouth and throat
- feeling dizzy when standing up
- crying with few or no tears and
- unusual sleepiness or fussiness

ROTAVIRUS VACCINES

Rotavirus vaccine is the best way to protect your child against rotavirus disease.

Most children (about 9 out of 10) who get the vaccine will be protected from severe rotavirus disease. About 7 out of 10 children will be protected from rotavirus disease of any severity. The following two rotavirus vaccines are currently licensed for infants in the United States:

- **RotaTeq®**. This is given in three doses at ages two months, four months, and six months.
- **Rotarix®**. This is given in two doses at ages two months and four months.

The first dose of either vaccine should be given before a child is 15 weeks of age. Children should receive all doses of rotavirus vaccine before they turn eight months old. Both vaccines are given by putting drops in the child's mouth.[1]

[1] "Rotavirus," Centers for Disease Control and Prevention (CDC), March 26, 2021. Available online. URL: https://www.cdc.gov/rotavirus/index.html. Accessed July 20, 2023.

Chapter 27 | Rubella

Rubella is a contagious disease caused by a virus. Most people who get rubella usually have a mild illness, with symptoms that can include a low-grade fever, sore throat, and a rash that starts on the face and spreads to the rest of the body. Rubella can cause a miscarriage or serious birth defects in a developing baby if a woman is infected while she is pregnant. The best protection against rubella is the measles, mumps, and rubella (MMR) vaccine.

RUBELLA IN THE UNITED STATES

Rubella is a contagious disease caused by a virus. It is also called "German measles," but it is caused by a different virus than measles. Rubella was eliminated from the United States in 2004. Rubella elimination is defined as the absence of continuous disease transmission for 12 months or more in a specific geographic area. Rubella is no longer endemic (constantly present) in the United States. However, rubella remains a problem in other parts of the world. It can still be brought into the United States by people who get infected in other countries.

Before the rubella vaccination program started in 1969, rubella was a common and widespread infection in the United States. During the last major rubella epidemic in the United States from 1964 to 1965, an estimated 12.5 million people got rubella; 11,000 pregnant women lost their babies; 2,100 newborns died; and 20,000 babies were born with congenital rubella syndrome. Once the vaccine became widely used, the number of people infected with rubella in the United States dropped dramatically.

Nowadays, less than 10 people in the United States are reported as having rubella each year. Since 2012, all rubella cases had evidence that they were infected when they were living or traveling outside the United States. To maintain rubella elimination, it is important that children and women of childbearing age are vaccinated against rubella.

SIGNS AND SYMPTOMS OF RUBELLA

In children, rubella is usually mild, with few noticeable symptoms. For children who do have symptoms, a red rash is typically the first sign. The rash generally first appears on the face and then spreads to the rest of the body and lasts about three days. Other symptoms that may occur one to five days before the rash appears include the following:

- a low-grade fever
- headache
- mild pink eye (redness or swelling of the white of the eye)
- general discomfort
- swollen and enlarged lymph nodes
- cough
- runny nose

Most adults who get rubella usually have a mild illness, with low-grade fever, sore throat, and a rash that starts on the face and spreads to the rest of the body. Some adults may also have a headache, pink eye, and general discomfort before the rash appears. About 25–50 percent of people infected with rubella will not experience any symptoms.

COMPLICATIONS OF RUBELLA

Up to 70 percent of women who get rubella may experience arthritis; this is rare in children and men. In rare cases, rubella can cause serious problems, including brain infections and bleeding problems.

The most serious complication of rubella infection is the harm it can cause to a pregnant woman's developing baby. If an unvaccinated pregnant woman gets infected with the rubella virus, she can have a miscarriage, or her baby can die just after birth. Also, she can pass the virus to her developing baby who can develop serious birth defects such as:

- heart problems
- loss of hearing and eyesight
- intellectual disability
- liver or spleen damage

Serious birth defects are more common if a woman is infected early in her pregnancy, especially in the first trimester. These severe birth defects are known as "congenital rubella syndrome."

TRANSMISSION OF RUBELLA

Rubella spreads when an infected person coughs or sneezes. Also, if a woman is infected with rubella while she is pregnant, she can pass it to her developing baby and cause serious harm.

A person with rubella may spread the disease to others up to one week before the rash appears and remain contagious up to seven days after. However, 25–50 percent of people infected with rubella do not develop a rash or have any symptoms, but they still spread it to others.

People infected with rubella should tell friends, family, and people they work with, especially pregnant women, if they have rubella. If your child has rubella, it is important to tell your child's school or day-care provider.

TREATMENT OF RUBELLA

There is no specific medicine to treat rubella or make the disease go away faster. In many cases, symptoms are mild. For others, mild symptoms can be managed with bed rest and medicines for fever, such as acetaminophen. If you are concerned about your symptoms or your child's symptoms, contact your doctor.[1]

[1] "Rubella (German Measles, Three-Day Measles)," Centers for Disease Control and Prevention (CDC), December 31, 2020. Available online. URL: www.cdc.gov/rubella/index.html. Accessed July 3, 2023.

Chapter 28 | Zika Virus Infection

Zika is spread mostly by the bite of an infected *Aedes* species mosquito (*Aedes aegypti* and *Aedes albopictus*). These mosquitoes bite during the day and night. Zika can be passed from a pregnant woman to her fetus. Infection during pregnancy can cause certain birth defects. There is no vaccine or medicine for Zika.

SYMPTOMS OF ZIKA

Many people infected with the Zika virus will not have symptoms or will only have mild symptoms. The most common symptoms of Zika are as follows:

- fever
- rash
- headache
- joint pain
- conjunctivitis (pink eyes)
- muscle pain

How Long Do Symptoms Last?

Zika is usually mild with symptoms lasting for several days to a week. People usually do not get sick enough to go to the hospital, and they very rarely die of Zika. For this reason, many people might not realize they have been infected. Symptoms of Zika are similar to other viruses spread through mosquito bites, like dengue and chikungunya.

How Soon Should You Be Tested?

Zika virus usually remains in the blood of an infected person for about a week. See your doctor or other health-care provider if you develop symptoms and you live in or have recently traveled to an area with risk of Zika. Your doctor or other health-care provider may order blood or urine tests to help determine if you have Zika. Once a person has been infected, he or she is likely to be protected from future infections.

When to See a Doctor or Health-Care Provider

See your doctor or other health-care provider if you have the symptoms described above and have visited an area with risk of Zika. This is especially important if you are pregnant. Be sure to tell your doctor or other health-care provider where you traveled.

HOW IS ZIKA TRANSMITTED?

Through Mosquito Bites

Zika virus is transmitted to people primarily through the bite of an infected Aedes species mosquito (*Ae. aegypti* and *Ae. albopictus*). These are the same mosquitoes that spread dengue and chikungunya viruses.

- These mosquitoes typically lay eggs in or near standing water in things such as buckets, bowls, animal dishes, flower pots, and vases. They prefer to bite people and live indoors and outdoors near people.
  - Mosquitoes that spread chikungunya, dengue, and Zika bite during the day and night.
- A mosquito gets infected with a virus when it bites an infected person during the period of time when the virus can be found in the person's blood, typically only through the first week of infection.
- Infected mosquitoes can then spread the virus to other people through bites.

From Mother to Child

- A pregnant woman can pass Zika virus to her fetus during pregnancy. Zika is a cause of microcephaly and other severe fetal brain defects. We are studying the full range of other potential health problems that Zika virus infection during pregnancy may cause.
- A pregnant woman already infected with Zika virus can pass the virus to her fetus during the pregnancy or around the time of birth.
- Zika virus has been found in breast milk. Possible Zika virus infections have been identified in breastfeeding babies, but Zika virus transmission through breast milk has not been confirmed. Additionally, we do not yet know the long-term effects of the Zika virus on young infants infected after birth. Because current evidence suggests that the benefits of breastfeeding outweigh the risk of the Zika virus spreading through breast milk, the Centers for Disease Control and Prevention (CDC) continues to encourage mothers to breastfeed, even if they were infected or lived in or traveled to an area with risk of Zika. The CDC continues to study the Zika virus and the ways it can spread and will update recommendations as new information becomes available.

Through Sex

- Zika can be passed through sex from a person who has Zika to his or her partners. Zika can be passed through sex, even if the infected person does not have symptoms at the time.
    - It can be passed from a person with Zika before their symptoms start while they have symptoms and after their symptoms end.
    - Though not well documented, the virus may also be passed by a person who carries the virus but never develops symptoms.

- Studies are underway to find out how long Zika stays in the semen and vaginal fluids of people who have Zika and how long it can be passed to sex partners. We know that Zika can remain in semen longer than in other body fluids, including vaginal fluids, urine, and blood.

Through Blood Transfusion

- To date, there have not been any confirmed blood transfusion transmission cases in the United States.
- There have been multiple reports of possible blood transfusion transmission cases in Brazil.
- During the French Polynesian outbreak, 2.8 percent of blood donors tested positive for Zika, and in previous outbreaks, the virus has been found in blood donors.

Through Laboratory and Health-Care Setting Exposure

- There are reports of laboratory-acquired Zika virus infections although the route of transmission was not clearly established in all cases.
- To date, no cases of Zika virus transmission in health-care settings have been identified in the United States. Recommendations are available for health-care providers to help prevent exposure to Zika virus in health-care settings.

TESTING FOR ZIKA

How Is Zika Diagnosed?

- To diagnose Zika, a doctor or other health-care provider will ask about any recent travel and any signs and symptoms.
- They may order blood or urine tests to help determine if you have Zika.

Remember to ask for your Zika test results even if you are feeling better.

Only Some People Need Zika Testing

Following the Zika virus outbreaks in 2016, the number of Zika cases reported from most parts of the world declined and is now very low. Therefore, very few people need Zika testing.

Testing is recommended if you have symptoms of Zika and have traveled to a country with a current Zika outbreak. Note: There are no countries or U.S. territories currently reporting an outbreak of Zika.

- Testing should take place as soon as possible while you still have symptoms.
- Testing may include a molecular test that looks for the presence of the virus in the body or serological testing that looks for antibodies your body makes to fight infection.
- If you have questions, talk to your health-care provider.

Testing is recommended if you are a pregnant woman with symptoms of Zika and have traveled to an area with risk of Zika outside of the United States and its territories based on the testing recommendations.

Testing is no longer routinely recommended if you are a pregnant woman with no symptoms of Zika but may be considered if you traveled to an area with risk of Zika.

- Upon your return from travel, testing should take place as soon as possible.

If You Have Tested Positive for Zika

- If you are pregnant, you can pass Zika to your fetus.
- You can pass Zika to your sex partner(s).
- You can pass Zika to mosquitoes, which can bite you, get infected with Zika virus, and spread the virus to other people.

Sexual Transmission and Testing

- A blood or urine test can help determine if you have Zika from sexual transmission; however, testing blood, semen, vaginal fluids, or urine is not recommended to determine how likely a person is to pass Zika virus through sex.

If You Think You May Have or Had Zika

- Treat the symptoms.
- Protect others from getting sick.

TREATMENT OF ZIKA VIRUS

There is no specific medicine or vaccine for the Zika virus.

- Treat the symptoms.
- Get plenty of rest.
- Drink fluids to prevent dehydration.
- Take medicine such as acetaminophen (Tylenol®) to reduce fever and pain.
- Do not take aspirin and other nonsteroidal anti-inflammatory drugs (NSAIDS) until dengue can be ruled out to reduce the risk of bleeding.
- If you are taking medicine for another medical condition, talk to your health-care provider before taking additional medication.

If You Are Caring for a Person with Zika

Take steps to protect yourself from exposure to the person's blood and body fluids (urine, stool, and vomit). If you are pregnant, you can care for someone with Zika if you follow these steps:

- Do not touch blood or body fluids or surfaces with these fluids on them with exposed skin.
- Wash hands with soap and water immediately after providing care.
- Immediately remove and wash clothes if they get blood or body fluids on them. Use laundry detergent and water temperature specified on the garment label. Using bleach is not necessary.

- Clean the sick person's environment daily using household cleaners according to label instructions.
- Immediately clean surfaces that have blood or other body fluids on them using household cleaners and disinfectants according to label instructions.

If you visit a family member or friend with Zika in a hospital, you should avoid contact with the person's blood and body fluids and surfaces with these fluids on them. Helping the person sit up or walk should not expose you. Make sure to wash your hands before and after touching the person.

PREVENTION OF ZIKA VIRUS

Use the tips below to protect yourself and others from Zika:

- Following these tips will help protect you, your partner, your family, your friends, and your community from Zika. The more steps you take, the more protected you are.
- If you are caring for a family member or friend with Zika, take steps to protect yourself from exposure to the person's blood and body fluids.

Prevent Mosquito Bites

- Zika virus is spread to people mainly through the bite of an infected mosquito.
- Mosquitoes that spread Zika and other viruses bite during the day and night.
- The best way to prevent Zika is to protect yourself from mosquito bites.
- Everyone, including pregnant and breastfeeding women, should take steps to prevent mosquito bites.
- When used as directed, EPA-registered insect repellents are proven safe and effective, even for pregnant and breastfeeding women.

Plan for Travel

- Outbreaks of Zika have occurred in different countries and territories.
- Zika virus will continue to infect people. It is difficult to know when and where Zika virus will occur in the future.

Protect Yourself during Sex

- Zika can be passed through sex from a person who has Zika to his or her sex partners.
- We know that Zika can remain in semen longer than in other body fluids, including vaginal fluids, urine, and blood.

WHAT YOU CAN DO

- Not having sex can eliminate the risk of getting Zika from sex.
- Condoms can reduce the chance of getting Zika from sex:
  - Condoms include male and female condoms.
  - To be effective, condoms should be used from start to finish, every time during vaginal, anal, and oral sex and the sharing of sex toys.
  - Dental dams (latex or polyurethane sheets) may also be used for certain types of oral sex (mouth to vagina or mouth to anus).

If You Have Zika, Protect Others

- During the first week of infection, Zika virus can be found in the blood and passed from an infected person to another mosquito through mosquito bites. An infected mosquito can then spread the virus to other people.
- Zika can be passed through sex from a person who has Zika to his or her partners. Sex includes vaginal, anal, and oral sex and the sharing of sex toys.

WHAT YOU CAN DO

- Take steps to prevent mosquito bites.
- Protect yourself during sex if your partner lives in or has traveled to an area with risk of Zika.[1]

[1] "Zika Virus," Centers for Disease Control and Prevention (CDC), May 20, 2019. Available online. URL: www.cdc.gov/zika/about/index.html. Accessed July 3, 2023.

Part 3 | Bacterial Contagious Diseases

Chapter 29 | Bacterial Meningitis

Bacterial meningitis is a serious infection. Some people with the infection die, and death can occur in as little as a few hours. However, most people recover from bacterial meningitis. Those who do recover can have permanent disabilities, such as brain damage, hearing loss, and learning disabilities.

CAUSES OF BACTERIAL MENINGITIS

Several types of bacteria can cause meningitis. Leading causes in the United States include the following:

- *Streptococcus pneumonia*
- group B *Streptococcus*
- *Neisseria meningitidis*
- *Haemophilus influenzae*
- *Listeria monocytogenes*
- *Escherichia coli*

Mycobacterium tuberculosis, which causes tuberculosis (TB), is a less common cause of bacterial meningitis (called "TB meningitis"). Many of these bacteria can also be associated with another serious illness, sepsis. Sepsis is the body's extreme response to infection. It is a life-threatening medical emergency. Sepsis happens when an infection triggers a chain reaction throughout your body. Without timely treatment, sepsis can quickly lead to tissue damage, organ failure, and death. Some causes of bacterial meningitis are more likely to affect certain age groups:

- **Newborns**. Group B *Streptococcus*, *S. pneumoniae*, *L. monocytogenes*, and *E. coli*.

- **Babies and young children**. *S. pneumoniae, N. meningitidis, H. influenzae*, group B *Streptococcus*, and *M. tuberculosis*.
- **Teens and young adults**. *N. meningitidis* and *S. pneumoniae*.
- **Older adults**. *S. pneumoniae, N. meningitidis, H. influenzae*, group B *Streptococcus*, and *L. monocytogenes*.

RISK FACTORS OF BACTERIAL MENINGITIS

Certain factors increase a person's risk of getting bacterial meningitis. These risk factors include the following:

- **Age**. Babies are at increased risk for bacterial meningitis compared to people in other age groups. However, people of any age can develop bacterial meningitis. See the previous section for which bacteria more commonly affect which age groups.
- **Group setting**. Infectious diseases tend to spread where large groups of people gather. For example, college campuses have reported outbreaks of meningococcal disease caused by *N. meningitidis*.
- **Certain medical conditions**. Certain medical conditions, medications, and surgical procedures put people at increased risk for meningitis. For example, having a human immunodeficiency virus (HIV) infection or a cerebrospinal fluid leak, or not having a spleen, can increase a person's risk for several types of bacterial meningitis.
- **Working with meningitis-causing pathogens**. Microbiologists routinely exposed to meningitis-causing bacteria are at increased risk for meningitis.
- **Travel**. Travelers may be at increased risk for meningococcal disease, caused by *N. meningitidis*, if they travel to certain places, such as:
    - the meningitis belt in sub-Saharan Africa, particularly during the dry season

- Mecca during the annual Hajj and Umrah pilgrimage

In many countries, TB is much more common than in the United States. Travelers should avoid close contact or prolonged time with known TB patients in crowded, enclosed environments (e.g., clinics, hospitals, prisons, or homeless shelters).

SIGNS AND SYMPTOMS OF BACTERIAL MENINGITIS

Meningitis symptoms include sudden onset of:

- fever
- headache
- stiff neck

There are often other symptoms, such as:

- nausea
- vomiting
- photophobia (eyes being more sensitive to light)
- altered mental status (confusion)

Newborns and babies may not have, or it may be difficult to notice the classic symptoms listed above. Instead, babies may:

- be slow or inactive
- be irritable
- vomit
- feed poorly
- have a bulging fontanelle (the "soft spot" on a baby's head)
- have abnormal reflexes

If you think your baby or child has any of these symptoms, call the doctor right away.

Typically, symptoms of bacterial meningitis develop within three to seven days after exposure; note that this is not true for TB meningitis, which can develop much later after exposure to the bacteria.

People with bacterial meningitis can have seizures, go into a coma, and even die. For this reason, anyone who thinks they may have meningitis should see a doctor as soon as possible.

HOW BACTERIAL MENINGITIS SPREADS

Certain germs that cause bacterial meningitis, such as *L. monocytogenes*, can spread through food. But most of these germs spread from one person to another.

How people spread the germs often depends on the type of bacteria. It is also important to know that people can have these bacteria in or on their bodies without being sick. These people are "carriers." Most carriers never become sick but can still spread the bacteria to others.

Here are some of the most common examples of how people spread each type of bacteria to each other:

- **Group B *Streptococcus* and *E. coli*.** Mothers can pass these bacteria to their babies during birth.
- ***H. influenzae, M. tuberculosis,* and *S. pneumoniae*.** People spread these bacteria by coughing or sneezing while in close contact with others who breathe in the bacteria.
- ***N. meningitidis*.** People spread these bacteria by sharing respiratory or throat secretions (saliva or spit). This typically occurs during close (coughing or kissing) or lengthy (living together) contact.
- ***E. coli*.** People can get these bacteria by eating food prepared by people who did not wash their hands well after using the toilet.

People usually get sick from *E. coli* and *L. monocytogenes* by eating contaminated food.

DIAGNOSIS OF BACTERIAL MENINGITIS

If a doctor suspects meningitis, they will collect samples of blood or cerebrospinal fluid (fluid near the spinal cord). A laboratory will test the samples to see what is causing the infection. Knowing the specific cause of meningitis helps doctors treat it.

TREATMENT FOR BACTERIAL MENINGITIS

Doctors treat bacterial meningitis with a number of antibiotics. It is important to start treatment as soon as possible.

PREVENTION OF BACTERIAL MENINGITIS

Vaccination

Vaccines are the most effective way to protect against certain types of bacterial meningitis. The following are the vaccines for four types of bacteria that can cause meningitis:

- **Meningococcal vaccines.** These vaccines help protect against *N. meningitidis.*
- **Pneumococcal vaccines.** These vaccines help protect against *S. pneumoniae.*
- ***H. influenzae* serotype b (Hib) vaccines.** These vaccines help protect against Hib.
- **Bacille Calmette-Guérin vaccine.** This vaccine helps protect against TB disease but is not widely used in the United States.

Make sure you and your child are vaccinated on schedule.

Like with any vaccine, these vaccines do not work 100 percent of the time. The vaccines also do not protect against infections from all the types (strains) of each of these bacteria. For these reasons, there is still a chance that vaccinated people can develop bacterial meningitis.[1]

[1] "Bacterial Meningitis," Centers for Disease Control and Prevention (CDC), July 15, 2021. Available online. URL: www.cdc.gov/meningitis/bacterial.html. Accessed July 19, 2023.

Chapter 30 | **Chancroid**

Chancroid prevalence has declined in the United States. When infection occurs, it is usually associated with sporadic outbreaks. Worldwide, chancroid appears to have decreased as well although infection might still occur in certain African regions and the Caribbean. Chancroid is a risk factor in human immunodeficiency virus (HIV) transmission and acquisition.

DIAGNOSTIC CONSIDERATIONS

A definitive diagnosis of chancroid requires identifying *Haemophilus ducreyi* (*H. ducreyi*) on special culture media that is not widely available from commercial sources; even when these media are used, sensitivity is less than 80 percent. No nucleic acid amplification test (NAAT) for *H. ducreyi* approved by the U.S. Food and Drug Administration (FDA) is available in the United States; however, such testing can be performed by clinical laboratories that have developed their own NAAT and have conducted Clinical Laboratory Improvement Amendments (CLIA) verification studies on genital specimens.

The combination of one or more deep and painful genital ulcers and tender suppurative inguinal adenopathy indicates the chancroid diagnosis; inguinal lymphadenitis typically occurs in less than 50 percent of cases. For both clinical and surveillance purposes, a probable diagnosis of chancroid can be made if all the following four criteria are met:

- The patient has one or more painful genital ulcers.
- The clinical presentation, appearance of genital ulcers, and, if present, regional lymphadenopathy are typical for chancroid.

- The patient has no evidence of *Treponema pallidum* infection by dark-field examination or NAAT (i.e., ulcer exudate or serous fluid) or by serologic tests for syphilis performed at least 7–14 days after the onset of ulcers.
- A herpes simplex virus 1 (HSV-1) or herpes simplex virus 2 (HSV-2) NAAT or HSV culture performed on the ulcer exudate or fluid is negative.

TREATMENT

Successful antimicrobial treatment for chancroid cures the infection, resolves the clinical symptoms, and prevents transmission to others. In advanced cases, genital scarring and rectal or urogenital fistulas from suppurative buboes can result despite successful therapy.

Recommended Regimens

- azithromycin: 1 g orally in a single dose
- ceftriaxone: 250 mg intramuscularly (IM) in a single dose
- ciprofloxacin: 500 mg orally two times/day for three days
- erythromycin base: 500 mg orally three times/day for seven days

Azithromycin and ceftriaxone offer the advantage of single-dose therapy. Worldwide, several isolates with intermediate resistance to either ciprofloxacin or erythromycin have been reported. However, because cultures are not routinely performed and chancroid is uncommon, data are limited regarding the prevalence of *H. ducreyi* antimicrobial resistance.

OTHER MANAGEMENT CONSIDERATIONS

Men who are uncircumcised and persons with HIV infection do not respond as well to treatment as persons who are circumcised or are HIV-negative. Patients should be tested for HIV at the time chancroid is diagnosed. If the initial HIV test results are negative, the provider can consider the benefits of offering more frequent testing and HIV pre-exposure prophylaxis (PrEP) to persons at increased risk for HIV infection.

FOLLOW-UP

Patients should be reexamined three to seven days after therapy initiation. If treatment is successful, ulcers usually improve symptomatically within three days and objectively within seven days after therapy. If no clinical improvement is evident, the clinician should consider whether:

- the diagnosis is correct
- another sexually transmitted infection (STI) is present
- the patient has an HIV infection
- the treatment was not used as instructed
- the *H. ducreyi* strain causing the infection is resistant to the prescribed antimicrobial

The time required for complete healing depends on the size of the ulcer; large ulcers might require greater than two weeks. In addition, healing can be slower for uncircumcised men who have ulcers under the foreskin. Clinical resolution of fluctuant lymphadenopathy is slower than that of ulcers and might require needle aspiration or incision and drainage despite otherwise successful therapy. Although needle aspiration of buboes is a simpler procedure, incision and drainage might be preferred because of the reduced need for subsequent drainage procedures.

MANAGEMENT OF SEX PARTNERS

Regardless of whether disease symptoms are present, sex partners of patients with chancroid should be examined and treated if they had sexual contact with the patient during the 10 days preceding the patient's symptom onset.

SPECIAL CONSIDERATIONS

Pregnancy

Data indicate ciprofloxacin presents a low risk to the fetus during pregnancy but has potential for toxicity during breastfeeding. Alternative drugs should be used if the patient is pregnant or lactating. No adverse effects of chancroid on pregnancy outcomes have been reported.

Human Immunodeficiency Virus Infection

Persons with HIV infection who have chancroid infection should be monitored closely because they are more likely to experience chancroid treatment failure and to have ulcers that heal slowly. Persons with HIV might require repeated or longer courses of therapy, and treatment failures can occur with any regimen. Data are limited concerning the therapeutic efficacy of the recommended single-dose azithromycin and ceftriaxone regimens among persons with HIV infection.

Children

Because sexual contact is the major primary transmission route among U.S. patients, diagnosis of chancroid ulcers among infants and children, especially in the genital or perineal region, is highly suspicious of sexual abuse. However, *H. ducreyi* is recognized as a major cause of nonsexually transmitted cutaneous ulcers among children in tropical regions and, specifically, countries where yaws is endemic. Acquisition of a lower-extremity ulcer attributable to *H. ducreyi* in a child without genital ulcers and reported travel to a region where yaws is endemic should not be considered evidence of sexual abuse.[1]

[1] "Chancroid," Centers for Disease Control and Prevention (CDC), July 22, 2021. Available online. URL: www.cdc.gov/std/treatment-guidelines/chancroid.htm. Accessed June 27, 2023.

Chapter 31 | Chlamydia and Lymphogranuloma Venereum

CHLAMYDIA

Chlamydia is a common sexually transmitted disease (STD) caused by infection with *Chlamydia trachomatis*. It can cause cervicitis, urethritis, and proctitis. In women, these infections can lead to:

- pelvic inflammatory disease (PID)
- tubal factor infertility
- ectopic pregnancy
- chronic pelvic pain

Lymphogranuloma venereum (LGV) is another type of STD caused by *C. trachomatis*. LGV is the cause of recent proctitis outbreaks among gay, bisexual, and other men who have sex with men (MSM) worldwide.

How Common Is Chlamydia?

The Centers for Disease Control and Prevention (CDC) estimates that there were 4 million chlamydial infections in 2018. Chlamydia is also the most frequently reported bacterial sexually transmitted infection (STI) in the United States. It is difficult to account for many cases of chlamydia. Most people with the infection have no symptoms and do not seek testing. Chlamydia is most common among young people. Two-thirds of new chlamydial infections occur among youth aged 15–24. Estimates show that 1 in 20 sexually active young women aged 14–24 has chlamydia.

Disparities persist among racial and ethnic minority groups. In 2021, chlamydia rates for African Americans/Blacks were six times that of Whites. Chlamydia is also common among MSM. Among MSM screened for rectal chlamydial infection, positivity ranges from 3.0 to 10.5 percent. Among MSM screened for pharyngeal chlamydial infection, positivity ranges from 0.5 to 2.3 percent.

How Do People Get Chlamydia?

Chlamydia spreads through vaginal, anal, or oral sex with someone with the infection. Semen does not have to be present to get or spread the infection.

Pregnant people can give chlamydia to their babies during childbirth. This can cause ophthalmia neonatorum (conjunctivitis) or pneumonia in some infants. Rectal or genital infection can persist one year or longer in infants infected at birth. However, sexual abuse should be a consideration among young children with vaginal, urethral, or rectal infections beyond the neonatal period. People treated for chlamydia can get the infection again if they have sex with a person with chlamydia.

Who Is at Risk for Chlamydia?

Sexually active people can get chlamydia through vaginal, anal, or oral sex without a condom with a partner who has chlamydia. It is a very common STD, especially among young people.

Sexually active young people are at high risk of getting chlamydia for behavioral, biological, and cultural reasons. Some do not always use condoms. Some may move from one monogamous relationship to another during the likely infectivity period of chlamydia. This can increase the risk of transmission. Teenage girls and young women may have cervical ectopy (where cells from the endocervix are present on the ectocervix). Cervical ectopy may increase susceptibility to chlamydial infection. High chlamydia prevalence among young people may also reflect barriers to accessing STD prevention services. These barriers can include lack of transportation, cost, and perceived stigma.

What Are the Symptoms of Chlamydia?

Some refer to chlamydia as a "silent" infection. This is because most people with the infection have no symptoms or abnormal physical exam findings. Studies find that the proportion of people with chlamydia who develop symptoms varies by setting and study methodology. Two modeling studies estimate that about 10 percent of men and 5–30 percent of women with a confirmed infection develop symptoms. The incubation period of chlamydia is unclear. Given the relatively slow replication cycle of the organism, symptoms may not appear until several weeks after exposure in people who develop symptoms.

In women, the bacteria initially infect the cervix. This may cause signs and symptoms of cervicitis (e.g., mucopurulent endocervical discharge, easily induced endocervical bleeding). It can also infect the urethra. This may cause signs and symptoms of urethritis (e.g., pyuria, dysuria, and urinary frequency). Infection can spread from the cervix to the upper reproductive tract (i.e., uterus, fallopian tubes), causing PID. PID may be asymptomatic ("subclinical PID") or acute, with typical symptoms of abdominal and/or pelvic pain. Signs of cervical motion tenderness and uterine or adnexal tenderness may also occur during the examination.

Men with symptoms typically have urethritis, with a mucoid or watery urethral discharge and dysuria. Some men develop epididymitis (with or without symptomatic urethritis) with unilateral testicular pain, tenderness, and swelling.

Chlamydia can infect the rectum in men and women. This can happen either directly (through receptive anal sex) or via spread from the cervix and vagina in a woman. While these infections often have no symptoms, they can cause symptoms of proctitis (e.g., rectal pain, discharge, and/or bleeding). Conjunctivitis can occur in both men and women through contact with infected genital secretions. While chlamydia can also spread to the throat by having oral sex, there are typically no symptoms. It also does not appear to be an important cause of pharyngitis.

What Health Problems Can Result from Chlamydia?

The initial damage that chlamydia causes is often unnoticed. However, infections can lead to serious health problems with both short- and long-term effects.

If a woman does not receive treatment, chlamydia can spread into the uterus or fallopian tubes, causing PID. Symptomatic PID occurs in about 10–15 percent of women who do not receive treatment. However, chlamydia can also cause subclinical inflammation of the upper genital tract ("subclinical PID"). Both acute and subclinical PID can cause long-term damage to the fallopian tubes, uterus, and surrounding tissues. The damage can lead to chronic pelvic pain, tubal factor infertility, and potentially fatal ectopic pregnancy.

Some patients with PID develop perihepatitis, or "Fitz-Hugh and Curtis syndrome." This syndrome includes inflammation of the liver capsule and surrounding peritoneum, which can cause right upper quadrant pain.

In pregnant women, untreated chlamydia can lead to preterm delivery, ophthalmia neonatorum (conjunctivitis), and pneumonia in the newborn. Reactive arthritis can occur in men and women following infection with or without symptoms. This is sometimes part of a triad of symptoms (with urethritis and conjunctivitis) formerly referred to as Reiter syndrome.

What about Chlamydia and Human Immunodeficiency Virus?

Untreated chlamydia may increase a person's chances of getting or transmitting the human immunodeficiency virus (HIV).

How Does Chlamydia Affect a Pregnant Woman and Her Baby?

In newborns, untreated chlamydia can cause:

- preterm delivery
- ophthalmia neonatorum (conjunctivitis)
- pneumonia

Prospective studies show that chlamydial conjunctivitis and pneumonia occur in 18–44 percent and 3–16 percent, respectively, of infants born to those with chlamydia. Neonatal prophylaxis against gonococcal conjunctivitis routinely performed at birth does not effectively prevent chlamydial conjunctivitis.

Screening for and treating chlamydia in pregnant people is the best way to prevent disease in infants. At the first prenatal visit and during the third trimester, screen:

- all pregnant people under the age of 25
- all pregnant people aged 25 and older at increased risk for chlamydia (e.g., those who have a new or more than one sex partner)

Retest those with infection four weeks and three months after they complete treatment.

Who Should Be Tested for Chlamydia?

Anyone with the following genital symptoms should not have sex until they see a health-care provider:

- a discharge
- a burning sensation when peeing
- unusual sores
- a rash

Anyone having oral, anal, or vaginal sex with a partner recently diagnosed with an STD should see a health-care provider.

Because chlamydia usually has no symptoms, screening is necessary to identify most infections. Screening programs can reduce rates of adverse sequelae in women. The CDC recommends yearly chlamydia screening of all sexually active women under the age of 25. The CDC also recommends screening for older women with risk factors, such as new or multiple partners or a sex partner who has an STI. Screen and treat those who are pregnant, as noted in "How Does Chlamydia Affect a Pregnant Person and Their Baby?" Women who are sexually active should discuss their risk factors with a health-care provider to determine if more frequent screening is necessary.

Routine screening is not necessary for men. However, consider screening sexually active young men in clinical settings with a high prevalence of chlamydia. This can include adolescent clinics, correctional facilities, and STD clinics. Consider this when resources permit and do not hinder screening efforts in women.

Screen sexually active MSM who have insertive intercourse for urethral chlamydial infection. Also, screen MSM who have receptive anal intercourse for rectal infection at least yearly. Screening for pharyngeal infection is not recommended. MSM, including those with HIV, should receive more frequent chlamydia screening at three- to six-month intervals if risk behaviors persist or if they or their sexual partners have multiple partners.

At the initial HIV care visit, providers should test all sexually active people for chlamydia. Test at least each year during HIV care. A patient's health-care provider might determine more frequent screening is necessary based on the patient's risk factors.

How Is Chlamydia Diagnosed?

Diagnose chlamydia with nucleic acid amplification tests (NAATs), cell culture, and other types of tests. NAATs are the most sensitive tests to use on easy-to-obtain specimens. This includes vaginal swabs (either clinician- or patient-collected) or urine.

To diagnose genital chlamydia in women using a NAAT, vaginal swabs are the optimal specimen. Urine is the specimen of choice for men. Urine is an effective alternative specimen type for women. Self-collected vaginal swab specimens perform as well as other approved specimens using NAATs. Patients may prefer self-collected vaginal swabs or urine-based screening to more invasive specimen collection. Adolescent girls may be good candidates for self-collected vaginal swab- or urine-based screening.

Diagnose rectal or pharyngeal infection by testing at the anatomic exposure site. While useful for these specimens, culture is not widely available. Additionally, NAATs have better sensitivity and specificity compared with culture for detecting *C. trachomatis* at nongenital sites. Most tests, including NAATs, are not approved by the U.S. Food and Drug Administration (FDA) for use with rectal or pharyngeal swab specimens. NAATs have better sensitivity and specificity compared with culture for the detection of *C. trachomatis* at rectal sites. However, some laboratories have met set requirements and have validated NAAT testing on rectal and pharyngeal swab specimens.

What Is the Treatment for Chlamydia?

Antibiotics can easily cure chlamydia. Treatment options are the same, whether a person also has HIV or not.

Patients treated with single-dose antibiotics should not have sex for seven days. Patients treated with a seven-day course of antibiotics should not have sex until they complete treatment and their symptoms are gone. This helps prevent the spreading of the infection to sex partners. It is important to take all medicine prescribed to cure chlamydia. Medicine should not be shared with anyone. Although treatment will cure the infection, it will not repair any long-term damage done by the disease. If a person's symptoms continue for more than a few days after receiving treatment, a health-care provider should reevaluate them.

Repeat infection with chlamydia is common. Women whose sex partners do not receive appropriate treatment are at high risk for reinfection. Having multiple chlamydial infections increases a woman's risk of serious reproductive health problems (e.g., PID and ectopic pregnancy). A health-care provider should retest those with chlamydia about three months after treatment of an initial infection. Retesting is necessary even if their partners receive successful treatment.

Infants with chlamydia may develop conjunctivitis and/or pneumonia. Health-care providers can treat infection in infants with antibiotics.

What about Partners?

People treated for chlamydia should tell their recent sex partners, so the partner can see a health-care provider. "Recent" partners include anyone the patient had anal, vaginal, or oral sex within the 60 days before symptom onset or diagnosis. This will help protect the partner from health problems and prevent reinfection.

In some states, health-care providers may give people with chlamydia extra medicine or prescriptions to give to their sex partner(s). This is called "expedited partner therapy" (EPT). Clinical trials comparing EPT to asking the patient to refer their partners in for treatment find that EPT leads to fewer reinfections in the index patient and more partner treatment. EPT is another strategy providers use to manage the partners of people with chlamydial infection. Partners should still seek medical care, regardless of whether they receive EPT.

How Can Chlamydia Be Prevented?

Condoms, when used correctly every time someone has sex, can reduce the risk of getting or giving chlamydia. The only way to completely avoid chlamydia is to not have vaginal, anal, and oral sex. Another option is being in a long-term, mutually monogamous relationship with a partner who has been tested and does not have chlamydia.[1]

LYMPHOGRANULOMA VENEREUM

Lymphogranuloma venereum is caused by *C. trachomatis* serovars L1, L2, or L3. LGV can cause severe inflammation and invasive infection, in contrast with *C. trachomatis* serovars A–K that cause mild or asymptomatic infection. Clinical manifestations of LGV can include genital ulcer disease (GUD), lymphadenopathy, or proctocolitis. Rectal exposure among MSM or women can result in proctocolitis, which is the most common presentation of LGV infection and can mimic inflammatory bowel disease (IBD) with clinical findings of mucoid or hemorrhagic rectal discharge, anal pain, constipation, fever, or tenesmus. Outbreaks of LGV proctocolitis have been reported among MSM with high rates of HIV infection. LGV proctocolitis can be an invasive, systemic infection and, if it is not treated early, can lead to chronic colorectal fistulas and strictures; reactive arthropathy has also been reported. However, reports indicate that rectal LGV can also be asymptomatic.

[1] "Chlamydia—CDC Detailed Fact Sheet," Centers for Disease Control and Prevention (CDC), April 11, 2023. Available online. URL: www.cdc.gov/std/chlamydia/stdfact-chlamydia-detailed.htm. Accessed June 27, 2023.

A common clinical manifestation of LGV among heterosexuals is tender inguinal or femoral lymphadenopathy that is typically unilateral. A self-limited genital ulcer or papule sometimes occurs at the site of inoculation. However, by the time persons seek care, the lesions have often disappeared. LGV-associated lymphadenopathy can be severe, with bubo formation from fluctuant or suppurative inguinal or femoral lymphadenopathy. Oral ulceration can occur and might be associated with cervical adenopathy. Persons with genital or colorectal LGV lesions can also experience secondary bacterial infection or can be infected with other sexually and nonsexually transmitted pathogens.

Diagnostic Considerations

A definitive LGV diagnosis can be made only with LGV-specific molecular testing (e.g., genotyping based on polymerase chain reaction (PCR)). These tests can differentiate LGV from non-LGV *C. trachomatis* in rectal specimens. However, these tests are not widely available, and results are not typically available in a time frame that would influence clinical management. Therefore, diagnosis is based on clinical suspicion, epidemiologic information, and a *C. trachomatis* NAAT at the symptomatic anatomic site, along with the exclusion of other etiologies for proctocolitis, inguinal lymphadenopathy, or genital, oral, or rectal ulcers. Genital or oral lesions, rectal specimens, and lymph node specimens (i.e., lesion swab or bubo aspirate) can be tested for *C. trachomatis* by NAAT or culture. NAAT is the preferred approach for testing because it can detect both LGV strains and non-LGV *C. trachomatis* strains. Therefore, all persons presenting with proctocolitis should be tested for chlamydia with a NAAT performed on rectal specimens. Severe symptoms of proctocolitis (e.g., bloody discharge, tenesmus, and rectal ulcers) indicate LGV. A rectal Gram stain with greater than 10 white blood cells (WBCs) has also been associated with rectal LGV.

Chlamydia serology (complement fixation or microimmunofluorescence) should not be used routinely as a diagnostic tool for LGV because the utility of these serologic methods has not been established, interpretation has not been standardized, and validation for clinical proctitis presentation has not been done. It might support an LGV diagnosis in cases of isolated inguinal or femoral lymphadenopathy for which diagnostic material for *C. trachomatis* NAAT cannot be obtained.

Treatment

At the time of the initial visit (before diagnostic NAATs for chlamydia are available), persons with a clinical syndrome consistent with LGV should be presumptively treated. Presumptive treatment for LGV is indicated among patients with symptoms or signs of proctocolitis (e.g., bloody discharge, tenesmus, or ulceration); in cases of severe inguinal lymphadenopathy with bubo formation, particularly if the patient has a recent history of a genital ulcer; or in the presence of a genital ulcer if other etiologies have been ruled out. The goal of treatment is to cure the infection and prevent ongoing tissue damage although tissue reaction to the infection can result in scarring. Buboes might require aspiration through intact skin or incision and drainage to prevent the formation of inguinal or femoral ulcerations.

RECOMMENDED REGIMEN FOR LYMPHOGRANULOMA VENEREUM

- doxycycline: 100 mg orally two times/day for 21 days

ALTERNATIVE REGIMENS

- azithromycin: 1 g orally once weekly for three weeks*
- erythromycin base: 500 mg orally four times/day for 21 days

**Because this regimen has not been validated, a test of cure with C. trachomatis NAAT four weeks after completion of treatment can be considered.*

The optimal treatment duration for symptomatic LGV has not been studied in clinical trials. The recommended 21-day course of doxycycline is based on long-standing clinical practice and is highly effective, with an estimated cure rate of greater than 98.5 percent.

Shorter courses of doxycycline might be effective on the basis of a small retrospective study of MSM with rectal LGV, 50 percent of whom were symptomatic, who received a 7- to 14-day course of doxycycline and had a 97 percent cure rate. Randomized prospective studies of shorter-course doxycycline for treating LGV are needed. Longer courses of therapy might be required in the setting of fistulas, buboes, and other forms of severe disease.

A small nonrandomized study from Spain involving patients with rectal LGV demonstrated cure rates of 97 percent with a regimen of azithromycin 1 g once weekly for three weeks. Pharmacokinetic data support this dosing strategy; however, this regimen has not been validated. Fluoroquinolone-based treatments might also be effective; however, the optimal duration of treatment has not been evaluated. The clinical significance of asymptomatic LGV is unknown, and it is effectively treated with a seven-day course of doxycycline.

Other Management Considerations

Patients should be followed clinically until signs and symptoms have resolved. Persons who receive an LGV diagnosis should be tested for other STIs, especially HIV, gonorrhea, and syphilis. Those whose HIV test results are negative should be offered HIV preexposure prophylaxis (PrEP).

Follow-Up

All persons who have been treated for LGV should be retested for chlamydia approximately three months after treatment. If retesting at three months is not possible, providers should retest at the patient's next visit for medical care within the 12-month period after initial treatment.

Management of Sex Partners

Persons who have had sexual contact with a patient who has LGV within the 60 days before the onset of the patient's symptoms should be evaluated, examined, and tested for chlamydial infection, depending on the anatomic site of exposure. Asymptomatic partners should be presumptively treated with a chlamydia regimen (doxycycline 100 mg orally two times/day for seven days).

Special Considerations

PREGNANCY

Use of doxycycline in pregnancy might be associated with discoloration of teeth; however, the risk is not well-defined. Doxycycline is compatible with breastfeeding. Azithromycin might prove useful for LGV treatment during pregnancy at a presumptive dose of 1 g weekly for three weeks; no published data are available regarding an effective dose and duration of treatment. Pregnant and lactating women with LGV can be treated with erythromycin although this regimen is associated with frequent gastrointestinal side effects. Pregnant women treated for LGV should have a test of cure performed four weeks after the initial *C. trachomatis* NAAT-positive test.

HUMAN IMMUNODEFICIENCY VIRUS INFECTION

Persons with LGV and HIV infection should receive the same regimens as those who do not have HIV. Prolonged therapy might be required because a delay in resolution of symptoms might occur.[2]

[2] "Lymphogranuloma Venereum (LGV)," Centers for Disease Control and Prevention (CDC), July 22, 2021. Available online. URL: www.cdc.gov/std/treatment-guidelines/lgv.htm. Accessed June 27, 2023.

Chapter 32 | Cholera

WHAT IS CHOLERA?

Cholera is an acute, diarrheal illness caused by infection of the intestine with the toxigenic bacterium *Vibrio cholerae* serogroup O1 or O139. An estimated 1.3–4 million people around the world get cholera each year, and 21,000–143,000 people die from it. People who get cholera often have mild symptoms or no symptoms, but cholera can be severe. Approximately 1 in 10 people who get sick with cholera will develop severe symptoms such as watery diarrhea, vomiting, and leg cramps. In these people, rapid loss of body fluids leads to dehydration and shock. Without treatment, death can occur within hours.

WHERE IS CHOLERA FOUND?

The cholera bacterium is usually found in water or in foods that have been contaminated by feces (poop) from a person infected with cholera bacteria. Cholera is most likely to occur and spread in places with inadequate water treatment, poor sanitation, and inadequate hygiene.

Cholera bacteria can also live in the environment in brackish rivers and coastal waters. Shellfish eaten raw have been a source of infection. Rarely, people in the United States have contracted cholera after eating raw or undercooked shellfish from the Gulf of Mexico.

HOW DOES A PERSON GET CHOLERA?

A person can get cholera by drinking water or eating food contaminated with cholera bacteria. In an epidemic, the source of the contamination is usually the feces of an infected person that contaminates water or food. The disease can spread rapidly in areas with inadequate treatment of sewage and drinking water. The infection is not likely to spread directly from one person to another; therefore, casual contact with an infected person is not a risk factor for becoming ill.

WHAT ARE THE SYMPTOMS OF CHOLERA?

Cholera infection is often mild or without symptoms but can be severe. Approximately 1 in 10 people who get sick with cholera will develop severe symptoms such as watery diarrhea, vomiting, and leg cramps. In these people, rapid loss of body fluids leads to dehydration and shock. Without treatment, death can occur within hours.

HOW LONG AFTER INFECTION DO THE SYMPTOMS APPEAR?

It usually takes two to three days for symptoms to appear after a person ingests cholera bacteria, but the time can range from a few hours to five days.

WHO IS MOST LIKELY TO GET CHOLERA?

Persons living in places with unsafe drinking water, poor sanitation, and inadequate hygiene are at the highest risk for cholera.

WHAT SHOULD YOU DO IF YOU OR SOMEONE YOU KNOW GETS SICK?

If you think you or a member of your family might have cholera, seek medical attention immediately. Dehydration can be rapid, so fluid replacement is essential. If you have an oral rehydration solution (ORS), start taking it immediately; it can save a life. Continue to drink ORS at home and while traveling to get medical treatment. If an infant has watery diarrhea, continue breastfeeding.

HOW IS CHOLERA DIAGNOSED?

To test for cholera, doctors must take a stool sample or a rectal swab and send it to a laboratory to look for the cholera bacteria.

WHAT IS THE TREATMENT FOR CHOLERA?

Cholera can be simply and successfully treated by immediate replacement of the fluid and salts lost through diarrhea. Patients can be treated with ORS, a prepackaged mixture of sugar and salts that is mixed with 1 liter of water and drunk in large amounts. This solution is used throughout the world to treat diarrhea. Severe cases also require intravenous (IV) fluid replacement. With prompt appropriate rehydration, fewer than 1 percent of cholera patients die.

Antibiotics shorten the course and diminish the severity of the illness, but they are not as important as rehydration. Persons who develop severe diarrhea and vomiting in countries where cholera occurs should seek medical attention promptly.

SHOULD YOU BE WORRIED ABOUT GETTING CHOLERA FROM OTHERS?

The disease is not likely to spread directly from one person to another; therefore, casual contact with an infected person is not a risk factor for becoming ill.

HOW CAN YOU AVOID GETTING SICK WITH CHOLERA?

Be aware of whether cholera cases have recently occurred in an area you plan to visit. However, the risk for cholera is very low for people visiting areas with epidemic cholera when simple prevention steps are taken. All visitors or residents in areas where cholera is occurring or has occurred should follow the following recommendations prevent getting sick:

- Drink only bottled, boiled, or chemically treated water and bottled or canned beverages. When using bottled drinks, make sure the seal has not been broken. Carbonated water may be safer than noncarbonated water. Avoid tap water, fountain drinks, and ice cubes.
- To disinfect your own water, choose one of the following options:
    - Boil it for one minute.
    - Filter it and add either half an iodine tablet or two drops of household bleach per liter/quart of water.

    - Use commercial water chlorination tablets according to the manufacturer's instructions.
- Wash your hands often with soap and clean water, especially before you eat or prepare food and after using the bathroom.
    - If no water and soap are available, use an alcohol-based hand sanitizer with at least 60 percent alcohol.
- Use bottled, boiled, or chemically treated water to wash dishes, brush teeth, wash and prepare food, and make ice.
- Eat foods that are packaged or that are freshly cooked and served hot.
    - Do not eat raw or undercooked meats and seafood or raw or undercooked fruits and vegetables unless they are peeled.
- Dispose of feces in a sanitary manner to prevent contamination of water and food sources.

IS A VACCINE AVAILABLE TO PREVENT CHOLERA?

A single-dose live oral cholera vaccine, called "Vaxchora" ("lyophilized CVD 103-HgR"), is approved by the U.S. Food and Drug Administration (FDA) for people aged 2–64 who are traveling to an area of active cholera transmission. Three other oral cholera vaccines are approved by the World Health Organization (WHO): Dukoral, ShanChol, and Euvichol-Plus/Euvichol. These vaccines are not available in the United States but may be available at your travel destination or if you are living outside the United States. Check the Travel Health Notices of the Centers for Disease Control and Prevention (CDC) website (wwwnc.cdc.gov/travel/notices) to identify areas with active cholera transmission. Visit a doctor or travel clinic to talk about vaccination if you will be traveling to or living in one of these areas.

WHAT IS THE RISK FOR CHOLERA IN THE UNITED STATES?

- Cholera was prevalent in the United States in the 1800s, but water-related spread has been eliminated by modern

water and sewage treatment systems. Very rarely, people in the United States get sick with cholera after eating raw or undercooked shellfish from the Gulf of Mexico.
- However, U.S. travelers to areas with epidemic cholera (e.g., parts of Africa, Asia, and Latin America) can be exposed to cholera bacteria and might develop illness after arriving home. Some travelers have brought contaminated seafood home from abroad, resulting in cholera.

WHERE CAN A TRAVELER GET INFORMATION ABOUT CHOLERA?

The global picture of cholera changes periodically, so travelers should seek updated information on countries of interest. The CDC has a Travelers' Health website (wwwnc.cdc.gov/travel/) with information on cholera and other diseases of concern to travelers.

WHAT IS THE U.S. GOVERNMENT DOING TO COMBAT CHOLERA?

- The U.S. and international public health authorities are working to enhance surveillance for cholera, investigate and respond to cholera outbreaks, and design and implement preventive measures across the globe. The CDC investigates epidemic cholera wherever it occurs at the invitation of the affected country and trains laboratory workers in proper techniques for the identification of *V. cholerae*. In addition, the CDC provides information on the diagnosis, treatment, and prevention of cholera to public health officials and educates the public about effective preventive measures.
- The World Health Organization (WHO) and the Global Task Force on Cholera Control (GTFCC), along with partners and various stakeholders, launched Ending Cholera—a Global Roadmap to 2030, which is an unprecedented initiative to fight and reduce cholera transmission globally. This comprehensive plan identifies priorities to reduce cholera deaths by 90 percent and stop transmission in up to 20 countries by 2030. The CDC supports the global strategy by participating in

task force working groups for water, sanitation, and hygiene (WASH), case management, epidemiology and surveillance, laboratory, and oral cholera vaccines.
- The U.S. Agency for International Development (USAID) sponsors some of the international U.S. government activities and provides medical supplies and water, sanitation, and hygiene supplies to affected countries.
- The FDA tests imported and domestic shellfish for *V. cholerae* and monitors the safety of U.S. shellfish beds through the shellfish sanitation program.[1]

[1] "Cholera—General Information," Centers for Disease Control and Prevention (CDC), September 30, 2022. Available online. URL: www.cdc.gov/cholera/general/index.html#one. Accessed June 27, 2023.

Chapter 33 | *Clostridium difficile* Infection

WHAT IS *CLOSTRIDIUM DIFFICILE*?

Clostridioides difficile (also known as "*C. diff*" or "*C. difficile*") is a germ (bacterium) that causes diarrhea and colitis (an inflammation of the colon). It is estimated to cause almost half a million infections in the United States each year. About one in six patients who get *C. diff* will get it again in the subsequent two to eight weeks. One in eleven people over age 65 diagnosed with a health-care-associated *C. diff* infection die within one month.

SYMPTOMS OF *CLOSTRIDIUM DIFFICILE*

Symptoms might develop within a few days after you begin taking antibiotics:

- diarrhea
- fever
- stomach tenderness or pain
- loss of appetite
- nausea

What If You Have Symptoms?

If you have been taking antibiotics recently and have symptoms of *C. diff*, you should see a health-care professional.

- Developing diarrhea is fairly common while on or after taking antibiotics, but in only a few cases will that diarrhea be caused by *C. diff*. If your diarrhea is severe, do not delay getting medical care.

- Your health-care professional will review your symptoms and order a lab test of a stool (poop) sample.
- If the test is positive, you will take a specific antibiotic (e.g., vancomycin or fidaxomicin) for at least 10 days. If you were already taking an antibiotic for another infection, your health-care professional might ask you to stop taking it if they think it is safe to do so.
- Your health-care team might decide to admit you to the hospital, in which case they will use certain precautions, such as wearing gowns and gloves, to prevent the spread of *C. diff* to themselves and to other patients.

YOUR RISK FOR *CLOSTRIDIUM DIFFICILE*

Clostridioides difficle bacteria are commonly found in the environment, but most cases of *C. diff* occur while you are taking antibiotics or not long after you have finished taking antibiotics. People are 7–10 times more likely to get *C. diff* while on antibiotics and during the month after.

That is because antibiotics that fight bacterial infections by killing bad germs can also get rid of the good germs that protect the body against harmful infections, such as *C. diff* infection. If you take antibiotics for more than a week, you could be even more at risk. Other *C. diff* risk factors include the following:

- older age (65 and older)
- recent stay at a hospital or nursing home
- a weakened immune system, such as people with human immunodeficiency virus/acquired immunodeficiency syndrome (HIV/AIDS), cancer, or organ transplant patients taking immunosuppressive drugs
- previous infection with *C. diff* or known exposure to the germs

You can still get *C. diff* even if you have none of these risk factors.

WHAT ARE THE COMPLICATIONS OF *CLOSTRIDIUM DIFFICILE*?

Common complications of *C. diff* are as follows:

- dehydration
- inflammation of the colon, known as "colitis"
- diarrhea

Rare complications of *C. diff* are as follows:

- serious intestinal conditions, such as toxic megacolon
- sepsis, the body's extreme response to an infection
- death

PREVENTING THE SPREAD OF *CLOSTRIDIUM DIFFICILE*

Information for Patients

C. diff germs are carried from person to person in poop. If someone with *C. diff* (or caring for someone with *C. diff*) does not clean their hands with soap and water after using the bathroom, they can spread the germs to people and things they touch. *C. diff* can also live on people's skin. People who touch an infected person's skin can pick up the germs on their hands. Taking a shower with soap and water can reduce the *C. diff* on your skin and lessen the chance of it spreading.

C. diff germs are so small relative to our size that if you were the size of the state of California, a germ would be the size of a baseball home plate. There is no way you can see *C. diff* germs on your hands, but that does not mean they are not there. Washing with soap and water is the best way to prevent the spread from person to person.

Remember: You can come in contact with *C. diff* germs—and even carry them on or in your body—and not get sick. But that does not mean you cannot spread the germs to others.

How Do You Kill *Clostridium difficile* Germs at Home?

Finding *C. diff* germs in the home is not unusual, even when no one in the home has been ill with *C. diff*. Most healthy adults who come in contact with *C. diff* in the home will not get sick. Hospitals use special cleaning products to kill *C. diff*, but you can make a cleaner at home. Mix one part bleach to nine parts water.

SURFACES

Focus on regularly cleaning items that are touched by hands. These include but are not limited to:

- doorknobs
- electronics (be careful because bleach can damage many electronics and plastics)
- refrigerator handles
- shared cups
- toilet flushers and toilet seats

LAUNDRY

If someone in your house has *C. diff*, wash items they touch before others use them. These include but are not limited to:

- bed linens
- towels
- household linens
- clothing, especially underwear

If these items have visible poop, rinse them well before washing. Then launder in a washer and dryer using the hottest water that is safe for those items. Use chlorine bleach if the items can be safely washed with it. Consider wearing gloves when handling dirty laundry and always wash your hands with soap and water after, even if you use gloves.

It is agreeable to take clothes to a dry cleaner that were worn by a patient infected with *C. diff*. However, dry cleaning is not as effective as other methods at killing the spores. Therefore, this option should be used only for clothes that cannot be machine washed.

LIFE AFTER *CLOSTRIDIUM DIFFICILE*

When Can You Go Back to Work? When Can Your Children Go Back to School?

You and your children should return to work or school only when your symptoms have stopped.

After Treatment, Can You Be Tested Again to Make Sure You Are Cured?

No, because once you recover from your *C. diff* infection, you could still be carrying the germs. A test would only show the germs are still there, but not whether you are likely to become sick again.

How Can You Avoid Getting *Clostridium difficile* Again?

The following are the best ways to be sure you do not get *C. diff* again:

- Work with your health-care professional to avoid taking unnecessary antibiotics.
- Tell your health-care professional if you have had a *C. diff* infection. This important information will help them make the best decisions when prescribing antibiotics in the future.
- Wash your hands with soap and water every time you use the bathroom and before you eat anything.[1]

[1] "*C. diff* (*Clostridioides difficile*)," Centers for Disease Control and Prevention (CDC), July 12, 2021. Available online. URL: www.cdc.gov/cdiff. Accessed June 29, 2023.

Chapter 34 | Diphtheria

WHAT IS DIPHTHERIA?

Diphtheria is a serious bacterial infection. You can catch it from a person who has the infection and coughs or sneezes. You can also get infected by coming in contact with an object, such as a toy, that has bacteria on it. Diphtheria usually affects the nose and throat.

Your doctor will diagnose it based on your signs and symptoms and a lab test. Getting treatment for diphtheria quickly is important. If your doctor suspects that you have it, you will start treatment before the lab tests come back. Treatment is with antibiotics.

Diphtheria, pertussis, and tetanus vaccines can prevent diphtheria, but their protection does not last forever. Children need another dose, or booster, at about age 12. Then, as adults, they should get a booster every 10 years. Diphtheria is very rare in the United States because of the vaccine.[1]

CAUSES OF DIPHTHERIA

Diphtheria is a serious infection caused by strains of bacteria called "*Corynebacterium diphtheriae*" that make a toxin. It is a toxin that can cause people to get very sick.

SIGNS AND SYMPTOMS OF DIPHTHERIA

Symptoms of diphtheria depend on the body part that is affected. People who are exposed to diphtheria usually start having symptoms in two to five days if they get sick. If a doctor thinks you have respiratory diphtheria, they will have you start treatment right away.

---

[1] MedlinePlus, "Diphtheria," National Institutes of Health (NIH), April 4, 2016. Available online. URL: https://medlineplus.gov/diphtheria.html. Accessed June 29, 2023.

Respiratory Diphtheria

The bacteria most commonly infect the respiratory system, which includes parts of the body involved in breathing. When the bacteria get into and attach to the lining of the respiratory system, it can cause:

- weakness
- sore throat
- mild fever
- swollen glands in the neck

The bacteria make a toxin that kills healthy tissues in the respiratory system. Within two to three days, the dead tissue forms a thick, gray coating that can build up in the throat or nose. Medical experts call this thick, gray coating a "pseudomembrane." It can cover tissues in the nose, tonsils, voice box, and throat, making it very hard to breathe and swallow. If the toxin gets into the bloodstream, it can cause heart, nerve, and kidney damage.

Diphtheria Skin Infection

The bacteria can also infect the skin, causing open sores or ulcers. However, diphtheria skin infections rarely result in severe disease.

HOW IT SPREADS

Diphtheria bacteria spread from person to person, usually through respiratory droplets, such as from coughing or sneezing. People can also get sick from touching infected open sores or ulcers. Those at increased risk of getting sick include the following:

- people in the same household
- people with a history of frequent, close contact with the patient
- people directly exposed to secretions from the suspected infection site (e.g., mouth and skin) of the patient

COMPLICATIONS OF DIPHTHERIA

Complications from respiratory diphtheria may include the following:

- airway blockage
- myocarditis (damage to the heart muscle)

- polyneuropathy (nerve damage)
- kidney failure

For some people, respiratory diphtheria can lead to death. Even with treatment, about 1 in 10 patients with respiratory diphtheria will die. Without treatment, up to half of patients can die from the disease.

DIAGNOSIS FOR DIPHTHERIA

Diphtheria can infect the respiratory tract (parts of the body involved in breathing) and skin. Diagnosis and treatment depend on the type of diphtheria someone has. If a doctor thinks you have respiratory diphtheria, they will have you start treatment right away.

Doctors usually decide if a person has diphtheria by looking for common signs and symptoms. They can swab the back of the throat or nose and test it for the bacteria that cause diphtheria. A doctor can also take a sample from an open sore or ulcer and try to grow the bacteria. If the bacteria grow and make the diphtheria toxin (refer to Figure 34.1), the doctor can be sure a patient has diphtheria. However, it takes time to grow the bacteria, so it is important to start treatment right away if a doctor suspects respiratory diphtheria.

TREATMENT FOR DIPHTHERIA

The following methods are involved in diphtheria treatment:

- **Using diphtheria antitoxin to stop the bacteria toxin from damaging the body**. This treatment is very important for respiratory diphtheria infections, but it is rarely used for diphtheria skin infections.
- **Using antibiotics to kill and get rid of the bacteria**. This is important for diphtheria infections in the respiratory system and on the skin and other parts of the body (e.g., eyes and blood).

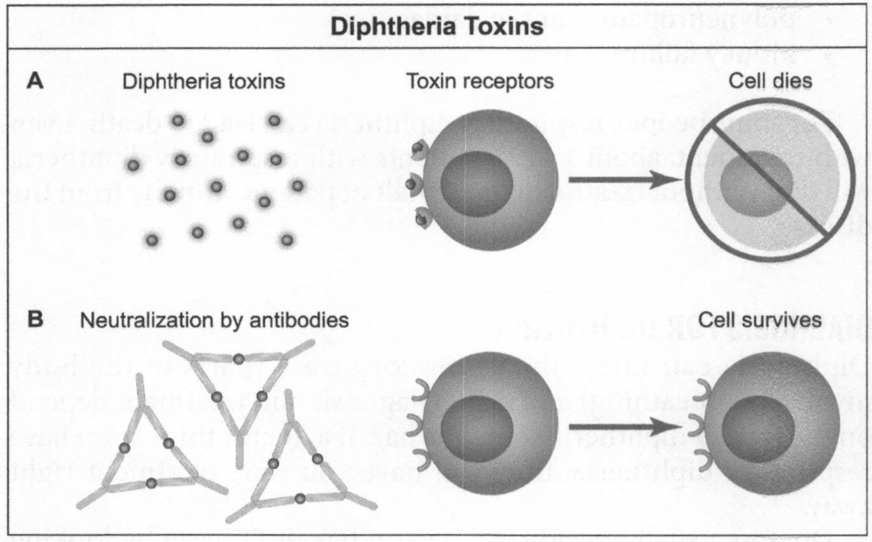

Figure 34.1. Diphtheria Toxins

Infobase

People with diphtheria are usually no longer able to infect others 48 hours after they begin taking antibiotics. However, it is important to finish taking the full course of antibiotics to make sure the bacteria are completely removed from the body. After the patient finishes the full treatment, the doctor will run tests to make sure the bacteria are not in the patient's body anymore.

PREVENTION OF DIPHTHERIA

Keeping up-to-date with recommended vaccines is the best protection against diphtheria.

Vaccination

In the United States, there are four vaccines used to prevent diphtheria: diphtheria, tetanus, and acellular pertussis (DTaP), tetanus, diphtheria, and acellular pertussis (Tdap), diphtheria and tetanus (DT), and tetanus and diphtheria (Td) vaccines. Each of these vaccines prevents diphtheria and tetanus; DTaP and Tdap also help prevent pertussis (whooping cough).

Antibiotics and Other Preventive Measures

The Centers for Disease Control and Prevention (CDC) recommends that close contacts* of someone with diphtheria receive antibiotics to prevent them from getting sick. Experts call this prophylaxis. In addition to getting antibiotics, close contact with someone with diphtheria should be:

- monitored for possible illness for 7–10 days from the time they were last exposed
- tested for diphtheria with a sample collected from the nose and throat
- given a diphtheria booster shot if they are not up-to-date with their vaccines

Health departments investigate each case of diphtheria to identify all close contacts and make sure they receive the right preventive measures.

**Close contacts are defined as all household members, people with a history of frequent and close contact with the patient, or people directly exposed to secretions from the suspected infection site of the patient.*[2]

[2] "About Diphtheria," Centers for Disease Control and Prevention (CDC), September 9, 2022. Available online. URL: www.cdc.gov/diphtheria/about/index.html. Accessed June 29, 2023.

Chapter 35 | *Haemophilus influenzae* Infections

WHAT IS *HAEMOPHILUS INFLUENZAE* DISEASE?

Haemophilus influenzae disease is a name for any infection caused by bacteria called "*H. influenzae*."

TYPES OF *HAEMOPHILUS INFLUENZAE* INFECTIONS

Haemophilus influenzae, a type of bacteria, can cause many different kinds of infections. These infections range from mild, such as ear infections, to serious, such as bloodstream infections.

Doctors consider some *H. influenzae* infections "invasive." Invasive disease happens when bacteria invade parts of the body that are normally free from germs. For example, *H. influenzae* can invade the fluid around the spine and brain, causing meningitis or bloodstream and causing bacteremia. Invasive disease is usually serious, requiring treatment in a hospital, and can sometimes result in death. The most common types of invasive disease caused by *H. influenzae* are as follows:

- pneumonia* (lung infection)
- bloodstream infection
- meningitis (swelling of the lining of the brain and spinal cord)
- epiglottitis (swelling in the throat)
- cellulitis (skin infection)
- infectious arthritis (inflammation of the joint)

H. influenzae can also be a common cause of ear infections in children and bronchitis in adults.

**Doctors consider pneumonia an invasive infection when* H. influenzae *also infects the blood or fluid surrounding the lungs.*

CAUSES OF *HAEMOPHILUS INFLUENZAE* DISEASE

Haemophilus influenzae disease is a name for any infection caused by bacteria called "*H. influenzae*." There are six distinct types of *H. influenzae* (named a through f), as well as other *H. influenzae* that are classified as non-typeable. The one that people are most familiar with is *H. influenzae* type b (Hib).

These bacteria live in a person's nose and throat and usually cause no harm. However, the bacteria can sometimes move to other parts of the body and cause infection.

Experts do not know how long it takes after *H. influenzae* enters a person's body for someone to get sick. However, it could take as little as a few days before symptoms appear.

SIGNS AND SYMPTOMS OF *HAEMOPHILUS INFLUENZAE*

Haemophilus influenzae can cause many different kinds of infections. Symptoms depend on the part of the body that is infected.

Pneumonia

Symptoms of pneumonia usually include the following:

- fever and chills
- cough
- shortness of breath or difficulty breathing
- sweating
- chest pain
- headache
- muscle pain or aches
- excessive tiredness

Bloodstream Infection

Symptoms of bloodstream infection usually include the following:

- fever and chills
- excessive tiredness
- pain in the belly

- nausea with or without vomiting
- diarrhea
- anxiety
- shortness of breath or difficulty breathing
- altered mental status (confusion)

A bloodstream infection from *H. influenzae* can occur with or without pneumonia.

Meningitis

Symptoms of meningitis typically include the following:

- fever
- headache
- stiff neck
- nausea with or without vomiting
- photophobia (eyes being more sensitive to light)
- altered mental status (confusion)

Babies with meningitis may:

- be irritable
- vomit
- feed poorly
- appear to be slow or inactive
- have abnormal reflexes

COMPLICATIONS OF *HAEMOPHILUS INFLUENZAE*

Even with appropriate treatment, some *H. influenzae* infections can result in long-term problems or death. For example, bloodstream infections can result in loss of limbs. Meningitis can cause brain damage or hearing loss.

Complications are rare and typically not severe for bronchitis and ear infections caused by *H. influenza*.

HOW IT SPREADS

People spread *H. influenzae*, including Hib, to others through respiratory droplets. People who are infected spread the bacteria by coughing or sneezing, which creates small respiratory droplets that contain the bacteria. Other people can get sick if they breathe in those droplets. People who are not sick but have the bacteria in their noses and throats can still spread the bacteria. That is how *H. influenzae* spreads most of the time. The bacteria can also spread to people who have close or lengthy contact with a person with *H. influenzae* disease.

PEOPLE AT INCREASED RISK

Haemophilus influenzae, including Hib, disease occurs mostly in children younger than age 5 and adults aged 65 or older. American-Indian people, Alaska Native people, and people with certain medical conditions are also at increased risk. Those medical conditions include the following:

- sickle cell disease
- asplenia (no spleen)
- human immunodeficiency virus (HIV) infection
- antibody and complement deficiency syndromes (rare conditions that affect the body's ability to fight infections)
- cancer requiring treatment with chemotherapy, radiation therapy, or bone marrow stem cell transplant

DIAGNOSIS OF *HAEMOPHILUS INFLUENZAE*

Doctors usually diagnose *H. influenzae* infection with one or more laboratory tests. The most common testing methods use a sample of blood or spinal fluid.

TREATMENT OF *HAEMOPHILUS INFLUENZAE*

People diagnosed with *H. influenzae* disease take antibiotics to treat the infection. Depending on how serious the infection is, people with *H. influenzae* disease may need care in a hospital. Other treatments may include the following:

- breathing support
- medication to treat low blood pressure
- wound care for parts of the body with damaged skin

When *H. influenzae* causes milder infections, such as bronchitis or ear infections, doctors may give antibiotics to prevent complications.

PREVENTION OF *HAEMOPHILUS INFLUENZAE*

Staying up-to-date with recommended vaccines and maintaining healthy habits, such as washing hands often and not having close contact with people who are sick, help prevent disease caused by *H. influenzae.*

Vaccine

Vaccines can prevent Hib disease. However, the Hib vaccine does not prevent disease caused by the other types of *H. influenzae.*

Reinfection

People can get *H. influenzae* more than once. A previous Hib infection might not protect you from future infection. Therefore, the Centers for Disease Control and Prevention (CDC) recommends Hib vaccination even if someone has had Hib disease in the past.

Preventive Antibiotics

H. influenzae can spread to people who have close or lengthy contact with a person with *H. influenzae* disease. In certain cases, close contacts of someone with *H. influenzae* disease should receive antibiotics to prevent them from getting sick. A doctor or local health department will make recommendations for who should receive preventive antibiotics.[1]

[1] "About *Haemophilus influenzae* Disease," Centers for Disease Control and Prevention (CDC), March 4, 2022. Available online. URL: www.cdc.gov/hi-disease/about/index.html. Accessed June 29, 2023.

Chapter 36 | **Hansen Disease**

WHAT IS HANSEN DISEASE?

Hansen disease (also known as "leprosy") is an infection caused by bacteria called "*Mycobacterium leprae*." These bacteria grow very slowly and may take up to 20 years to develop signs of the infection.

The disease can affect the nerves, skin, eyes, and lining of the nose (nasal mucosa). The bacteria attack the nerves, which can become swollen under the skin. This can cause the affected areas to lose the ability to sense touch and pain, which can lead to injuries such as cuts and burns. Usually, the affected skin changes color and becomes:

- lighter or darker, often dry or flaky, with a loss of feeling
- reddish due to inflammation of the skin

Early diagnosis and treatment usually prevent disability that can result from the disease, and people with Hansen disease can continue to work and lead an active life. Once treatment is started, the person is no longer contagious. However, it is very important to finish the entire course of treatment as directed by the doctor.

Each year, about 150 people in the United States and 250,000 around the world get the illness. In the past, Hansen disease was feared as a highly contagious, devastating disease, but now we know that it is hard to spread, and it is easily treatable once recognized. Still, a lot of stigma and prejudice remains about the disease, and those suffering from it are isolated and discriminated against in many places where the disease is seen. Continued commitment to fighting the stigma through education and improving access to treatment will lead to a world free of this completely treatable disease.

SIGNS AND SYMPTOMS OF HANSEN DISEASE

Symptoms mainly affect the skin, nerves, and mucous membranes (the soft, moist areas just inside the body's openings). The following are the symptoms caused by the disease on the skin:

- discolored patches of skin, usually flat that may be numb and look faded (lighter than the skin around)
- growths (nodules) on the skin
- thick, stiff, or dry skin
- painless ulcers on the soles of feet
- painless swelling or lumps on the face or earlobes
- loss of eyebrows or eyelashes

The following are the symptoms caused by damage to the nerves:

- numbness of affected areas of the skin
- muscle weakness or paralysis (especially in the hands and feet)
- enlarged nerves (especially those around the elbow and knee and in the sides of the neck)
- eye problems that may lead to blindness (when facial nerves are affected)

The following are the symptoms caused by the disease in the mucous membranes:

- a stuffy nose
- nosebleeds

Since Hansen disease affects the nerves, loss of feeling or sensation can occur. When loss of sensation occurs, injuries such as burns may go unnoticed. Because you may not feel the pain that can warn you of harm to your body, take extra caution to ensure the affected parts of your body are not injured. If left untreated, the signs of advanced leprosy can include the following:

- paralysis and crippling of hands and feet
- shortening of toes and fingers due to reabsorption

- chronic nonhealing ulcers on the bottoms of the feet
- blindness
- loss of eyebrows
- nose disfigurement

The following are other complications that may sometimes occur:

- painful or tender nerves
- redness and pain around the affected area
- burning sensation in the skin

TRANSMISSION OF HANSEN DISEASE

How Do People Get Hansen Disease?

It is not known exactly how Hansen disease spreads between people. Scientists currently think it may happen when a person with Hansen disease coughs or sneezes and a healthy person breathes in the droplets containing the bacteria. Prolonged, close contact with someone with untreated leprosy over many months is needed to catch the disease. You cannot get leprosy from casual contact with a person who has Hansen disease, such as:

- shaking hands or hugging
- sitting next to each other on the bus
- sitting together at a meal

Hansen disease is also not passed on from a mother to her unborn baby during pregnancy, and it is also not spread through sexual contact.

Due to the slow-growing nature of the bacteria and the long time it takes to develop signs of the disease, it is often very difficult to find the source of infection.

In the southern United States, some armadillos are naturally infected with the bacteria that cause Hansen disease in people, and it may be possible that they can spread it to people. However, the risk is very low, and most people who come into contact with armadillos are unlikely to get Hansen disease.

For general health reasons, avoid contact with armadillos whenever possible. If you had contact with an armadillo and are worried about getting Hansen disease, talk to your health-care provider. Your doctor will follow up with you over time and perform periodic skin examinations to see if you develop the disease. In the unlikely event that you have Hansen disease, your doctor can help you get treatment.

Who Is at Risk?

In the United States, Hansen disease is rare. Around the world, as many as 2 million people are permanently disabled as a result of Hansen disease.

Overall, the risk of getting Hansen disease for any adult around the world is very low. That is because more than 95 percent of all people have natural immunity to the disease.

You may be at risk for the disease if you live in a country where the disease is widespread. Countries that reported more than 1,000 new cases of Hansen disease to the World Health Organization (WHO) between 2011 and 2015 are as follows:

- **Africa**. Democratic Republic of Congo, Ethiopia, Madagascar, Mozambique, Nigeria, and the United Republic of Tanzania.
- **Asia**. Bangladesh, India, Indonesia, Myanmar, Nepal, Philippines, and Sri Lanka.
- **Americas**. Brazil.

You may also be at risk if you are in prolonged close contact with people who have untreated Hansen disease. If they have not been treated, you could get the bacteria that cause Hansen disease. However, as soon as patients start treatment, they are no longer able to spread the disease.

DIAGNOSIS OF HANSEN DISEASE

Hansen disease can be recognized by the appearance of patches of skin that may look lighter or darker than normal skin. Sometimes, the affected skin areas may be reddish. Loss of feeling in these skin patches is common. You may not feel a light touch or a prick with a needle.

To confirm the diagnosis, your doctor will take a sample of your skin or nerve (through a skin or nerve biopsy) to look for the bacteria under the microscope and may also do tests to rule out other skin diseases.

TREATMENT OF HANSEN DISEASE

Hansen disease is treated with a combination of antibiotics. Typically, two or three antibiotics are used at the same time. These are dapsone with rifampicin, and clofazimine is added for some types of the disease. This is called "multidrug therapy." This strategy helps prevent the development of antibiotic resistance by the bacteria, which may otherwise occur due to the length of the treatment.

Treatment usually lasts between one and two years. The illness can be cured if treatment is completed as prescribed. If you are treated for Hansen disease, it is important to do the following:

- Tell your doctor if you experience numbness or a loss of feeling in certain parts of the body or in patches on the skin. This may be caused by nerve damage from the infection. If you have numbness and loss of feeling, take extra care to prevent injuries that may occur, such as burns and cuts.
- Take the antibiotics until your doctor says your treatment is complete. If you stop earlier, the bacteria may start growing again, and you may get sick again.
- Tell your doctor if the affected skin patches become red and painful, nerves become painful or swollen, or you develop a fever, as these may be complications of Hansen disease that may require more intensive treatment with medicines that can reduce inflammation.

If left untreated, the nerve damage can result in paralysis and crippling of hands and feet. In very advanced cases, the person may have multiple injuries due to lack of sensation, and eventually, the body may reabsorb the affected digits over time, resulting in the apparent loss of toes and fingers. Corneal ulcers or blindness can also occur if facial nerves are affected due to loss of sensation of the cornea (outside) of the eye. Other signs of advanced leprosy may include loss of eyebrows and saddlenose deformity resulting from damage to the nasal septum.

Antibiotics used during the treatment will kill the bacteria that cause leprosy. But, while the treatment can cure the disease and prevent it from getting worse, it does not reverse nerve damage or physical disfiguration that may have occurred before the diagnosis. Thus, it is very important that the disease be diagnosed as early as possible before any permanent nerve damage occurs.[1]

[1] "What Is Hansen's Disease?" Centers for Disease Control and Prevention (CDC), February 10, 2017. Available online. URL: www.cdc.gov/leprosy/about/about.html. Accessed June 29, 2023.

Chapter 37 | Methicillin-Resistant *Staphylococcus aureus* Infection

WHAT IS METHICILLIN-RESISTANT *STAPHYLOCOCCUS AUREUS*?

Methicillin-resistant *Staphylococcus aureus* (MRSA) is a type of bacteria that is resistant to several antibiotics.

Outside Health-Care Settings

In the community (where you live, work, shop, and go to school), MRSA most often causes skin infections. In some cases, it causes pneumonia (lung infection) and other infections. If left untreated, MRSA infections can become severe and cause sepsis—the body's extreme response to an infection.

In Health-Care Settings

In places such as a hospital or nursing home, MRSA can cause severe problems such as:

- bloodstream infections
- pneumonia
- surgical site infections

WHO IS AT RISK?

Anyone can get MRSA. The risk increases with activities or places that involve crowding, skin-to-skin contact, and shared equipment or supplies. Some of the people who carry MRSA can go on to get an MRSA infection. Non-intact skin, such as when there are abrasions or incisions, is often the site of an MRSA infection. Athletes, day care and school students, military personnel in barracks, and those who receive inpatient medical care or have surgery or medical devices inserted in their bodies are at higher risk of MRSA infection.

HOW COMMON IS METHICILLIN-RESISTANT *STAPHYLOCOCCUS AUREUS*?

Approximately 5 percent of patients in U.S. hospitals carry MRSA in their noses or on their skin.

SYMPTOMS OF METHICILLIN-RESISTANT *STAPHYLOCOCCUS AUREUS* INFECTION

The symptoms of an MRSA infection depend on the part of the body that is infected. For example, people with MRSA skin infections often can get swelling, warmth, redness, and pain in infected skin. In most cases, it is hard to tell if an infection is due to MRSA or another type of bacteria without laboratory tests that your doctor can order. Some MRSA skin infections can have a fairly typical appearance and can be confused with a spider bite. However, unless you actually see the spider, the irritation is likely not a spider bite. Most *S. aureus* skin infections, including MRSA, appear as a bump or infected area on the skin that might be:

- red
- swollen
- painful
- warm to the touch
- full of pus or other drainage
- accompanied by a fever

WHAT SHOULD YOU DO IF YOU SEE THESE SYMPTOMS?

You cannot tell by looking at the skin if it is a staph infection (including MRSA). Getting medical care early makes it less likely that the infection will become serious. If you or someone in your family experiences the signs and symptoms of MRSA, you may have to do the following:

- Contact your health-care provider, especially if the symptoms are accompanied by a fever.
- Do not pick at or pop the sore.
- Cover the area with clean, dry bandages until you can see a health-care provider.
- Clean your hands often.

HOW IS METHICILLIN-RESISTANT *STAPHYLOCOCCUS AUREUS* SPREAD?

Methicillin-resistant *S. aureus* is usually spread in the community by contact with infected people or things that are carrying the bacteria. This includes contact with a contaminated wound or by sharing personal items, such as towels or razors, that have touched infected skin.

The opioid epidemic may also be connected to the rise of staph infections in communities. People who inject drugs are 16 times more likely to develop a serious staph infection.

HOW DO YOU PREVENT THE SPREAD OF METHICILLIN-RESISTANT *STAPHYLOCOCCUS AUREUS* INFECTION?

- Cover your wounds with clean, dry bandages until healed. Follow your health-care provider's instructions about proper care of the wound. Pus from infected wounds can contain MRSA.
- Do not pick at or pop a sore.
- Throw away bandages and tape with the regular trash.
- Clean your hands often. You, your family, and others in close contact should wash your hands often with soap and water or use an alcohol-based hand rub, especially:
    - after changing a bandage
    - after touching an infected wound
    - after touching dirty clothes

- Do not share personal items such as towels, washcloths, razors, and clothing, including uniforms.
- Wash laundry before use by others and clean your hands after touching dirty clothes.[1]

[1] "Methicillin-Resistant *Staphylococcus aureus* (MRSA)," Centers for Disease Control and Prevention (CDC), June 26, 2019. Available online. URL: www.cdc.gov/mrsa/community/index.html. Accessed July 3, 2023.

Chapter 38 | Pneumonia

WHAT IS PNEUMONIA?

Pneumonia is an infection that affects one or both lungs. It causes the air sacs, or alveoli, of the lungs to fill up with fluid or pus. Bacteria, viruses, or fungi may cause pneumonia. Symptoms can range from mild to serious and may include a cough with or without mucus (a slimy substance), fever, chills, and trouble breathing. How serious your pneumonia is depends on your age, your overall health, and what caused your infection.

To diagnose pneumonia, your health-care provider will review your medical history, perform a physical exam, and order diagnostic tests such as a chest x-ray. This information can help determine what type of pneumonia you have.

Treatment for pneumonia may include antibiotic, viral, or fungal medicines. It may take several weeks to recover from pneumonia. If your symptoms get worse, you should see a health-care provider right away. If you have severe pneumonia, you may need to go to the hospital for antibiotics given through an intravenous (IV) line and oxygen therapy. Some types of pneumonia can be prevented by vaccines. Good hygiene and heart-healthy living can also lower your risk for pneumonia.

CAUSES AND RISK FACTORS OF PNEUMONIA

Most of the time, your body filters germs out of the air that you breathe. Sometimes, germs, such as bacteria, viruses, or fungi, get into your lungs and cause infections.

When these germs get into your lungs, your immune system, which is your body's natural defense against germs, goes into action. Immune cells attack the germs and may cause inflammation of your air sacs, or alveoli. Inflammation can cause your air sacs to fill up with fluid and pus and cause pneumonia symptoms.

Causes of Pneumonia

BACTERIA

Bacteria are a common cause of pneumonia in adults. Many types of bacteria can cause pneumonia, but *Streptococcus pneumoniae* (also called "pneumococcus bacteria") is the most common cause in the United States.

Some bacteria cause pneumonia with different symptoms or other characteristics than the usual pneumonia. This infection is called "atypical pneumonia." For example, *Mycoplasma pneumoniae* causes a mild form of pneumonia, often called "walking pneumonia." *Legionella pneumophila* causes a severe type of pneumonia called "Legionnaires' disease." Bacterial pneumonia can develop on its own or after you have a cold or the flu.

VIRUSES

Viruses that infect your lungs and airways can cause pneumonia. The flu (influenza virus) and the common cold (rhinovirus) are the most common causes of viral pneumonia in adults. Respiratory syncytial virus (RSV) is the most common cause of viral pneumonia in young children.

Many other viruses can cause pneumonia, including severe acute respiratory syndrome coronavirus 2 (SARS-CoV-2), the virus that causes coronavirus disease (COVID-19).

FUNGI

Fungi such as *Pneumocystis jirovecii* may cause pneumonia, especially for people who have weakened immune systems. Some fungi found in the soil in the southwestern United States and in the Ohio and Mississippi River valleys can also cause pneumonia.

Risk Factors of Pneumonia

Your risk for pneumonia may be higher because of your age, environment, lifestyle habits, and other medical conditions.

AGE

Pneumonia can affect people of all ages. However, the following two age groups are at higher risk of developing pneumonia and having more serious pneumonia:

- **Babies and children aged two or younger.** This age group is at higher risk because their immune systems are still developing. This risk is higher for premature babies.
- **Older adults aged 65 or older**. This age group is also at higher risk because their immune systems generally weaken as people age. Older adults are also more likely to have other chronic (long-term) health conditions that raise the risk of pneumonia.

Babies, children, and older adults who do not get the recommended vaccines to prevent pneumonia have an even higher risk.

ENVIRONMENT OR OCCUPATION

Most people get pneumonia when they catch an infection from someone else in their community. Your chance of getting pneumonia is higher if you live or spend a lot of time in crowded places, such as military barracks, prisons, homeless shelters, or nursing homes. Your risk is also higher if you regularly breathe in air pollution or toxic fumes.

Some germs that cause pneumonia can infect birds and other animals. You are most likely to encounter these germs if you work in a chicken or turkey processing center, pet shop, or veterinary clinic.

LIFESTYLE HABITS

- **Smoking cigarettes**. This habit can make you less able to clear mucus from your airways.
- **Using drugs or alcohol**. This habit can weaken your immune system. You are also more likely to accidentally breathe in saliva or vomit into your windpipe if you are sedated or unconscious from an overdose.

OTHER MEDICAL CONDITIONS

You may have an increased risk of pneumonia if you have any of the following medical conditions:

- Brain disorders, such as a stroke, a head injury, dementia, or Parkinson disease (PD), can affect your ability to cough or swallow. This can lead to food, drink, vomit, or saliva going down your windpipe instead of your esophagus and getting into your lungs.
- Conditions that weaken your immune system may also increase your risk. These include pregnancy, human immunodeficiency virus (HIV)/acquired immunodeficiency syndrome (AIDS), or an organ or bone marrow transplant. Chemotherapy, which is used to treat cancer, and long-term use of steroid medicines can also weaken your immune system.
- Critical diseases that require hospitalization, including receiving treatment in a hospital intensive care unit (ICU), can raise your risk of hospital-acquired pneumonia. Your risk is higher if you cannot move around much or are sedated or unconscious. Using a ventilator raises the risk of a type called "ventilator-associated pneumonia."
- Lung diseases, such as asthma, bronchiectasis, cystic fibrosis, or chronic obstructive pulmonary disease (COPD), also increase your pneumonia risk.
- Other serious conditions, such as malnutrition, diabetes, heart failure, sickle cell disease (SCD), or liver or kidney disease, are additional risk factors.

SYMPTOMS OF PNEUMONIA

The symptoms of pneumonia can be mild or serious. Young children, older adults, and people who have serious health conditions are at risk for developing more serious pneumonia or life-threatening complications. The symptoms of pneumonia may include the following:

- chest pain when you breathe or cough
- chills

- cough with or without mucus
- fever
- low oxygen levels in your blood, measured with a pulse oximeter
- shortness of breath

You may also have other symptoms, including a headache, muscle pain, extreme tiredness, nausea (feeling sick to your stomach), vomiting, and diarrhea.

Older adults and people who have serious illnesses or weakened immune systems may not have the typical symptoms. They may have a lower-than-normal temperature instead of a fever. Older adults who have pneumonia may feel weak or suddenly confused. Sometimes, babies do not have typical symptoms either. They may vomit, have a fever or cough, or appear restless or tired and without energy. Babies may also show the following signs of breathing problems:

- bluish tone to the skin and lips
- grunting
- pulling inward of the muscles between the ribs when breathing
- rapid breathing
- widening of the nostrils with each breath

DIAGNOSIS OF PNEUMONIA

Your health-care provider will diagnose pneumonia based on your medical history, a physical exam, and test results. Sometimes, pneumonia is hard to diagnose because your symptoms may be the same as a cold or flu. You may not realize that your condition is more serious until it lasts longer than these other conditions.

Medical History and Physical Exam

Your provider will ask about your symptoms and when they began. They will also ask whether you have any risk factors for pneumonia. You may also be asked about:

- exposure to sick people at home, school, or work or in a hospital

- flu or pneumonia vaccinations
- medicines you take
- past and current medical conditions and whether any have gotten worse recently
- recent travel
- exposure to birds and other animals
- smoking

During your physical exam, your provider will check your temperature and listen to your lungs with a stethoscope.

Diagnostic Tests and Procedures

If your provider thinks you have pneumonia, he or she may do one or more of the following tests:

- **Chest x-ray**. This looks for inflammation in your lungs. A chest x-ray is often used to diagnose pneumonia.
- **Blood tests**. These tests, such as a complete blood count (CBC), see whether your immune system is fighting an infection.
- **Pulse oximetry**. This measures how much oxygen is in your blood. Pneumonia can keep your lungs from getting enough oxygen into your blood. To measure the levels, a small sensor called a "pulse oximeter" is attached to your finger or ear.

If you are in the hospital, have serious symptoms, are older, or have other health problems, your provider may do the following other tests to diagnose pneumonia:

- **Blood gas test**. This test may be done if you are very sick. For this test, your provider measures your blood oxygen levels using a blood sample from an artery, usually in your wrist. This is called an "arterial blood gas" (ABG) test.
- **Sputum test**. This test that uses a sample of sputum (spit) or mucus from your cough may be used to find out what germ is causing your pneumonia.

- **Blood culture test**. This test can identify the germ causing your pneumonia and also show whether a bacterial infection has spread to your blood.
- **Polymerase chain reaction (PCR) test**. This test quickly checks your blood or sputum sample to find the deoxyribonucleic acid (DNA) of germs that cause pneumonia.
- **Bronchoscopy**. This procedure looks inside your airways. If your treatment is not working well, this procedure may be needed. At the same time, your doctor may also collect samples of your lung tissue and fluid from your lungs to find the cause of your pneumonia.
- **Chest computed tomography (CT) scan**. This scan can show how much of your lungs are affected by pneumonia. It can also show whether you have complications such as lung abscesses or pleural disorders. A CT scan shows more detail than a chest x-ray.
- **Thoracentesis**. A pleural fluid culture can be taken using this procedure, which is when a doctor uses a needle to take a sample of fluid from the pleural space between your lungs and chest wall. The fluid is then tested for bacteria.

TREATMENT OF PNEUMONIA

Treatment for pneumonia depends on your risk factors and how serious your pneumonia is. Many people who have pneumonia are prescribed medicine and recover at home. You may need to be treated in the hospital or an ICU if your pneumonia is serious.

Medicines

Your health-care provider may prescribe some of the following medicines to treat your pneumonia at home or at the hospital, depending on how sick you are.

Management at Home

If your pneumonia is mild, your provider may prescribe medicines or suggest over-the-counter (OTC) medicines to treat it at home.

- **Antibiotics**. These medicines may be prescribed for bacterial pneumonia. Most people begin to feel better after one to three days of antibiotic treatment. However, you should take antibiotics as your doctor prescribes. If you stop too soon, your pneumonia may come back.
- **Antiviral medicines**. These medicines are sometimes prescribed for viral pneumonia. However, these medicines do not work against every virus that causes pneumonia.
- **Antifungal medicines**. These medicines are prescribed for fungal pneumonia.
- **OTC medicines**. These medicines may be recommended to treat your fever and muscle pain or help you breathe easier. Talk to your provider before taking a cough or cold medicine.

Management at the Hospital

If your pneumonia is serious, you may be treated in a hospital, so you can get antibiotics and fluids through an IV line inserted into your vein. You may also get oxygen therapy to increase the amount of oxygen in your blood. If your pneumonia is very serious, you may need to be put on a ventilator.

Procedures

You may need a procedure or surgery to remove seriously infected or damaged parts of your lung. This may help you recover and may prevent your pneumonia from coming back.

PREVENTION OF PNEUMONIA

Pneumonia can be very serious and even life-threatening. You can take a few steps to try and prevent it.

Vaccines can help prevent some types of pneumonia. Good hygiene (washing your hands often), quitting smoking, and keeping your immune system strong by getting regular physical activity and eating healthy are other ways to lower your risk of getting pneumonia.

Vaccines

Vaccines can help prevent pneumonia caused by pneumococcus bacteria or the flu virus. Vaccines cannot prevent all cases of pneumonia. However, compared to people who do not get vaccinated, those who are vaccinated and still get pneumonia tend to have:

- fewer serious complications
- milder infections
- pneumonia that does not last as long

PNEUMOCOCCUS VACCINES

Two vaccines are available to prevent infections from the pneumococcus bacteria, the most common type of bacteria that causes pneumonia. Pneumococcus vaccines are especially important for people at high risk of pneumonia, including the following:

- adults aged 65 or older
- children aged two or younger
- people who have chronic (ongoing) diseases, serious long-term health problems, or weak immune systems. This may include people who have cancer, HIV, asthma, SCD, or damaged or removed spleens
- people who smoke

FLU (INFLUENZA) VACCINE

Your yearly flu vaccine can help prevent pneumonia caused by the flu. The flu vaccine is usually given in September through October before flu season starts.

HAEMOPHILUS INFLUENZAE TYPE B VACCINE

Haemophilus influenzae type b (Hib) is a type of bacteria that can cause pneumonia and meningitis. The Hib vaccine is recommended for all children under age five in the United States. The vaccine is often given to infants starting when they are two months old.

Other Ways to Prevent Pneumonia

You can take the following steps to prevent pneumonia:

- Wash your hands with soap and water or alcohol-based hand sanitizers to kill germs.
- Do not smoke. Smoking prevents your lungs from properly filtering out and defending your body against germs.
- Keep your immune system strong. Get plenty of physical activity and follow a healthy eating plan.
- If you have problems swallowing, eat smaller meals of thickened food and sleep with the head of your bed raised up. These steps can help you avoid getting food, drink, or saliva into your lungs.
- If you have a planned surgery, your provider may recommend that you do not eat for eight hours or drink liquids for two hours before your surgery. This can help prevent food or drink from getting into your airway while you are sedated.
- If your immune system is impaired or weakened, your provider may recommend you take antibiotics to prevent bacteria from growing in your lungs.[1]

[1] "What Is Pneumonia?" National Heart, Lung, and Blood Institute (NHLBI), March 24, 2022. Available online. URL: www.nhlbi.nih.gov/health/pneumonia. Accessed July 3, 2023.

Chapter 39 | Salmonellosis

Salmonella are a group of bacteria that can cause gastrointestinal illness and fever called "salmonellosis." *Salmonella* can be spread by food handlers who do not wash their hands and/or the surfaces and tools they use between food preparation steps and when people eat raw or undercooked foods.

Salmonella can also spread from animals to people. People who have direct contact with certain animals, including poultry and reptiles, can spread the bacteria from the animals to food if they do not practice proper handwashing hygiene before handling food. Pets can also spread the bacteria within the home environment if they eat food contaminated with *Salmonella*.

SYMPTOMS OF *SALMONELLA*

Most people infected with *Salmonella* will begin to develop symptoms 12–72 hours after infection. The illness, salmonellosis, usually lasts four to seven days, and most people recover without treatment.

Most people with salmonellosis develop diarrhea, fever, and abdominal cramps. More severe cases of salmonellosis may include a high fever, aches, headaches, lethargy, a rash, and blood in the urine or stool, and in some cases, salmonellosis may become fatal. The U.S. Centers for Disease Control and Prevention (CDC) estimated that approximately 450 persons in the United States die each year from acute salmonellosis.

Due to the range in severity of illness, people should consult their health-care provider if they suspect that they have developed symptoms that resemble a *Salmonella* infection.

AT-RISK GROUPS

Children under age five, the elderly, and people with weakened immune systems are more likely to have severe salmonellosis infections.

FOODS LINKED TO THE U.S. OUTBREAKS OF SALMONELLOSIS

Past U.S. outbreaks of salmonellosis have been associated with meat products, poultry products, raw or undercooked eggs and dough, dairy products, fruits, leafy greens, raw sprouts, fresh vegetables, nut butters and spreads, and pet foods and treats.

PREVENTING FOODBORNE ILLNESS AT HOME

Consumers should follow the following steps:

- Wash the inside walls and shelves of the refrigerator, cutting boards and countertops, and utensils that may have contacted contaminated foods; then sanitize them with a solution of one tablespoon of chlorine bleach to one gallon of hot water; and dry with a clean cloth or paper towel that has not been previously used.
- Wash and sanitize surfaces used to serve or store potentially contaminated products.
- Wash hands with warm water and soap following the cleaning and sanitation process.
- Children, the elderly, pregnant women, and persons with weakened immune systems should avoid eating raw sprouts of any kind.
- People with pets should take special care to avoid cross-contamination when preparing their pet's food. Be sure to pick up and thoroughly wash food dishes as soon as pets are done eating and prevent children, the elderly, and any other people with weak immune systems from handling or being exposed to the food or pets that have eaten potentially contaminated food.
- Consumers can also submit a voluntary report, a complaint, or an adverse event (illness or serious allergic reaction) related to a food product.

ADVICE FOR RESTAURANTS AND RETAILERS

In the event that retailers and/or other food service operators are found to have handled recalled or other potentially contaminated food in their facilities, they should follow the following steps:

- Contact their local health department and communicate to their customers regarding possible exposure to *Salmonella*.
- Wash the inside walls and shelves of the refrigerator, cutting boards and countertops, and utensils that may have contacted contaminated foods; then sanitize them with a solution of one tablespoon of chlorine bleach to one gallon of hot water; and dry with a clean cloth or paper towel that has not been previously used.
- Wash and sanitize display cases and surfaces used to potentially store, serve, or prepare potentially contaminated foods.
- Wash hands with warm water and soap following the cleaning and sanitation process.
- Conduct regular frequent cleaning and sanitizing of cutting boards and utensils used in processing to help minimize the likelihood of cross-contamination.[1]

DIAGNOSIS AND TREATMENT OF *SALMONELLA*

Salmonella infection is diagnosed when a laboratory test detects *Salmonella* bacteria in a person's poop (stool), body tissue, or fluids. Most people recover without specific treatment. Antibiotics are typically used only to treat people with severe illness. Patients should drink extra fluids as long as the diarrhea lasts. In some cases, diarrhea may be so severe that the person needs to be hospitalized.

In rare cases, infection may spread from the intestines to the bloodstream and then to other parts of the body. In these people, *Salmonella* can cause death unless the person is treated promptly with antibiotics.

[1] "*Salmonella* (Salmonellosis)," U.S. Food and Drug Administration (FDA), March 29, 2019. Available online. URL: www.fda.gov/food/foodborne-pathogens/salmonella-salmonellosis. Accessed July 11, 2023.

Diagnostic and Public Health Testing

Diagnosing *Salmonella* infection requires testing a specimen (sample), such as stool (poop) or blood. Testing can help guide treatment decisions.

Following are the steps involved in laboratory testing and reporting *Salmonella* infection:

- Infection is diagnosed when a laboratory test detects *Salmonella* bacteria in stool, body tissue, or fluids. The test could be a culture that isolates the bacteria or a culture-independent diagnostic test (CIDT) that detects the genetic material of the bacteria.
  - The CDC encourages laboratories to culture specimens with positive CIDT results. This process is called "reflex culturing."
- Clinical diagnostic laboratories report the test results to the doctor and submit *Salmonella* isolates to state public health laboratories for serotyping and deoxyribonucleic acid (DNA) fingerprinting.
- Public health laboratories report the results to the CDC's laboratory-based enteric disease surveillance and to PulseNet.
- Public health laboratories forward unusual serotypes to the CDC's National *Salmonella* Reference Laboratory for further characterization or confirmation.

SALMONELLA SEROTYPES

Salmonella are divided into serotypes according to the structures on their surface. Some serotypes are only found in one kind of animal or in a single place. Others are found in many different animals and all over the world. A few serotypes can cause especially severe illnesses; most typically cause milder illnesses.

Serotyping has played an important role for decades in understanding the epidemiologic and molecular characterization of *Salmonella*. Today, modern genetic subtyping methods provide scientists with additional information that is used to determine the serotypes and to identify, investigate, and trace outbreaks.

PULSENET

State public health laboratories routinely subtype *Salmonella* isolates by serotyping and by subtyping based on whole genome sequencing (WGS). The laboratories submit results from WGS to a dynamic database maintained by PulseNet, a national network of public health and food regulatory agency laboratories coordinated by the CDC.

PulseNet includes state health departments, local health departments, agricultural laboratories, and federal agencies (the CDC, the Food Safety and Inspection Service (FSIS) of the U.S. Department of Agriculture (USDA), and the U.S. Food and Drug Administration (FDA)).

PulseNet data are available to participating health departments for comparing WGS profiles. Finding a group of infections with the same or very similar profiles could indicate an outbreak. Finding the same profile in a food could help link illness to a specific food source.

PREVENTION OF *SALMONELLA*

Five Fast Facts

Do not let *Salmonella* make you or your loved ones sick. Take a look at the following five facts and the CDC's tips for lowering your chance of getting a *Salmonella* infection:

- You can get a *Salmonella* infection from a variety of foods. *Salmonella* can be found in many foods, including sprouts and other vegetables, eggs, chicken, pork, fruits, and even processed foods, such as nut butters, frozen pot pies, chicken nuggets, and stuffed chicken entrees. Contaminated foods usually look and smell normal, which is why it is important to know how to prevent infection.
- *Salmonella* can also spread from animals to people and from people to people. Always wash your hands after contact with animals. Also, wash your hands after using the toilet, changing diapers, or helping someone with diarrhea clean up after using the toilet. If you have a

Salmonella infection, you should not prepare food or drinks for others until you no longer have diarrhea.
- *Salmonella* illness is more common in the summer. Warmer weather and unrefrigerated foods create ideal conditions for *Salmonella* to grow. Be sure to refrigerate or freeze perishables (foods likely to spoil or go bad quickly), prepared foods, and leftovers within two hours (or one hour if the temperature outside is 90 °F (32 °C) or hotter).
- *Salmonella* illness can be serious and is more dangerous for certain people. Anyone can get a *Salmonella* infection, but some people are more likely to develop a serious illness, including children under age five, older adults, and people with immune systems weakened from medical conditions, such as diabetes, liver or kidney disease, and cancer or its treatment.
- *Salmonella* causes far more illnesses than you might suspect. For every person with a *Salmonella* illness confirmed by a laboratory test, there are about 30 more people with *Salmonella* illnesses that are not reported. Most people who get food poisoning do not go to a doctor or submit a sample to a laboratory, so we never learn what germ made them sick.

Play Safe around Animals

Pets and other healthy animals, including those at petting zoos, farms, fairs, and even schools and day cares, can carry *Salmonella* and other germs that make people sick. The following tips will help you stay safe when it comes to our feathery, furry, and scaly friends:
- Wash your hands thoroughly with running water and soap after touching pets and other animals or their food, water, poop, belongings (such as toys and bowls), or habitats (such as beds, cages, tanks, coops, stalls, and barns).
- Do not put your hands in your mouth after petting or playing with animals. Keep other items that have come into contact with animals out of your mouth.

- Do not kiss cats, dogs, chickens, turtles, lizards, or other pets or animals.
- Do not let children under age five, people with weakened immune systems, or older adults touch high-risk animals (such as turtles, frogs, chickens, or ducks) or their belongings or habitats.
- Never eat or drink around high-risk animals or in areas where they live and roam.
- Clean your pet's bed, cage, terrarium, or aquarium and its contents (such as food and water bowls) outdoors. If you must clean your pet's habitat indoors, use a bathtub or large sink that can be cleaned and disinfected. Avoid using a kitchen sink, if possible.
- Take your pet to the veterinarian regularly. By keeping your pet healthy, you also help keep yourself and your family healthy.[2]

[2] "Diagnosis and Treatment," Centers for Disease Control and Prevention (CDC), April 8, 2019. Available online. URL: www.cdc.gov/salmonella/general/diag-testing-salmonella.html. Accessed July 11, 2023.

Chapter 40 | Shigellosis

Shigella bacteria cause an infection called "shigellosis." *Shigella* can spread easily from one person to another—and it only takes a small amount of *Shigella* to cause illness.

SYMPTOMS OF SHIGELLOSIS

People with *Shigella* infection (shigellosis) usually start experiencing symptoms one to two days after contact with the germ. These symptoms include the following:

- diarrhea that can be bloody or prolonged (lasting more than three days)
- fever
- stomach pain
- feeling the need to pass stool (poop) even when the bowels are empty

Some people will not have any symptoms. Symptoms usually last five to seven days, but some people may experience symptoms anywhere from a few days to four or more weeks. In some cases, it may take several months before bowel habits (i.e., how often someone passes stool and the consistency of their stool) are entirely normal.

When to Contact Your Doctor

People with diarrhea should contact their doctor if they have any of the following symptoms:

- fever
- bloody or prolonged diarrhea
- severe stomach cramping or tenderness
- dehydration

People who are in poor health or whose immune systems are weakened from diseases (such as human immunodeficiency virus (HIV)) or medical treatments (such as chemotherapy for cancer) are more likely to get sick for a longer period of time. Contact your doctor if you are in one of these groups and have symptoms of *Shigella* infection (shigellosis).

RARE RISKS FROM *SHIGELLA* INFECTION (SHIGELLOSIS)

Reactive Arthritis

About 2 percent of people who are infected with certain types of *Shigella*, most commonly *Shigella flexneri*, will experience reactive arthritis after infection, which can cause joint pain, eye irritation, and painful urination. The syndrome typically occurs in people who have a specific genetic makeup that puts them at risk. It usually lasts for three to five months, but occasionally, it can last for years and lead to chronic arthritis. Reactive arthritis can also occur in people who get sick from *Shigella sonnei* but is less common in other types of *Shigella* called "*Shigella boydii*" and "*Shigella dysenteriae*."

Bloodstream Infections

Around 0.4–7.3 percent of people with *Shigella* infection (shigellosis) develop bloodstream infections caused by *Shigella* germs or by other germs in the gut that get into the bloodstream when *Shigella* damage intestinal linings. Bloodstream infections are most common among patients with weakened immune systems, such as those with HIV, diabetes, cancer, or severe malnutrition, and are more commonly seen in children. Bloodstream infections are most commonly seen in infections caused by *S. flexneri* and *S. dysenteriae*. Shigellosis patients with bloodstream infections are at a higher risk of death compared to those without bloodstream infections.

Seizures

Generalized seizures have been reported among young children with *Shigella* infection (shigellosis) but usually go away without treatment. Children with *Shigella* infection who experience seizures typically have a high fever, low blood sugar, or abnormal blood electrolytes (salts). However, health-care professionals have not been able to definitively explain why these seizures occur.

Hemolytic Uremic Syndrome

Hemolytic uremic syndrome (HUS) is a rare complication of *Shigella* infections (shigellosis) that also most commonly occurs in children. HUS occurs when bacteria enter the digestive system and produce a toxin that destroys red blood cells, which block the kidneys' filtering function and can lead to kidney failure. Patients with HUS often have bloody diarrhea, and it can be a deadly complication. In patients with shigellosis, HUS is associated with Shiga-toxin-producing *Shigella*, most often occurring with *S. dysenteriae*. HUS can occur when antimicrobial-resistant drugs are used to treat the infection or when treatment is started after four days of symptoms, and it is the leading cause of death in *S. dysenteriae* outbreaks.

DIAGNOSIS OF SHIGELLOSIS

Infection is diagnosed when a laboratory identifies *Shigella* bacteria in the stool (poop) of an ill person. The test could be a culture that isolates the bacteria or a rapid diagnostic test that detects the genetic material of the bacteria.

TREATMENT OF SHIGELLOSIS

Contact your health-care provider if you or one of your family members has bloody or prolonged diarrhea (diarrhea lasting more than three days) or severe stomach cramping or tenderness, especially if you also have a fever or feel very sick. Tell your health-care provider if you have other medical conditions or a weakened immune system—for example, because of an HIV infection or chemotherapy treatment. If you have a weakened immune system, you may be more likely to become severely ill.

- People with *Shigella* infection should drink plenty of fluids to prevent dehydration.
- People with bloody diarrhea should not use antidiarrheal medicines, such as loperamide

(Imodium) or diphenoxylate with atropine (Lomotil). These medicines may make symptoms worse.
- Antibiotics can shorten the time you have fever and diarrhea by about two days.
- Ciprofloxacin and azithromycin are two recommended oral antibiotics.

If your health-care provider prescribes an antibiotic, take it exactly as directed and finish taking all the pills even if you feel better.

PREVENTION OF *SHIGELLA* INFECTION

Shigella germs can spread easily from one person to another, and it takes only a small amount of *Shigella* to make someone sick.

Take Steps to Avoid Getting Sick

People can get a *Shigella* infection (shigellosis) after putting something in their mouth or swallowing something that has come into contact with the stool (poop) of someone with a *Shigella* infection. The following tips can reduce your chance of getting *Shigella* infection:

- Carefully wash your hands with soap and water during key times:
  - before any sexual activity
  - before preparing food or eating
  - after going to the bathroom, changing a diaper, or cleaning up after someone who went to the bathroom
- Take care when changing diapers and perform the following steps:
  - As soon as you change a diaper, throw it away in a covered, lined garbage can.
  - Clean up any leaks or spills from the diaper right away.
  - Wash your hands and the child's hands with soap and water right away.

- Avoid swallowing water from ponds, lakes, or swimming pools.
- When traveling internationally, follow safe food and water habits and wash hands often with soap and water.
- If you or your partner has been diagnosed with shigellosis, do not have sex. To reduce the chance of *Shigella* spreading, wait at least two weeks after the diarrhea ends to have sex.

Help Prevent the Spread of *Shigella* Infection to Others When You Are Sick

- Wash hands often, especially:
  - before eating or preparing food
  - after using the bathroom or changing diapers
- Do not prepare food if you are sick or share food with anyone.
- Do not swim.
- Do not have sex for at least two weeks after you no longer have diarrhea.
- Stay home from school or from health-care, food service, or childcare jobs while sick or until your health department says it is safe to return.[1]

[1] "*Shigella* – Shigellosis," Centers for Disease Control and Prevention (CDC), February 24, 2023. Available online. URL: www.cdc.gov/shigella/index.html. Accessed July 11, 2023.

Chapter 41 | **Staph Infections: Group A**

Chapter Contents

Section 41.1 | Staphylococcal Infections

WHAT ARE STAPHYLOCOCCAL INFECTIONS?

Staphylococcus (staph) is a group of bacteria. There are more than 30 types. A type called "*Staphylococcus aureus*" causes most infections. Staph bacteria can cause many different types of infections, including the following:

- skin infections, which are the most common types of staph infections
- bacteremia, an infection of the bloodstream, which can lead to sepsis, a very serious immune response to infection
- bone infections
- endocarditis, an infection of the inner lining of the heart chambers and valves
- food poisoning
- pneumonia
- toxic shock syndrome (TSS), a life-threatening condition caused by toxins from certain types of bacteria

WHAT CAUSES STAPH INFECTIONS?

Some people carry staph bacteria on their skin or in their noses, but they do not get an infection. But, if they get a cut or wound, the bacteria can enter the body and cause an infection.

Staph bacteria can spread from person to person. They can also spread through objects, such as towels, clothing, door handles, athletic equipment, and remotes. If you have staph and do not handle food properly when you are preparing it, you can also spread staph to others.

WHAT ARE THE SYMPTOMS OF STAPH INFECTIONS?

The symptoms of a staph infection depend on the following types of infections:

- **Skin infections**. These infections can look like pimples or boils. They may be red, swollen, and painful.

Sometimes, there is pus or other drainage. They can turn into impetigo, which turns into a crust on the skin, or cellulitis, a swollen, red area of skin that feels hot.
- **Bone infections**. These infections can cause pain, swelling, warmth, and redness in the infected area. You may also have chills and a fever.
- **Endocarditis**. This causes some flu-like symptoms: fever, chills, and fatigue. It also causes symptoms such as rapid heartbeat, shortness of breath, and fluid buildup in your arms or legs.
- **Food poisoning**. This infection typically causes nausea and vomiting, diarrhea, and fever. If you lose too many fluids, you may also become dehydrated.
- **Pneumonia symptoms**. The symptoms include a high fever, chills, and cough that do not get better. You may also have chest pain and shortness of breath.
- **TSS**. It causes high fever, sudden low blood pressure, vomiting, diarrhea, and confusion. You may have a sunburn-like rash somewhere on your body. TSS can lead to organ failure.

WHO IS MORE LIKELY TO GET A STAPH INFECTION?

Anyone can develop a staph infection, but certain people are more likely to get one, including those who:
- have a chronic condition, such as diabetes, cancer, vascular disease, eczema, and lung disease
- have a weakened immune system, such as from human immunodeficiency virus (HIV), medicines to prevent organ rejection, or chemotherapy
- had surgery
- are in the hospital
- use a catheter, breathing tube, or feeding tube
- have an implanted device, such as a pacemaker, artificial joint, or heart valve

- have burns, especially if they are deep or cover a large area of the body
- are on dialysis
- inject illegal drugs
- do contact sports since you may have skin-to-skin contact with others or share equipment

HOW ARE STAPH INFECTIONS DIAGNOSED?

Your health-care provider will do a physical exam and ask about your symptoms. Often, providers can tell if you have a staph skin infection by looking at it. To check for other types of staph infections, providers may do a culture with a skin scraping, tissue sample, stool sample, or throat or nasal swabs. There may be other tests, such as imaging tests, depending on the type of infection.

WHAT ARE THE TREATMENTS FOR STAPH INFECTIONS?

Treatment for staph infections is antibiotics. Depending on the type of infection, the antibiotics might be a cream, ointment, medicines (to swallow), or intravenous (IV) medicine. If you have an infected wound, your provider might drain it. Sometimes, you may need surgery for bone infections.

Some staph infections, such as methicillin-resistant *Staphylococcus aureus* (MRSA), are resistant to many antibiotics. There are still certain antibiotics that can treat these infections.

CAN STAPH INFECTIONS BE PREVENTED?

The following steps can help prevent staph infections:

- Use good hygiene, including washing your hands often.
- Do not share towels, sheets, or clothing with someone who has a staph infection.
- It is best not to share athletic equipment. If you do need to share, make sure that it is properly cleaned and dried before you use it.

- Practice food safety, including not preparing food for others when you have a staph infection.
- If you have a cut or wound, keep it covered.[1]

Section 41.2 | Vancomycin-Intermediate/Vancomycin-Resistant *Staphylococcus aureus* Infections

Vancomycin-intermediate *Staphylococcus aureus* (VISA) and vancomycin-resistant *Staphylococcus aureus* (VRSA) are specific types of antimicrobial-resistant bacteria. However, as of October 2010, all VISA and VRSA isolates have been susceptible to other drugs approved by the U.S. Food and Drug Administration (FDA). Persons who develop this type of staph infection may have underlying health conditions (such as diabetes and kidney disease), tubes going into their bodies (such as catheters), previous infections with methicillin-resistant *Staphylococcus aureus* (MRSA), and recent exposure to vancomycin and other antimicrobial agents.

WHAT IS *STAPHYLOCOCCUS AUREUS*?

Staphylococcus aureus is a bacterium commonly found on the skin and in the nose of about 30 percent of individuals. Most of the time, staph does not cause any harm. These infections can look like pimples, boils, or other skin conditions, and most are able to be treated. Sometimes, staph bacteria can get into the bloodstream and cause serious infections that can be fatal, including the following:

- bacteremia or sepsis when bacteria spread to the bloodstream, usually as a result of using catheters or having surgery
- pneumonia that predominantly affects people with underlying lung disease, including those on mechanical ventilators

[1] MedlinePlus, "Staphylococcal Infections," National Institutes of Health (NIH), April 4, 2023. Available online. URL: https://medlineplus.gov/staphylococcalinfections.html. Accessed July 11, 2023.

- endocarditis (infection of the heart valves), which can lead to heart failure
- osteomyelitis (bone infection), which can be caused by staph bacteria traveling in the bloodstream or put there by direct contact such as following trauma (puncture wound of foot or intravenous (IV) drug abuse)

HOW DO VISA AND VRSA GET THEIR NAMES?

Staph bacteria are classified as VISA or VRSA based on laboratory tests. Laboratories perform tests to determine if staph bacteria are resistant to antimicrobial agents that might be used for the treatment of infections. For vancomycin and other antimicrobial agents, laboratories determine how much of the agent it requires to inhibit the growth of the organism in a test tube. The result of the test is usually expressed as a minimum inhibitory concentration (MIC) or the minimum amount of antimicrobial agent that inhibits bacterial growth in the test tube. Therefore, staph bacteria are classified as VISA if the MIC for vancomycin is 4–8 μg/ml and classified as VRSA if the MIC for vancomycin is greater than 16 μg/ml.

ARE VISA AND VRSA TREATABLE?

Yes. As of October 2010, all VISA and VRSA isolates have been susceptible to several FDA-approved drugs.

HOW CAN THE SPREAD OF VISA AND VRSA INFECTIONS BE PREVENTED?

The use of appropriate infection control practices (such as wearing gloves before and after contact with infectious body substances and adherence to hand hygiene) by health-care personnel can reduce the spread of VISA and VRSA.

WHAT SHOULD A PERSON DO IF A FAMILY MEMBER OR CLOSE FRIEND HAS VISA OR VRSA?

Vancomycin-intermediate *S. aureus* and VRSA are types of antibiotic-resistant staph bacteria. Therefore, as with all staph bacteria, spread occurs among people having close physical contact with infected patients or contaminated material, such as bandages. Persons having close physical contact with infected patients while they are outside the health-care setting should keep their hands clean by washing thoroughly with soap and water and avoid contact with other people's wounds or material contaminated from wounds. If they go to the hospital to visit a friend or family member who is infected with VISA or VRSA, they must follow the hospital's recommended precautions.

WHAT IS THE CDC DOING TO ADDRESS VISA AND VRSA?

In addition to providing guidance for clinicians and infection control personnel, the Centers for Disease Control and Prevention (CDC) is also working with state and local health agencies, healthcare facilities, and clinical microbiology laboratories to ensure that laboratories are using proper methods to detect VISA and VRSA.[2]

[2] "VISA/VRSA in Health Care Settings," Centers for Disease Control and Prevention (CDC), November 24, 2010. Available online. URL: www.cdc.gov/hai/organisms/visa_vrsa/visa_vrsa.html. Accessed July 11, 2023.

Chapter 42 | **Streptococcal Infections: Group A**

Chapter Contents

Section 42.1 | Impetigo

Impetigo is a bacterial infection of the skin that is most common in young children. Doctors use antibiotics to treat impetigo. Antibiotics can also help protect others from getting sick.

TWO BACTERIA CAN CAUSE IMPETIGO

Impetigo is a skin infection caused by one or both of the following bacteria: group A *Streptococcus* and *Staphylococcus aureus*. Here, the focus is on impetigo caused by group A *Streptococcus* (group A strep). Another name for impetigo is infantigo.

HOW YOU GET IMPETIGO

Group A strep bacteria are very contagious. When group A strep bacteria infect the skin, they cause sores. The bacteria can spread to others if someone touches those sores or comes into contact with fluid from the sores.

It usually takes 10 days for sores to appear after someone is exposed to group A strep bacteria.

SYMPTOMS

In general, impetigo is a mild infection that can occur anywhere on the body. It most often affects exposed skin, such as:

- around the nose and mouth
- on the arms or legs

Symptoms include red, itchy sores that break open and leak a clear fluid or pus for a few days. Next, a crusty yellow or "honey-colored" scab forms over the sore, which then heals without leaving a scar.

SOME PEOPLE ARE AT INCREASED RISK

Anyone can get impetigo, but some factors increase someone's risk of getting this infection.

Age

Impetigo is most common in children aged two to five.

Infections or Injuries That Break the Skin

People with scabies infection are at increased risk for impetigo. Participating in activities where cuts or scrapes are common can also increase someone's risk of impetigo.

Group Settings

Close contact with another person with impetigo is the most common risk factor for illness. For example, if someone has impetigo, the bacteria often spread to other people in their household.

Infectious illnesses also tend to spread wherever large groups of people gather. Crowded conditions can increase the risk of spreading impetigo. These settings include the following:

- schools
- day care centers
- military training facilities

Climate

Impetigo is more common in areas with hot, humid summers and mild winters (subtropics) or wet and dry seasons (tropics), but it can occur anywhere.

Poor Personal Hygiene

Lack of proper handwashing, body washing, and facial cleanliness can increase someone's risk of getting impetigo.

DOCTORS DIAGNOSE IMPETIGO BY APPEARANCE

Doctors typically diagnose impetigo by looking at the sores during a physical examination. Lab tests are not needed.

IMPETIGO TREATMENT INVOLVES ANTIBIOTICS

Doctors treat impetigo with antibiotics, such as:

- topical antibiotics (medicine rubbed onto the sores)
- oral antibiotics (medicine taken by mouth)

A doctor might recommend a topical ointment for only a few sores. Oral antibiotics can be used when there are more sores. Use the prescription exactly as the doctor says to. Once the sores heal, someone with impetigo is usually not able to spread the bacteria to others.

When to Return to Work or School after Illness

People with impetigo can return to work, school, or day care if they:

- have started antibiotic treatment
- keep all sores on exposed skin covered

SERIOUS COMPLICATIONS ARE VERY RARE

Very rarely, impetigo complications can include the following:

- kidney problems (post-streptococcal glomerulonephritis)
- rheumatic fever (a disease that can affect the heart, joints, brain, and skin)

If someone has post-streptococcal glomerulonephritis, it usually starts one to two weeks after the skin sores go away.

PREVENT IMPETIGO

People can get impetigo more than once. Having impetigo does not protect someone from getting it again in the future. There are no vaccines to prevent group A strep infections, but there are things you can do to help protect yourself and others. To help prevent group A step infections, you should:

- clean and care for wounds
- wash your hands and laundry often
- take antibiotics, if prescribed

Clean and Care for Wounds

- **Wash hands often**. Wash hands often with soap and water or use an alcohol-based hand rub if washing is not possible.
- **Clean wounds**. Clean all minor cuts and injuries that break the skin (such as blisters and scrapes) with soap and water.
- **Bandage wounds**. Clean and cover draining or open wounds with clean, dry bandages until they heal.
- **See a doctor**. See a doctor for punctures and other deep or serious wounds.
- **Protect wounds and infections**. If you have an open wound or skin infection, avoid spending time in:
    - hot tubs
    - swimming pools
    - natural bodies of water (e.g., lakes, rivers, and oceans)

Wash Hands and Laundry Often

Appropriate personal hygiene and frequent body and hair washing with soap and clean, running water is important to help prevent impetigo.

You should wash the clothes, linens, and towels of anyone who has impetigo every day. These items should not be shared with anyone else. After they have been washed, these items are safe for others to use.

The best way to keep from getting or spreading group A strep bacteria is to wash your hands often. This is especially important after coughing or sneezing.

Take Antibiotics, If Prescribed

Antibiotics help prevent someone with impetigo from spreading the bacteria to others.[1]

---

[1] "Impetigo: All You Need to Know," Centers for Disease Control and Prevention (CDC), June 27, 2022. Available online. URL: www.cdc.gov/groupastrep/diseases-public/impetigo.html. Accessed July 12, 2023.

Section 42.2 | Scarlet Fever

WHAT CAUSES SCARLET FEVER?

Bacteria called "group A *Streptococcus*" (group A strep) cause scarlet fever. These bacteria are also the cause of strep throat. The bacteria sometimes make a toxin (poison), which causes a rash—the "scarlet" of scarlet fever.

HOW YOU GET SCARLET FEVER

Group A strep bacteria are very contagious. Generally, people spread the bacteria to others through:

- respiratory droplets
- direct contact

Rarely, people can spread group A strep bacteria through food that is not handled properly.

It usually takes two to five days for someone exposed to group A strep bacteria to become sick with strep throat or scarlet fever.

Respiratory Droplets

Group A strep bacteria often live in the nose and throat. People who are infected spread the bacteria by talking, coughing, or sneezing, which creates respiratory droplets that contain the bacteria.

People can get sick if they:

- breathe in respiratory droplets that contain the bacteria
- touch something with those droplets on it and then touch their mouth or nose
- drink from the same glass or eat from the same plate as a person infected with group A strep

Direct Contact

People can also spread group A strep bacteria from infected sores on their skin. Other people can get sick if they touch sores on the skin caused by group A strep (impetigo) or come into contact with fluid from the sores.

People Are Contagious Even with No Symptoms

Some people infected with group A strep do not have symptoms or seem sick. People who are sick with strep throat are more contagious than those who do not have symptoms.

RASH AND FEVER ARE COMMON SYMPTOMS

In general, scarlet fever is a mild disease. The illness usually begins with a fever and sore throat.

General Symptoms

Some symptoms of scarlet fever are common to other infections, too. These may include the following:

- fever (101 °F (38 °C) or higher) or chills
- sore throat and pain when swallowing
- headache or body aches
- stomach pain
- nausea or vomiting

Physical Signs

Some physical signs are typical of scarlet fever (refer to Figures 42.1 and 42.2).

TONGUE, THROAT, AND NECK

The following are the signs in these areas:

- whitish coating on the tongue early in the illness
- "strawberry" (red and bumpy) tongue
- very red throat
- red and swollen tonsils
- white patches or streaks of pus on the tonsils
- tiny, red spots on the roof of the mouth, called "petechiae"
- swollen lymph nodes in the front of the neck

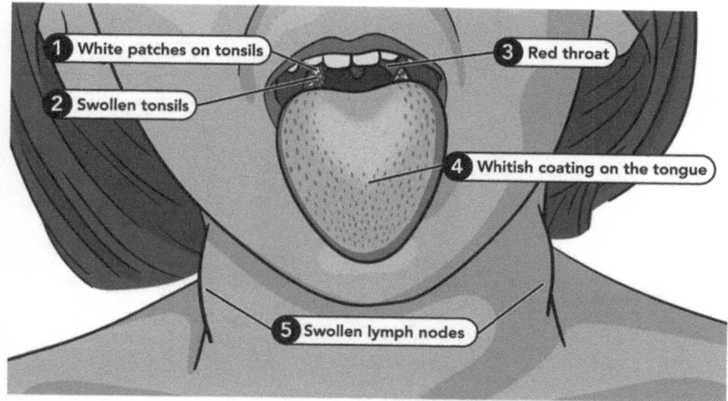

Figure 42.1. Scarlet Fever with White Tongue
Centers for Disease Control and Prevention (CDC)

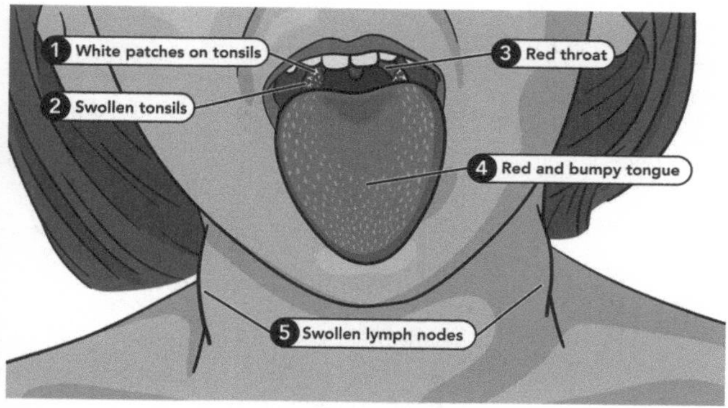

Figure 42.2. Scarlet Fever with Strawberry Tongue
Centers for Disease Control and Prevention (CDC)

SKIN

The following are the signs of scarlet fever rash (refer to Figure 42.3):

- red rash that feels rough like sandpaper
- brighter red skin in the creases of the underarm, elbow, and groin
- a pale area around the mouth
- skin peeling as the rash fades

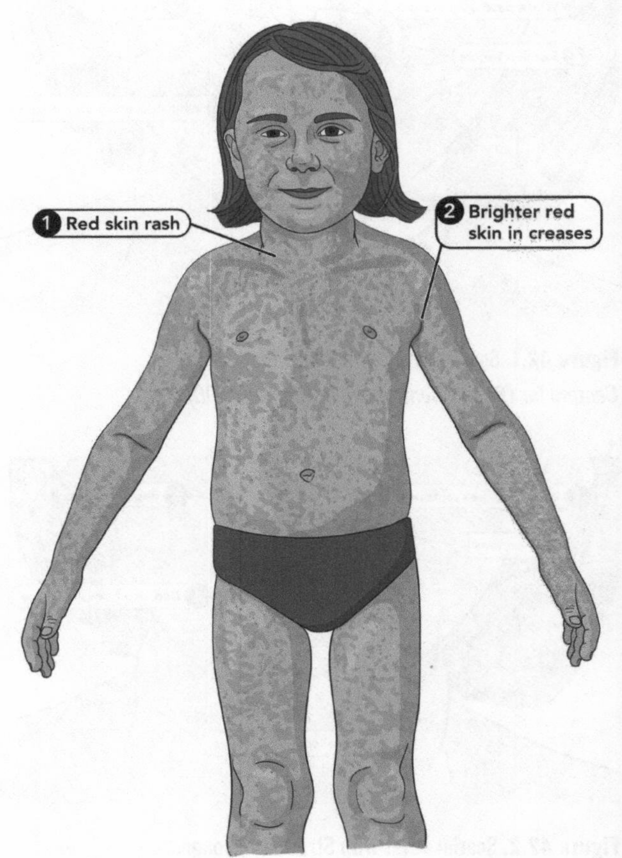

Figure 42.3. Scarlet Fever Rash

Centers for Disease Control and Prevention (CDC)

One to two days after the illness begins, a red rash usually appears. However, the rash can appear before illness or up to seven days later.

The rash may first appear on the neck, underarm, and groin (the area where your stomach meets your thighs). Over time, the rash spreads over the body. The rash usually begins as small, flat blotches that slowly become fine bumps that feel like sandpaper.

Although the cheeks might look flushed (rosy), there may be a pale area around the mouth. Underarm, elbow, and groin skin creases may become brighter red than the rest of the rash.

The rash from scarlet fever fades in about seven days. As the rash fades, the skin may peel around the fingertips, toes, and groin area. This peeling can last up to several weeks.

WHO IS AT INCREASED RISK?

Anyone can get scarlet fever, but there are some factors that can increase the risk of getting this infection.

Age

Scarlet fever, such as strep throat, is more common in children than adults. It is most common in children aged 5–15. It is rare in children under age three. Adults who are at increased risk for scarlet fever include the following:

- parents of school-aged children
- adults who are often in contact with children

Group Settings

Close contact with another person with scarlet fever is the most common risk factor for illness. For example, if someone has scarlet fever, the bacteria often spread to other people in their household.

Infectious illnesses tend to spread wherever large groups of people gather. Crowded settings can increase the risk of getting a group A strep infection. These settings include the following:

- schools
- day care centers
- military training facilities

DIAGNOSIS OF SCARLET FEVER

Many viruses and bacteria can cause an illness that includes a red rash and sore throat. A doctor will determine what type of illness you have by asking about symptoms and doing a physical exam. If they think you might have scarlet fever, they will swab your throat to test for strep throat. There are two types of tests for strep throat: a rapid strep test and a throat culture.

Rapid Strep Test

A rapid strep test involves swabbing the throat and running a test on the swab. The test quickly shows if group A strep bacteria are causing the illness.

- If the test is positive, doctors can prescribe antibiotics.
- If the test is negative, but a doctor still suspects scarlet fever, then the doctor can take a throat culture swab.

Throat Culture

A throat culture takes time to see if group A strep bacteria grow from the swab. While it takes more time, a throat culture sometimes finds infections that the rapid strep test misses.

Culture is important to use in children and teens since they can get rheumatic fever from an untreated scarlet fever infection. For adults, it is usually not necessary to do a throat culture following a negative rapid strep test. Adults are generally not at risk of getting rheumatic fever following scarlet fever.

TREATMENT FOR SCARLET FEVER

Doctors treat scarlet fever with antibiotics. The benefits of antibiotics include the following:

- decreasing how long someone is sick
- decreasing symptoms (feeling better)
- preventing the bacteria from spreading to others
- preventing serious complications such as rheumatic fever

Antibiotic Dos and Don'ts

- Do take the prescription exactly as the doctor says to.
- Do not stop taking the medicine, even if you or your child feels better, unless the doctor says to stop.

LONG-TERM HEALTH PROBLEMS ARE NOT COMMON

Complications can occur after having scarlet fever. This can happen if the bacteria spread to other parts of the body. Complications can include the following:

- abscesses (pockets of pus) around the tonsils
- swollen lymph nodes in the neck
- ear, sinus, and skin infections
- pneumonia (lung infection)
- rheumatic fever (a disease that can affect the heart, joints, brain, and skin)
- post-streptococcal glomerulonephritis (a kidney disease)
- arthritis (joint inflammation)

Treatment with antibiotics can prevent most of these health problems.

PROTECTING YOURSELF AND OTHERS

People can get scarlet fever more than once. Having scarlet fever does not protect someone from getting it again in the future. While there is no vaccine to prevent scarlet fever, there are things people can do to protect themselves and others.

Good Hygiene

The best way to keep from getting or spreading group A strep is to wash your hands often. This is especially important after coughing or sneezing and before preparing foods or eating.

To prevent group A strep infections, you should:

- cover your mouth and nose with a tissue when you cough or sneeze
- put your used tissue in the wastebasket
- cough or sneeze into your upper sleeve or elbow, not your hands, if you do not have a tissue
- wash your hands often with soap and water for at least 20 seconds
- use an alcohol-based hand rub if soap and water are not available

You should also wash glasses, utensils, and plates after someone who is sick uses them. These items are safe for others to use once washed.

Antibiotics

Antibiotics help prevent someone with strep throat from spreading the bacteria to others.[2]

Section 42.3 | Strep Throat

WHAT CAUSES STREP THROAT?

Viruses cause most sore throats. However, strep throat is an infection in the throat and tonsils caused by bacteria called "group A *Streptococcus*" (group A strep).

HOW YOU GET STREP THROAT

Group A strep bacteria are very contagious. Generally, people spread the bacteria to others through:

- respiratory droplets
- direct contact

Rarely people can spread group A strep bacteria through food that is not handled properly.

It usually takes two to five days for someone exposed to group A strep bacteria to become ill with strep throat.

Respiratory Droplets

Group A strep bacteria often live in the nose and throat. People who are infected spread the bacteria by talking, coughing, or sneezing, which creates respiratory droplets that contain the bacteria.

[2] "Scarlet Fever: All You Need to Know," Centers for Disease Control and Prevention (CDC), May 10, 2023. Available online. URL: www.cdc.gov/groupastrep/diseases-public/scarlet-fever.html. Accessed July 12, 2023.

People can get sick if they:

- breathe in respiratory droplets that contain the bacteria
- touch something with those droplets on it and then touch their mouth or nose
- drink from the same glass or eat from the same plate as a person infected with group A strep bacteria

Direct Contact

People can also spread group A strep bacteria from infected sores on their skin. Other people can get sick if they:

- touch sores on the skin caused by group A strep bacteria (impetigo) or come into contact with fluid from the sores

People Are Contagious Even with No Symptoms

Some people infected with group A strep do not have symptoms or seem sick. People who are sick with strep throat are more contagious than those who do not have symptoms.

SYMPTOMS OF STREP THROAT

In general, strep throat is a mild disease, but it can be very painful. Common symptoms may include the following:

- fever
- pain when swallowing
- sore throat that can start very quickly and may look red
- red and swollen tonsils
- white patches or streaks of pus on the tonsils
- tiny, red spots on the roof of the mouth, called "petechiae"
- swollen lymph nodes in the front of the neck

Less Common Symptoms May Include Vomiting and Headache

Some people, especially children, may have other symptoms, too. Other symptoms may include the following:

- headache
- stomach pain

- nausea or vomiting
- rash (scarlet fever)

Symptoms Do Not Include Cough or Runny Nose

The following symptoms suggest a virus is the cause of the illness instead of strep throat:

- cough
- runny nose
- hoarseness (changes in your voice that make it sound breathy, raspy, or strained)
- pink eye (conjunctivitis)

WHO ARE AT INCREASED RISK?

Age

Strep throat is more common in children than adults. It is most common in children aged 5–15. It is very rare in children under age three.

Adults who are at increased risk for strep throat include the following:

- parents of school-aged children
- adults who are often in contact with children

Group Settings

Close contact with another person with strep throat is the most common risk factor for illness. For example, if someone has strep throat, the bacteria often spread to other people in their household.

Infectious illnesses tend to spread wherever large groups of people gather. Crowded settings can increase the risk of getting a group A strep infection. These settings include the following:

- schools
- day care centers
- military training facilities

Strep Throat: More Common in Children

- Up to 3 in 10 children with a sore throat have strep throat.
- About 1 in 10 adults with a sore throat has strep throat.

DIAGNOSIS OF STREP THROAT

A doctor will determine what type of illness you have by asking about symptoms and doing a physical exam. If they think you might have strep throat, they will swab your throat to test for strep throat. There are two types of tests for strep throat: a rapid strep test and a throat culture.

Rapid Strep Test

A rapid strep test involves swabbing the throat and running a test on the swab. The test quickly shows if group A strep bacteria are causing the illness.

- If the test is positive, doctors can prescribe antibiotics.
- If the test is negative, but a doctor still suspects strep throat, then the doctor can take a throat culture swab.

Throat Culture

A throat culture takes time to see if group A strep bacteria grow from the swab. While it takes more time, a throat culture sometimes finds infections that the rapid strep test misses.

Culture is important to use in children and teens since they can get rheumatic fever from an untreated strep throat infection. For adults, it is usually not necessary to do a throat culture following a negative rapid strep test. Adults are generally not at risk of getting rheumatic fever following a strep throat infection.

TREATMENT FOR STREP THROAT

Doctors treat strep throat with antibiotics. The benefits of antibiotics include the following:

- decreasing how long someone is sick
- decreasing symptoms (feeling better)
- preventing the bacteria from spreading to others
- preventing serious complications such as rheumatic fever

Someone with strep throat should start feeling better in just a day or two after starting antibiotics. Call the doctor if you or your child is not feeling better after taking antibiotics for 48 hours.

When to Return to Work or School

People with strep throat should stay home from work, school, or day care until they:

- no longer have a fever
- have taken antibiotics for at least 12–24 hours (Ask the doctor how long you should stay home after starting antibiotics.)

Use Antibiotics Properly

- Take the prescription exactly as the doctor says to.
- Keep taking the medicine even if you or your child feels better. Do not stop unless the doctor says to stop.

WHO NEEDS ANTIBIOTICS?

Someone who tests positive for strep throat but has no symptoms (called a "carrier") usually does not need antibiotics. They are less likely to spread the bacteria to others and very unlikely to get complications.

If a carrier gets a sore throat illness caused by a virus, the rapid strep test can be positive. In these cases, it can be hard to know what is causing the sore throat.

If someone keeps getting a sore throat after taking the right antibiotics, they may be a strep carrier and have a viral throat infection. Talk to a doctor if you think you or your child may be a strep carrier.

SERIOUS COMPLICATIONS ARE NOT COMMON

Complications can occur after a strep throat infection. This can happen if the bacteria spread to other parts of the body.

Complications can include the following:

- abscesses (pockets of pus) around the tonsils or in the neck
- swollen lymph nodes in the neck
- sinus infections
- ear infections

- rheumatic fever (a disease that can affect the heart, joints, brain, and skin)
- post-streptococcal glomerulonephritis (a kidney disease)

PROTECTING YOURSELF AND OTHERS

People can get strep throat more than once. Having strep throat does not protect someone from getting it again in the future. While there is no vaccine to prevent strep throat, there are things people can do to protect themselves and others.

Good Hygiene

The best way to keep from getting or spreading group A strep is to wash your hands often. This is especially important after coughing or sneezing and before preparing foods or eating.

To prevent group A strep infections, you should:

- cover your mouth and nose with a tissue when you cough or sneeze
- put your used tissue in the wastebasket
- cough or sneeze into your upper sleeve or elbow, not your hands, if you do not have a tissue
- wash your hands often with soap and water for at least 20 seconds
- use an alcohol-based hand rub if soap and water are not available

You should also wash glasses, utensils, and plates after someone who is sick uses them. These items are safe for others to use once washed.

Antibiotics

Antibiotics help prevent someone with strep throat from spreading the bacteria to others.[3]

[3] "Strep Throat: All You Need to Know," Centers for Disease Control and Prevention (CDC), January 6, 2023. Available online. URL: www.cdc.gov/groupastrep/diseases-public/strep-throat.html. Accessed July 12, 2023.

Chapter 43 | Streptococcal Infections: Group B

Chapter Contents

Section 43.1 | Group B *Streptococcus* Infection

Group B *Streptococcus* (group B strep or GBS) can cause serious illness in people of all ages, especially newborns. Pregnant women can take steps to help protect their babies from this potentially deadly illness.

CAUSES AND HOW IT SPREADS

Group B strep bacteria commonly live in people's bodies and usually are not harmful. Babies can be exposed to GBS bacteria during delivery. How other people are exposed to these bacteria is not completely known.

Causes

GBS bacteria cause GBS disease. GBS bacteria commonly live in people's gastrointestinal and genital tracts. The gastrointestinal tract is the part of the body that digests food and includes the stomach and intestines. The genital tract is the part of the body involved in reproduction and includes the vagina in women.

Most of the time, the bacteria are not harmful and do not make people feel sick or have any symptoms. Sometimes, the bacteria invade the body and cause certain infections, which are known as "GBS disease."

How It Spreads

How people spread GBS bacteria to others is generally unknown. However, experts know that pregnant women can pass the bacteria to their babies during delivery. Most babies who get GBS disease in the first week of life are exposed to the bacteria this way. It can be hard to figure out how babies who develop GBS disease later get the bacteria. The bacteria may have come from the mother during birth or from another source.

Other people who live with someone who has GBS bacteria, including other children, are not at increased risk of getting sick.

PEOPLE AT INCREASED RISK

Anyone can get GBS disease, but some people are at greater risk than others. Being a certain age or having certain medical conditions can put you at increased risk for GBS disease.

Newborns

GBS disease is most common in newborns. There are factors that can increase a pregnant woman's risk of having a baby who will develop GBS disease, including the following:

- testing positive for GBS bacteria late in pregnancy
- developing a fever during labor
- having 18 hours or more pass between when their water breaks and when their baby is born

About one in every four pregnant women carry GBS bacteria in their body.

Adults

In adults, most cases of GBS disease are among those who have other medical conditions. Other medical conditions that put adults at increased risk include the following:

- diabetes
- heart disease
- congestive heart failure
- cancer or history of cancer
- obesity

The risk for serious GBS disease increases as people get older. Adults aged 65 or older are at increased risk compared to adults under age 65.

TYPES OF INFECTIONS

Group B strep bacteria can cause many types of infections. Some of these infections can be life-threatening. The following are the types of infections caused by GBS bacteria:

- bacteremia (a bloodstream infection)

- sepsis (the body's extreme response to an infection)
- bone and joint infections
- urinary tract infections (UTIs; infections of the urinary tract)
- meningitis (an infection of the lining of the brain and spinal cord)
- pneumonia (a lung infection)
- skin and soft tissue infections

Most Common Infections

GBS bacteria most commonly cause bacteremia, sepsis, pneumonia, and meningitis in newborns. It is very uncommon for GBS bacteria to cause meningitis in adults.

Some of these infections are "invasive." Invasive disease means that germs invade parts of the body that are normally free from germs. When this happens, the disease is usually very severe, requiring care in a hospital and even causing death in some cases.

SIGNS AND SYMPTOMS OF GROUP B *STREPTOCOCCUS*

Group B strep disease can include many different types of infections. Symptoms depend on the part of the body that is infected. Symptoms of GBS disease are different in newborns compared to people of other ages who get GBS disease.

Newborns

The symptoms of GBS disease can seem like other health problems in newborns and babies. Symptoms include the following:

- fever
- difficulty feeding
- irritability or lethargy (limpness or hard to wake up the baby)
- difficulty breathing
- blueish color to the skin

Most newborns who get sick in the first week of life have symptoms on the day of birth. In contrast, babies who develop disease later can appear healthy at birth and during their first week of life.

Pregnant Women Who Test Positive

Some women test positive for GBS bacteria during routine screening toward the end of their pregnancy. Those women usually do not feel sick or have any symptoms.

Others

Symptoms depend on the part of the body that is infected. The following are symptoms associated with the most common infections caused by GBS bacteria in adults. Symptoms of bacteremia (bloodstream infection) and sepsis (the body's extreme response to an infection) include the following:

- fever
- chills
- low alertness

Symptoms of pneumonia (lung infection) include the following:

- fever
- chills
- cough
- rapid breathing or difficulty breathing
- chest pain

Skin and soft tissue infections often appear as a bump or infected area on the skin that may be:

- red
- swollen or painful
- warm to the touch
- full of pus or other drainage

People with skin infections may also have a fever. Bone and joint infections often appear as pain in the infected area and might also include the following:

- fever
- chills

- swelling
- stiffness or inability to use the affected limb or joint

DIAGNOSIS OF GROUP B *STREPTOCOCCUS*

Group B strep disease is often serious. Early diagnosis and treatment are very important.

If doctors suspect someone has GBS disease, they do the following:

- Take samples of sterile body fluids such as blood and spinal fluid. Doctors look to see if GBS bacteria grow from the samples (culture). It can take a few days to get these results since the bacteria need time to grow.
- Order a chest x-ray to help determine if someone has GBS disease.

Sometimes, GBS bacteria can cause UTIs or bladder infections. Doctors use a sample of urine to diagnose UTIs.

TREATMENT OF GROUP B *STREPTOCOCCUS*

Doctors usually treat GBS disease with antibiotics. Sometimes, people with soft tissue and bone infections may need additional treatment, such as surgery. Treatment will depend on the kind of infection caused by GBS bacteria. It is important to start treatment as soon as possible.

COMPLICATIONS OF GROUP B *STREPTOCOCCUS*

Babies

Babies may have long-term problems, such as deafness and developmental disabilities, due to having GBS disease. Babies who have had meningitis are especially at risk for having long-term problems.

EVEN WITH GOOD CARE, BABIES CAN STILL DIE

Care for sick babies has improved a lot in the United States. However, 2–3 in every 50 babies (4–6%) who develop GBS disease will die.

GBS bacteria may be one of many different factors that can cause some miscarriages, stillbirths, and preterm deliveries. Most of the time, the cause of these events is not known.

Adults

Serious GBS infections, such as bacteremia, sepsis, and pneumonia, can also be deadly for adults. On average, about 1 in 20 nonpregnant women with serious GBS infections will die. The risk of death is lower among younger adults and adults who do not have other medical conditions.[1]

Section 43.2 | Group B Strep in Newborns and Pregnant Women

Rates of serious group B strep (GBS) infections are higher among newborns, but anyone can get GBS disease. The following are some other important facts about GBS disease in babies, pregnant women, and others.

GROUP B STREP DISEASE CAN BE VERY SERIOUS, ESPECIALLY FOR BABIES

- In the United States, GBS bacteria are a leading cause of meningitis and bloodstream infections in a newborn's first three months of life.
- Newborns are at increased risk for GBS disease if their mother tests positive for the bacteria late in pregnancy.
- Two to three in every fifty babies (4–6%) who develop GBS disease die.

[1] "About Group B Strep," Centers for Disease Control and Prevention (CDC), October 18, 2022. Available online. URL: www.cdc.gov/groupbstrep/index.html. Accessed July 13, 2023.

PREGNANT WOMEN SHOULD GET TESTED FOR GROUP B STREP BACTERIA

- About one in four pregnant women carry GBS bacteria in their bodies.
- Doctors and midwives should test pregnant women for GBS bacteria when they are 36–37 weeks pregnant.
- Giving pregnant women who carry GBS bacteria antibiotics through the vein (intravenous (IV)) during labor can prevent most cases of GBS disease in newborns during the first week of life.

NONPREGNANT ADULTS CAN GET SERIOUS GROUP B STREP DISEASE

- The most common GBS infections among nonpregnant adults include bloodstream infections, pneumonia, and skin and bone infections.
- The rate of serious GBS disease increases with age.
- On average, about 1 in 20 nonpregnant adults with serious GBS infections will die.[2]

PREVENTING GROUP B STREP DISEASE

There are currently no vaccines to prevent GBS disease, but they are under development. There are things doctors and midwives can do to prevent GBS disease during the first week of a newborn's life. Unfortunately, experts have not yet identified effective ways to prevent GBS disease in babies older than one week.

Preventing Illness in Newborns

The two best ways to prevent GBS disease during the first week of a newborn's life are as follows:

- testing pregnant women for GBS bacteria
- giving antibiotics, during labor, to women at increased risk

[2] "Fast Facts," Centers for Disease Control and Prevention (CDC), October 18, 2022. Available online. URL: www.cdc.gov/groupbstrep/about/fast-facts.html. Accessed July 13, 2023.

TESTING PREGNANT WOMEN

The American College of Obstetricians and Gynecologists (ACOG) and the American College of Nurse-Midwives (ACNM) recommend women get tested for GBS bacteria when they are 36–37 weeks pregnant. The test is simple and does not hurt. Doctors and midwives use a sterile swab ("Q tip") to collect a sample from the vagina and the rectum. They send the sample to a laboratory for testing.

Women who test positive for GBS bacteria are not sick. However, they are at increased risk of passing the bacteria to their babies during birth. GBS bacteria come and go naturally in people's bodies. A woman may test positive for the bacteria at some times and not others. That is why women get tested late in their pregnancy, close to the time of delivery.

ANTIBIOTICS DURING LABOR

Doctors and midwives give antibiotics to women who are at increased risk of having a baby who will develop GBS disease. The antibiotics help protect babies from infection, but only if given during labor. Antibiotics cannot be given before labor begins because the bacteria can grow back quickly.

Doctors and midwives give the antibiotic by IV (through the vein). They most commonly prescribe a type of antibiotic called "beta-lactam," which includes penicillin and ampicillin. However, they can also give other antibiotics to women who are severely allergic to these antibiotics. Antibiotics are very safe. For example, about 1 in 10 women has mild side effects from receiving penicillin. There is a rare chance (about 1 in 10,000 women) of having a severe allergic reaction that requires emergency treatment. Antibiotics are very effective at preventing GBS disease in newborns. Consider the following examples:

- Tanya tested positive for GBS bacteria and got antibiotics during labor. Her baby has a 1 in 4,000 chance of developing GBS disease.
- Emma tested positive for GBS bacteria and did not get antibiotics during labor. Her baby has a 1 in 200 chance

of developing GBS disease. Because Emma did not get antibiotics during labor, her baby is 20 times more likely to get GBS disease compared to Tanya's baby.

STRATEGIES PROVEN NOT TO WORK

The following strategies are not effective at preventing GBS disease in babies:

- taking antibiotics by mouth
- taking antibiotics before labor begins
- using birth canal washes with the disinfectant chlorhexidine[3]

[3] "About Group B Strep," Centers for Disease Control and Prevention (CDC), October 18, 2022. Available online. URL: www.cdc.gov/groupbstrep/index.html. Accessed August 18, 2023.

Chapter 44 | Syphilis

Syphilis is a sexually transmitted disease (STD) caused by the bacterium *Treponema pallidum*. Syphilis can cause serious health effects without adequate treatment.

HOW COMMON IS SYPHILIS?

Syphilis case reports have continued to increase since reaching a historic low in 2000 and 2001. In 2021, there were 176,713 new cases of syphilis (all stages). Gay, bisexual, and other men who have sex with men (MSM) are experiencing extreme effects of syphilis. They account for 36 percent of all primary and secondary (P&S) syphilis cases in the 2021 STD Surveillance Report (www.cdc.gov/std/statistics/2021/overview.htm#Syphilis). They also account for 47 percent of all male P&S cases.

However, case rates have increased among heterosexual men and women in recent years. Congenital syphilis continues to be a concern in the United States. Congenital syphilis occurs when a pregnant person passes syphilis to their baby. Final 2021 data show more than 2,800 cases of congenital syphilis.

HOW DO PEOPLE GET SYPHILIS?

Syphilis spreads from person to person by direct contact with a syphilitic sore, known as a "chancre." Chancres can occur in, on, or around the penis, vagina, anus, rectum, and lips or mouth. Syphilis can spread during vaginal, anal, or oral sex. Pregnant people with syphilis can also transmit the infection to their unborn child.

HOW QUICKLY DO SYMPTOMS APPEAR AFTER INFECTION?

The average time between the acquisition of syphilis and the start of the first symptom is 21 days. However, this can range from 10 to 90 days.

WHAT ARE THE SIGNS AND SYMPTOMS IN ADULTS?

Many refer to syphilis as "the great pretender," as its symptoms can look like many other diseases. However, syphilis typically follows a progression of stages that can last for weeks, months, or even years.

Primary Stage

A single chancre marks the onset of the primary (first) stage of syphilis, but there may be multiple sores. The chancre is usually (but not always) firm, round, and painless. It appears at the location where syphilis enters the body. These painless chancres can occur in locations that make them difficult to notice (e.g., the vagina or anus). The chancre lasts three to six weeks and heals regardless of whether a person receives treatment. However, the infection will progress to the secondary stage if the person with syphilis does not receive treatment.

Secondary Stage

Skin rashes and/or mucous membrane lesions (sores in the mouth, vagina, or anus) mark the second stage of symptoms. This stage typically starts with the development of a rash on one or more areas of the body. Rashes during the secondary stage:

- can appear when the primary chancre is healing or several weeks after the chancre heals
- usually does not cause itching
- may appear as rough, red, or reddish-brown spots on the palms of the hands and bottoms of the feet (However, rashes with a different appearance may occur on other parts of the body. Sometimes, they resemble rashes caused by other diseases.)
- may be so faint they are hard to notice

Condyloma lata are large, raised, and gray to white lesions. They may develop in warm, moist areas such as the mouth, underarm, or groin region. In addition to rashes, signs and symptoms of secondary syphilis may include the following:

- fever
- swollen lymph nodes
- sore throat
- patchy hair loss
- headaches
- weight loss
- muscle aches
- fatigue

The symptoms of secondary syphilis will go away with or without treatment. However, without treatment, the infection will progress to the latent and possibly tertiary stage of the disease.

Latent Stage

The latent (hidden) stage of syphilis is a period when there are no visible signs or symptoms of syphilis. Without treatment, syphilis will remain in the body even though there are no signs or symptoms. Early latent syphilis is latent syphilis, where infection occurs within the past 12 months. Late latent syphilis is latent syphilis, where infection occurred more than 12 months ago. Latent syphilis of unknown duration is when there is not enough evidence to confirm initial infection was within the past 12 months. Latent syphilis can last for years.

Tertiary Syphilis

Tertiary syphilis is rare and develops in a subset of untreated syphilis infections. It can appear 10–30 years after a person gets the infection, and it can be fatal. Tertiary syphilis can affect multiple organ systems, including the:

- brain
- nerves
- eyes

- heart
- blood vessels
- liver
- bones
- joints

Symptoms of tertiary syphilis vary depending on the organ system affected.

Neurosyphilis, Ocular Syphilis, and Otosyphilis

At any stage of infection, syphilis can invade the:

- nervous system (neurosyphilis)
- visual system (ocular syphilis)
- auditory and/or vestibular system (otosyphilis)

These infections can cause a wide range of symptoms.

Signs and symptoms of neurosyphilis can include the following:

- severe headache
- trouble with muscle movements
- muscle weakness or paralysis (not able to move certain parts of the body)
- numbness
- changes in mental status (trouble focusing, confusion, and personality change) and/or dementia (problems with memory, thinking, and/or making decisions)

Signs and symptoms of ocular syphilis can include the following:

- eye pain or redness
- floating spots in the field of vision ("floaters")
- sensitivity to light
- changes in vision (blurry vision or even blindness)

Signs and symptoms of otosyphilis may include the following:

- hearing loss
- ringing, buzzing, roaring, or hissing in the ears ("tinnitus")
- balance difficulties
- dizziness or vertigo

Health-care providers should be aware of neurosyphilis, ocular syphilis, and otosyphilis, as well as how to diagnose and manage these infections.

HOW DOES SYPHILIS AFFECT A PREGNANT PERSON AND THEIR BABY?

When a pregnant person has syphilis, the infection can spread to their unborn baby. All pregnant people should receive testing for syphilis at the first prenatal visit. Some people will need testing again during the third trimester (28 weeks gestation) and at delivery. This includes people who live in areas with high syphilis rates or are at risk for getting syphilis during pregnancy. Risk factors for getting syphilis during pregnancy include the following:

- sex with multiple partners
- sex in conjunction with drug use or transactional sex
- late entry to prenatal care (i.e., first visit during the second trimester or later) or no prenatal care
- methamphetamine or heroin use
- incarceration of pregnant women or their partner
- unstable housing or homelessness

Also, assess the risk for reinfection by discussing ongoing risk behavior and treatment of sex partners. Any person who delivers a stillborn infant after 20 weeks gestation should also receive testing for syphilis. Depending on how long a pregnant person has had syphilis, they may be at high risk of having a stillbirth. The baby could also die shortly after birth. Untreated syphilis in pregnant people results in infant death in up to 40 percent of cases.

A baby born alive with syphilis may not have any signs or symptoms of the disease. However, if treatment is not immediate, the baby may develop serious problems within a few weeks. Babies who do not receive treatment may have developmental delays, seizures, or die. Babies born to those who test positive for syphilis during pregnancy should receive congenital syphilis screening and a thorough exam. Health-care providers should only use penicillin therapy to treat syphilis and prevent passing it to the baby. Treatment with penicillin is extremely effective (success rate of 98%) in preventing transmission to the baby. Pregnant people who are allergic to penicillin should see a specialist for desensitization to penicillin.

HOW CAN HEALTH-CARE PROVIDERS DIAGNOSE SYPHILIS?

Treponemal tests detect antibodies that are specific for syphilis. These tests include *Treponema pallidum* particle agglutination assay (TP-PA), various enzyme immunoassays (EIAs), chemiluminescence immunoassays, immunoblots, and rapid treponemal assays. Treponemal antibodies appear earlier than nontreponemal antibodies. They usually remain detectable for life, even after successful treatment. If using a treponemal test for screening and the results are positive, perform a nontreponemal test with titer. This will confirm the diagnosis and guide patient management decisions. The results may require further treponemal testing. For further guidance, please refer to the 2021 Sexually Transmitted Infections (STI) Treatment Guidelines (www.cdc.gov/std/treatment-guidelines/syphilis.htm). This sequence of testing (treponemal, then nontreponemal test) is the "reverse" sequence testing algorithm. Reverse sequence testing can identify people previously treated for syphilis and those with untreated syphilis. False-positive results can occur in those with a low likelihood of infection with reverse sequence testing as well.

Special note: Untreated syphilis in pregnant people can infect their developing baby. This is why every pregnant patient should have a blood test for syphilis. Health-care providers should screen all pregnant people at their first prenatal visit. Some patients should receive a second test during the third trimester (at 28 weeks) and again at delivery.

Babies born to someone with reactive nontreponemal and treponemal test results should be evaluated for congenital syphilis. Perform a quantitative nontreponemal test on infant serum. If reactive, examine the infant thoroughly for evidence of congenital syphilis. Examine suspicious lesions, body fluids, or tissues (e.g., umbilical cord and placenta) by dark-field microscopy, polymerase chain reaction (PCR) testing, and/or special stains. Other recommended evaluations may include the following:

- analysis of cerebrospinal fluid by venereal disease research laboratory (VDRL)
- cell count and protein
- complete blood count (CBC) with differential and platelet count
- long-bone radiographs

WHAT IS THE LINK BETWEEN SYPHILIS AND HUMAN IMMUNODEFICIENCY VIRUS?

In the United States, about half of MSM with P&S syphilis also have human immunodeficiency virus (HIV). Additionally, MSM who are HIV-negative and diagnosed with P&S syphilis are more likely to get HIV in the future. Genital sores caused by syphilis make it easier to transmit and acquire HIV infection sexually. The risk of acquiring HIV increases if exposure to that infection occurs when syphilis is present. Furthermore, syphilis and other STDs might indicate ongoing behaviors and exposures that place a person at greater risk for acquiring HIV.

WHAT IS THE TREATMENT FOR SYPHILIS?

For detailed treatment recommendations, refer to the 2021 STI Treatment Guidelines (www.cdc.gov/std/treatment-guidelines/syphilis.htm). The recommended treatment for adults and adolescents with primary, secondary, or early latent syphilis is:

- benzathine penicillin G: 2.4 million units administered intramuscularly in a single dose

The treatment recommendation for adults and adolescents with late latent syphilis or latent syphilis of unknown duration is:

- benzathine penicillin G: 7.2 million units total, administered as three doses of 2.4 million units administered intramuscularly each at weekly intervals

The treatment recommendation for neurosyphilis, ocular syphilis, or otosyphilis is:

- aqueous crystalline penicillin G: 18–24 million units per day, administered as 3–4 million units intravenously every four hours or continuous infusion for 10–14 days

Treatment will prevent disease progression, but it might not repair damage already done. The selection of the appropriate penicillin preparation is important to properly treat and cure syphilis. Combinations of some penicillin preparations are not appropriate replacements for benzathine penicillin, for example, Bicillin C-R, a combination of benzathine penicillin and procaine penicillin. These combinations provide inadequate doses of penicillin.

Data to support the use of alternatives to penicillin are limited. Options for nonpregnant patients who are allergic to penicillin may include the following:

- doxycycline
- tetracycline
- potentially ceftriaxone (for neurosyphilis)

Health-care providers should use these therapies only in conjunction with close clinical and laboratory follow-ups. This ensures appropriate serological response and cure. People receiving syphilis treatment should not have sex with new partners until syphilis sores completely heal. People with syphilis should notify their sex partners, so they can also receive testing and treatment if necessary.

WHO SHOULD RECEIVE SYPHILIS TESTING?

Any person with signs or symptoms suggestive of syphilis should receive a test for syphilis. Also, anyone with an oral, anal, or vaginal sex partner who receives a recent syphilis diagnosis should receive testing. Some people should receive testing (screening) for syphilis even if they do not have symptoms or know of a sex partner who has syphilis. Anyone who is sexually active should discuss their risk factors with a health-care provider. They should ask their health-care provider about testing for syphilis or other

STDs. In addition, health-care providers should routinely test for syphilis in people who:

- are pregnant
- are sexually active MSM
- are living with HIV and are sexually active
- are taking pre-exposure prophylaxis (PrEP) for HIV prevention

WILL SYPHILIS RECUR?

After appropriate treatment, evaluating clinical and serologic response to treatment is necessary. However, even following successful treatment, reinfection can occur. People who experience reinfection or treatment failure likely:

- have signs or symptoms that persist or recur
- have a continuous fourfold increase in nontreponemal test titer

Asymptomatic chancres can be present in the vagina, rectum, or mouth. Therefore, it may not be obvious that a sex partner has syphilis.

HOW CAN SOMEONE PREVENT SYPHILIS?

Condoms, when used correctly every time someone has sex, can reduce the risk of getting or giving syphilis. Condoms offer protection when the condom covers the infected area or site of potential exposure. However, syphilis transmission can occur with lesions not covered by a condom. The only way to completely avoid syphilis is to not have vaginal, anal, or oral sex. Another option is to be in a long-term, mutually monogamous relationship with a partner who does not have syphilis. Partner-based interventions include partner notification—a critical component in preventing the spread of syphilis. Sexual partners of patients with syphilis are at risk and should receive treatment per the 2021 STI Treatment Guidelines (www.cdc.gov/std/treatment-guidelines/syphilis.htm).[1]

---

[1] "Syphilis—CDC Detailed Fact Sheet," Centers for Disease Control and Prevention (CDC), April 11, 2023. Available online. URL: www.cdc.gov/std/syphilis/stdfact-syphilis-detailed.htm. Accessed July 13, 2023.

Chapter 45 | Tuberculosis

Tuberculosis (TB) is caused by a bacterium called "*Mycobacterium tuberculosis.*" The bacteria usually attack the lungs, but TB bacteria can attack any part of the body, such as the kidney, spine, and brain. Not everyone infected with TB bacteria becomes sick. As a result, two TB-related conditions exist: latent TB infection (LTBI) and TB disease. If not treated properly, TB disease can be fatal.

HOW TUBERCULOSIS SPREADS

Tuberculosis bacteria are spread through the air from one person to another. The TB bacteria are put into the air when a person with TB disease of the lungs or throat coughs, speaks, or sings. People nearby may breathe in these bacteria and become infected.

TB is not spread by:

- shaking someone's hand
- sharing food or drink
- touching bed linens or toilet seats
- sharing toothbrushes
- kissing

When a person breathes in TB bacteria, the bacteria can settle in the lungs and begin to grow. From there, they can move through the blood to other parts of the body, such as the kidney, spine, and brain.

TB disease in the lungs or throat can be infectious. This means that the bacteria can be spread to other people. TB in other parts of the body, such as the kidney or spine, is usually not infectious. People with TB disease are most likely to spread it to people they spend time with every day. This includes family members, friends, and coworkers or schoolmates.

LATENT TUBERCULOSIS INFECTION AND TUBERCULOSIS DISEASE

Not everyone infected with TB bacteria becomes sick. As a result, two TB-related conditions exist: LTBI and TB disease.

Latent Tuberculosis Infection

TB bacteria can live in the body without making you sick. This is called "latent TB infection." In most people who breathe in TB bacteria and become infected, the body is able to fight the bacteria to stop them from growing. People with latent TB infection:

- have no symptoms
- do not feel sick
- cannot spread TB bacteria to others
- usually have a positive TB skin test (TST) reaction or a positive TB blood test
- may develop TB disease if they do not receive treatment for LTBI

Many people who have LTBI never develop TB disease. In these people, the TB bacteria remain inactive for a lifetime without causing disease. But, in other people, especially people who have a weak immune system, the bacteria become active, multiply, and cause TB disease.

Tuberculosis Disease

TB bacteria become active if the immune system cannot stop them from growing. When TB bacteria are active (multiplying in your body), this is called "TB disease." People with TB disease are sick. They may also be able to spread the bacteria to people they spend time with every day.

Many people who have LTBI never develop TB disease. Some people develop TB disease soon after becoming infected (within weeks) before their immune system can fight the TB bacteria. Other people may get sick years later when their immune system becomes weak for another reason.

For people whose immune systems are weak, especially those with human immunodeficiency virus (HIV) infection, the risk of developing TB disease is much higher than for people with normal immune systems. Table 45.1 shows the difference between LTBI and TB disease.

Table 45.1. Difference between Latent Tuberculosis Infection and Tuberculosis Disease

A Person with Latent Tuberculosis Infection	A Person with Tuberculosis Disease
Has no symptoms	Has symptoms that may include: • a bad cough that lasts three weeks or longer • pain in the chest • coughing up blood or sputum • weakness or fatigue • weight loss • no appetite • chills • fever • sweating at night
Does not feel sick	Usually feels sick
Cannot spread TB bacteria to others	May spread TB bacteria to others
Usually has a skin test or blood test result indicating TB infection	Usually has a skin test or blood test result indicating TB infection
Has a normal chest x-ray and a negative sputum smear	May have an abnormal chest x-ray, a positive sputum smear, or a culture
Needs treatment for LTBI to prevent TB disease	Needs treatment for TB disease

SIGNS AND SYMPTOMS OF TUBERCULOSIS

Symptoms of TB disease depend on where in the body the TB bacteria are growing. TB bacteria usually grow in the lungs (pulmonary TB). TB disease in the lungs may cause symptoms such as:

- a bad cough that lasts three weeks or longer
- pain in the chest
- coughing up blood or sputum (phlegm from deep inside the lungs)

Other symptoms of TB disease are:

- weakness or fatigue
- weight loss

- no appetite
- chills
- fever
- sweating at night

Symptoms of TB disease in other parts of the body depend on the area affected. People who have LTBI:

- do not feel sick
- do not have any symptoms
- cannot spread TB to others

TUBERCULOSIS RISK FACTORS

Some people develop TB disease soon after becoming infected (within weeks) before their immune system can fight the TB bacteria. Other people may get sick years later when their immune system becomes weak for another reason.

Overall, about 5–10 percent of infected persons who do not receive treatment for LTBI will develop TB disease at some time in their lives. For persons whose immune systems are weak, especially those with HIV infection, the risk of developing TB disease is much higher than for persons with normal immune systems. Generally, persons at high risk for developing TB disease fall into the following two categories.

Persons Who Have Been Recently Infected with Tuberculosis Bacteria

This includes:

- close contact with a person with infectious TB disease
- persons who have immigrated from areas of the world with high rates of TB
- children under the age of five who have a positive TB test
- groups with high rates of TB transmission, such as homeless persons, injection drug users, and persons with HIV infection
- persons who work or reside with people who are at high risk for TB in facilities or institutions, such as hospitals,

homeless shelters, correctional facilities, nursing homes, and residential homes for those with HIV

Persons with Medical Conditions That Weaken the Immune System

Babies and young children often have weak immune systems. Other people can have weak immune systems too, especially people with any of the following conditions:

- HIV infection (the virus that causes acquired immunodeficiency syndrome (AIDS))
- substance abuse
- silicosis
- diabetes mellitus
- severe kidney disease
- low body weight
- organ transplants
- head and neck cancer
- medical treatments, such as corticosteroids or organ transplant
- specialized treatment for rheumatoid arthritis (RA) or Crohn's disease

EXPOSURE TO TUBERCULOSIS

What to Do If You Have Been Exposed to Tuberculosis

You may have been exposed to TB bacteria if you spent time near someone with TB disease. The TB bacteria are put into the air when a person with active TB disease of the lungs or throat coughs, sneezes, speaks, or sings. You cannot get TB from:

- clothes
- drinking glasses
- eating utensils
- handshakes
- toilets
- other surfaces

If you think you have been exposed to someone with TB disease, you should contact your doctor or local health department about getting a TST or a special TB blood test. Be sure to tell the doctor or nurse when you have spent time with a person who has TB disease.

It is important to know that a person who is exposed to TB bacteria is not able to spread the bacteria to other people right away. Only persons with active TB disease can spread TB bacteria to others. Before you would be able to spread TB to others, you would have to breathe in TB bacteria and become infected. Then, the active bacteria would have to multiply in your body and cause active TB disease. At this point, you could possibly spread TB bacteria to others. People with TB disease are most likely to spread the bacteria to people they spend time with every day, such as family members, friends, coworkers, or schoolmates.

Some people develop TB disease soon (within weeks) after becoming infected before their immune system can fight the TB bacteria. Other people may get sick years later when their immune system becomes weak for another reason. Many people with TB infection never develop TB disease.

TUBERCULOSIS TESTING AND DIAGNOSIS

Testing

There are two kinds of tests used to detect TB bacteria in the body: the TST and TB blood tests. A positive TST or TB blood test only tells that a person has been infected with TB bacteria. It does not tell whether the person has LTBI or has progressed to TB disease. Other tests, such as a chest x-ray and a sample of sputum, are needed to see whether the person has TB disease.

Diagnosis

If a person is infected with TB bacteria, other tests are needed to see if the person has LTBI or TB disease.

WHO SHOULD BE TESTED FOR TUBERCULOSIS INFECTION?

Certain people should be tested for TB infection because they are at higher risk for being infected with TB bacteria, including:

- people who have spent time with someone who has TB disease

- people from a country where TB disease is common (most countries in Latin America, the Caribbean, Africa, Asia, Eastern Europe, and Russia)
- people who live or work in high-risk settings (e.g., correctional facilities, long-term care facilities or nursing homes, and homeless shelters)
- health-care workers who care for patients at increased risk for TB disease
- infants, children, and adolescents exposed to adults who are at increased risk for LTBI or TB disease

TESTING FOR TUBERCULOSIS INFECTION

There are two types of tests for TB infection: the TST and the TB blood test. A person's health-care provider should choose which TB test to use. Factors in selecting which test to use include the reason for testing, test availability, and cost. Generally, it is not recommended to test a person with both a TST and a TB blood test.

Tuberculosis Skin Test

ADMINISTERING THE TUBERCULOSIS SKIN TEST

The TST is also called the "Mantoux tuberculin skin test" (TST). A TST requires two visits with a health-care provider.

On the first visit, the test is placed; on the second visit, the health-care provider reads the test.

- The TST is performed by injecting a small amount of fluid (called "tuberculin") into the skin on the lower part of the arm.
- A person given the tuberculin skin test must return within 48–72 hours to have a trained health-care worker look for a reaction on the arm.
- The result depends on the size of the raised, hard area or swelling.

A positive skin test means the person's body was infected with TB bacteria. Additional tests are needed to determine if the person has LTBI or TB disease.

A negative skin test means the person's body did not react to the test and that LTBI or TB disease is not likely.

There is no problem in repeating a TST. If repeated, the additional test should be placed in a different location on the body (e.g., other arm). The TST is the preferred TB test for children under age five.

Tuberculosis Blood Test

The TB blood tests are also called "interferon-gamma release assays" (IGRAs).

Two TB blood tests are approved by the U.S. Food and Drug Administration (FDA) and are available in the United States: the QuantiFERON®-TB Gold Plus (QFT-Plus) and the T-SPOT®.TB test (T-Spot). A health-care provider will draw a patient's blood and send it to a laboratory for analysis and results.

- **Positive TB blood test.** This means that the person has been infected with TB bacteria. Additional tests are needed to determine if the person has LTBI or TB disease.
- **Negative TB blood test.** This means that the person's blood did not react to the test and that LTBI or TB disease is not likely.

TB blood tests are the preferred TB test for:

- people who have received the TB vaccine bacille Calmette-Guérin (BCG)
- people who have a difficult time returning for a second appointment to look for a reaction to the TST

Testing in Bacille Calmette-Guérin-Vaccinated Persons

Many people born outside the United States have been given a vaccine called "BCG." People who were previously vaccinated with BCG may receive a TST to test for TB infection. Vaccination with BCG may cause a false positive reaction to a TST. A positive reaction to a TST may be due to the BCG vaccine itself or due to infection with TB bacteria.

The TB blood tests (IGRAs), unlike the TST, are not affected by prior BCG vaccination and are not expected to give a false-positive result in people who have received BCG. TB blood tests are the preferred method of TB testing for people who have received the BCG vaccine.

TREATMENT FOR LATENT TUBERCULOSIS INFECTION AND TUBERCULOSIS DISEASE

Not everyone infected with TB bacteria becomes sick. As a result, two TB-related conditions exist: LTBI and TB disease. Both LTBI and TB disease can be treated.

Without treatment, LTBI can progress to TB disease. If not treated properly, TB disease can be fatal. Directly observed therapy (DOT) helps people with TB complete treatment.

Treatment Regimens for Latent Tuberculosis Infection

There are several treatment regimens recommended in the United States for LTBI. The medications used to treat LTBI include the following:

- isoniazid (INH)
- rifapentine (RPT)
- rifampin (RIF)

The Centers for Disease Control and Prevention (CDC) and the National Tuberculosis Controllers Association (NTCA) preferentially recommend short-course, rifamycin-based, three- or four-month LTBI treatment regimens over six- or nine-month isoniazid monotherapy. Short-course regimens include the following:

- three months of once-weekly isoniazid plus rifapentine (3HP)
- four months of daily rifampin (4R)
- three months of daily isoniazid plus rifampin (3HR)

Short-course treatment regimens, such as 3HP and 4R, are effective and safe and have higher completion rates than longer six to nine months of isoniazid monotherapy (6H/9H). Shorter, rifamycin-based treatment regimens generally have a lower risk of hepatotoxicity than 6H and 9H.

If short-course treatment regimens are not a feasible or available option, 6H and 9H are alternative, effective LTBI treatment regimens. Although effective, 6H and 9H have higher toxicity risk and lower treatment completion rates than most short-term treatment regimens.

All treatments must be modified if the patient is in contact with an individual with drug-resistant TB disease. Clinicians should choose the appropriate treatment regimen based on drug susceptibility results of the presumed source case (if known), coexisting medical conditions (e.g., HIV), and potential for drug–drug interactions. Consultation with a TB expert is advised if the known source of TB infection has drug-resistant TB.

PREVENTION OF TUBERCULOSIS

Preventing Latent Tuberculosis Infection from Progressing to Tuberculosis Disease

Many people who have LTBI never develop TB disease. But some people who have LTBI are more likely to develop TB disease than others. Those at high risk for developing TB disease include the following:

- people with HIV infection
- people who became infected with TB bacteria in the last two years
- babies and young children
- people who inject illegal drugs
- people who are sick with other diseases that weaken the immune system
- elderly people
- people who were not treated correctly for TB in the past

If you have LTBI and you are in one of these high-risk groups, you should take medicine to keep from developing TB disease. There are several treatment options for LTBI. You and your health-care provider must decide which treatment is best for you. If you take your medicine as instructed, it can keep you from developing TB disease. Because there are fewer bacteria, treatment for LTBI is much easier than treatment for TB disease. A person with TB disease has a large amount of TB bacteria in the body. Several drugs are needed to treat TB disease.

Preventing Exposure to Tuberculosis Disease While Traveling Abroad

In many countries, TB is much more common than in the United States. Travelers should avoid close contact or prolonged time with known TB patients in crowded, enclosed environments (e.g., clinics, hospitals, prisons, or homeless shelters).

Although multidrug-resistant (MDR) and extensively drug-resistant (XDR) TB are occurring globally, they are still rare. HIV-infected travelers are at greatest risk if they come in contact with a person with MDR or XDR TB.

Air travel itself carries a relatively low risk of infection with TB of any kind. Travelers who will be working in clinics, hospitals, or other health-care settings where TB patients are likely to be encountered should consult infection control or occupational health experts. They should ask about administrative and environmental procedures for preventing exposure to TB. Once those procedures are implemented, additional measures could include using personal respiratory protective devices.

Travelers who anticipate possible prolonged exposure to people with TB (e.g., those who expect to come in contact routinely with clinic, hospital, prison, or homeless shelter populations) should have a TST or a TB blood test before leaving the United States. If the test reaction is negative, they should have a repeat test 8–10 weeks after returning to the United States. Additionally, annual testing may be recommended for those who anticipate repeated or prolonged exposure or an extended stay over a period of years. Because people with HIV infection are more likely to have an impaired response to TB tests, travelers who are HIV positive should tell their physicians about their HIV infection status.

VACCINES FOR TUBERCULOSIS

Tuberculosis Vaccine

BCG is a vaccine for TB disease. This vaccine is not widely used in the United States, but it is often given to infants and small children in other countries where TB is common. BCG does not always protect people from getting TB.

Bacille Calmette-Guérin Recommendations

In the United States, BCG should be considered only for very selected people who meet specific criteria and in consultation with a TB expert. Health-care providers who are considering BCG vaccination for their patients are encouraged to discuss this intervention with the TB control program in their area.

Children

BCG vaccination should only be considered for children who have a negative TB test and who are continually exposed, and they cannot be separated from adults who:

- are untreated or ineffectively treated for TB disease, and the child cannot be given long-term primary preventive treatment for TB infection
- have TB disease caused by strains resistant to isoniazid and rifampin

Health-Care Workers

BCG vaccination of health-care workers should be considered on an individual basis in settings in which:

- a high percentage of TB patients are infected with TB strains resistant to both isoniazid and rifampin
- there is an ongoing transmission of drug-resistant TB strains to health-care workers, and subsequent infection is likely
- comprehensive TB infection-control precautions have been implemented but have not been successful

Health-care workers considered for BCG vaccination should be counseled regarding the risks and benefits associated with both BCG vaccination and the treatment of LTBI.

Testing for Tuberculosis in Bacille Calmette-Guérin-Vaccinated People

Many people born outside the United States have been BCG-vaccinated. People who were previously vaccinated with BCG may receive a TST to test for TB infection. Vaccination with BCG may cause a positive reaction to a TST. A positive reaction to a TST may be due to the BCG vaccine itself or due to infection with TB bacteria.

Tuberculosis blood tests (IGRAs), unlike the TST, are not affected by prior BCG vaccination and are not expected to give a false-positive result in people who have received BCG.

For children under age five, the TST is preferred over TB blood tests. A positive TST or TB blood test only tells that a person has been infected with TB bacteria. It does not tell whether the person has LTBI or has progressed to TB disease. Other tests, such as a chest x-ray and a sample of sputum, are needed to see whether the person has TB disease.[1]

[1] "Basic TB Facts," Centers for Disease Control and Prevention (CDC), May 3, 2022. Available online. URL: www.cdc.gov/tb/topic/basics/default.htm. Accessed July 13, 2023.

Chapter 46 | Typhoid and Paratyphoid Fever

WHAT IS TYPHOID FEVER?

Typhoid fever and paratyphoid fever are similar diseases caused by bacteria. *Salmonella* Typhi bacteria cause typhoid fever. *Salmonella* Paratyphi bacteria cause paratyphoid fever.

People infected with these bacteria can spread them to others. This typically happens when an infected person uses the bathroom and does not wash their hands. The bacteria can stay on their hands and contaminate everything that the person touches, including food and drinks.

In countries with poor sanitation, the water used to rinse and prepare food and beverages, including tap water, can also be contaminated with these bacteria. Travelers who eat foods or drink beverages contaminated with these bacteria can then get sick.

Typhoid fever and paratyphoid fever cause similar symptoms. People with these diseases usually have a fever that can be as high as 103–104 °F (39–40 °C). They may also have weakness, stomach pain, headache, diarrhea or constipation, cough, and loss of appetite. Some people have a rash of flat, rose-colored spots. Internal bleeding and death can occur but are rare.

WHO IS AT RISK?

Typhoid and paratyphoid fever are most common in parts of the world where water and food may be unsafe and sanitation is poor. Travelers to Eastern and Southern Asia (especially Pakistan, India, and Bangladesh), Africa, the Caribbean, Central and South America, and the Middle East are at increased risk for typhoid and paratyphoid fever.

People visiting friends or relatives are more likely than other travelers to get typhoid fever because they may stay in the country longer, may be less cautious about the food they eat or the beverages they drink because they eat local food prepared in people's homes, and may not think about getting vaccinated before traveling.

In the United States each year, about 425 people are diagnosed with typhoid fever, and about 125 people are diagnosed with paratyphoid fever each year. Most of these people traveled internationally.

WHAT CAN TRAVELERS DO TO PREVENT TYPHOID FEVER?

Getting vaccinated, choosing food and drinks carefully, and washing your hands are the best ways to avoid getting typhoid. Check if the typhoid fever vaccination is recommended for your destination. Two typhoid vaccines are available in the United States. Visit your doctor or a travel clinic at least one month before traveling to discuss your options.

- **Pill vaccine**. People aged six and older can take the pill vaccine. Finish taking all four pills (one pill every other day) at least one week before travel.
- **Shot vaccine**. People aged two and older can get the shot vaccine. Get one shot (or a booster shot) at least two weeks before travel.

Typhoid vaccines are only 50–80 percent effective, so you should still be careful about what you eat and drink to lower your risk of getting typhoid fever. Also, there is no vaccine that protects against paratyphoid fever. For these reasons, it is very important that you also take the following steps to prevent typhoid.

Choose Food and Drinks Carefully

- Only eat foods that are cooked and served hot.
- Avoid food that has been sitting on a buffet.
- Eat raw fruits and vegetables only if you have washed them in clean water or peeled them.
- Only drink beverages from factory-sealed containers.

Typhoid and Paratyphoid Fever

- Avoid ice because it may have been made from unsafe water.
- Only drink pasteurized milk.

Wash Your Hands

- Wash hands often with soap and water for 20 seconds, especially after using the bathroom and before eating.
- If soap and water are not readily available, use an alcohol-based hand sanitizer with at least 60 percent alcohol.
- Keep your hands away from your face and mouth.[1]

[1] "Typhoid Fever," Centers for Disease Control and Prevention (CDC), June 2, 2023. Available online. URL: wwwnc.cdc.gov/travel/diseases/typhoid. Accessed July 13, 2023.

Chapter 47 | Vaginal and Reproductive Tract Infections

WHAT IS BACTERIAL VAGINOSIS?

Bacterial vaginosis (BV) is a condition caused by changes in the amount of certain types of bacteria in your vagina. BV can develop when your vagina has more harmful bacteria than good bacteria.

Who Gets Bacterial Vaginosis?

BV is the most common vaginal condition in women aged 15–44. But women of any age can get it, even if they have never had sex. You may be more at risk for BV if you:

- have a new sex partner
- have multiple sex partners
- douche
- do not use condoms or dental dams
- are pregnant (BV is common during pregnancy. About one in four pregnant women get BV. The risk for BV is higher for pregnant women because of the hormonal changes that happen during pregnancy.)
- are African American (BV is twice as common in African-American women as in White women.)
- have an intrauterine device (IUD), especially if you also have irregular bleeding

How Do You Get Bacterial Vaginosis?

Researchers are still studying how women get BV. You can get BV without having sex, but BV is more common in women who are sexually active. Having a new sex partner or multiple sex partners, as well as douching, can upset the balance of good and harmful bacteria in your vagina. This raises your risk of getting BV.

What Are the Symptoms of Bacterial Vaginosis?

Many women have no symptoms. If you do have symptoms, they may include the following:

- unusual vaginal discharge, which can be white (milky) or gray and may also be foamy or watery (Some women report a strong fish-like odor, especially after sex.)
- burning when urinating
- itching around the outside of the vagina
- vaginal irritation

These symptoms may be similar to vaginal yeast infections and other health problems. Only your doctor or nurse can tell you for sure whether you have BV.

How Is Bacterial Vaginosis Diagnosed?

There are tests to find out if you have BV. Your doctor or nurse takes a sample of vaginal discharge. Your doctor or nurse may then look at the sample under a microscope, use an in-office test, or send it to a lab to check for harmful bacteria. Your doctor or nurse may also see signs of BV during an exam. Before you see a doctor or nurse for a test:

- do not douche or use vaginal deodorant sprays as they might cover odors that can help your doctor diagnose BV and can also irritate your vagina
- make an appointment for a day when you do not have your period

How Is Bacterial Vaginosis Treated?

BV is treated with antibiotics prescribed by your doctor. If you get BV, your male sex partner will not need to be treated. But, if you are female and have a female sex partner, she might also have BV. If your current partner is female, she needs to see her doctor. She may also need treatment.

It is also possible to get BV again. Learn how to lower your risk for BV. BV and vaginal yeast infections are treated differently. BV is treated with antibiotics prescribed by your doctor. Yeast infections can be treated with over-the-counter (OTC) medicines. But you cannot treat BV with OTC yeast infection medicine.

What Should You Do If You Have Bacterial Vaginosis?

BV is easy to treat. If you think you have BV, do the following:

- See a doctor or nurse. Antibiotics will treat BV.
- Take all of your medicine. Even if symptoms go away, you need to finish all of the antibiotics.
- Tell your sex partner(s) if she is female, so she can be treated.
- Avoid sexual contact until you finish your treatment.
- See your doctor or nurse again if you have symptoms that do not go away within a few days after finishing the antibiotic.

How Can You Lower Your Risk of Bacterial Vaginosis?

Researchers do not know exactly how BV spreads. Steps that might lower your risk of BV include the following:

- **Keeping your vaginal bacteria balanced.** Use warm water only to clean the outside of your vagina. You do not need to use soap. Even mild soap can cause irritate your vagina. Always wipe front to back from your vagina to your anus. Keep the area cool by wearing cotton or cotton-lined underpants.
- **Not douching.** Douching upsets the balance of good and harmful bacteria in your vagina. This may raise your risk of BV. It may also make it easier to get BV again after treatment. Doctors do not recommend douching.

- **Not having sex.** Researchers are still studying how women get BV. You can get BV without having sex, but BV is more common in women who have sex.
- **Limiting your number of sex partners.** Researchers think that your risk of getting BV goes up with the number of partners you have.[1]

WHAT IS PELVIC INFLAMMATORY DISEASE?

Pelvic inflammatory disease (PID) is an infection of a woman's reproductive organs. The reproductive organs include the uterus (womb), fallopian tubes, ovaries, and cervix. PID can be caused by many different types of bacteria. Usually, PID is caused by bacteria from sexually transmitted infections (STIs). Sometimes, PID is caused by normal bacteria found in the vagina.

Who Gets Pelvic Inflammatory Disease?

PID affects about 5 percent of women in the United States. Your risk for PID is higher if you:

- have had an STI
- have had PID before
- are under age 25 and have sex (PID is most common in women 15–24 years old.)
- have more than one sex partner or have a partner who has multiple sexual partners
- douche (Douching can push bacteria into the reproductive organs and cause PID. Douching can also hide the signs of PID.)
- recently had an IUD inserted (The risk of PID is higher for the first few weeks only after insertion of an IUD, but PID is rare after that. Getting tested for STIs before the IUD is inserted lowers your risk for PID.)

[1] Office on Women's Health (OWH), "Bacterial Vaginosis," U.S. Department of Health and Human Services (HHS), May 31, 2022. Available online. URL: www.womenshealth.gov/a-z-topics/bacterial-vaginosis. Accessed July 14, 2023.

How Do You Get Pelvic Inflammatory Disease?

A woman can get PID if bacteria move up from her vagina or cervix and into her reproductive organs. Many different types of bacteria can cause PID. Most often, PID is caused by infection from two common STIs: gonorrhea and chlamydia. The number of women with PID has dropped in recent years. This may be because more women are getting tested regularly for chlamydia and gonorrhea.

You can also get PID without having an STI. Normal bacteria in the vagina can travel into a woman's reproductive organs and can sometimes cause PID. Sometimes, the bacteria travel up to a woman's reproductive organs because of douching. Do not douche. No doctor or nurse recommends douching.

What Are the Signs and Symptoms of Pelvic Inflammatory Disease?

Many women do not know they have PID because they do not have any signs or symptoms. When symptoms do happen, they can be mild or more serious. Signs and symptoms include the following:

- pain in the lower abdomen (which is the most common symptom)
- fever (100.4 °F (38 °C) or higher)
- vaginal discharge that may smell foul
- painful sex
- pain when urinating
- irregular menstrual periods
- pain in the upper right abdomen (this is rare)

PID can come on fast, with extreme pain and fever, especially if it is caused by gonorrhea.

How Is Pelvic Inflammatory Disease Diagnosed?

To diagnose PID, doctors usually do a physical exam to check for signs of PID and test for STIs. If you think that you may have PID, see a doctor or nurse as soon as possible. If you have pain in your lower abdomen, your doctor or nurse will check for:

- unusual discharge from your vagina or cervix
- an abscess (collection of pus) near your ovaries or fallopian tubes
- tenderness or pain in your reproductive organs

Your doctor may do tests to find out whether you have PID or a different problem that looks like PID. These can include the following:

- tests for STIs, especially gonorrhea and chlamydia, which can cause PID
- a test for a urinary tract infection or other conditions that can cause pelvic pain
- ultrasound or another imaging test, so your doctor can look at your internal organs for signs of PID

A Papanicolaou (Pap) test is not used to detect PID.

How Is Pelvic Inflammatory Disease Treated?

Your doctor or nurse will give you antibiotics to treat PID. Most of the time, at least two antibiotics are used that work against many different types of bacteria. You must take all of your antibiotics, even if your symptoms go away. This helps make sure the infection is fully cured. See your doctor or nurse again two to three days after starting the antibiotics to make sure they are working.

Your doctor or nurse may suggest going to the hospital to treat your PID if:

- you are very sick
- you are pregnant
- your symptoms do not go away after taking the antibiotics or if you cannot swallow pills (If this is the case, you will need IV antibiotics.)
- you have an abscess in a fallopian tube or ovary

If you still have symptoms or if the abscess does not go away after treatment, you may need surgery. Problems caused by PID, such as chronic pelvic pain and scarring, are often hard to treat. But sometimes, they get better after surgery.

How Can You Prevent Pelvic Inflammatory Disease?

You may not be able to prevent PID. It is not always caused by an STI. Sometimes, normal bacteria in your vagina can travel up to your reproductive organs and cause PID. But you can lower your risk of PID by not douching. You can also prevent STIs by not having vaginal, oral, or anal sex. If you do have sex, lower your risk of getting an STI with the following steps:

- **Use condoms.** Condoms are the best way to prevent STIs when you have sex. Because a man does not need to ejaculate (come) to give or get STIs, make sure to put the condom on before the penis touches the vagina, mouth, or anus. Other methods of birth control, such as birth control pills, shots, implants, or diaphragms, will not protect you from STIs.
- **Get tested.** Be sure you and your partner are tested for STIs. Talk to each other about the test results before you have sex.
- **Be monogamous.** Having sex with just one partner can lower your risk for STIs. After being tested for STIs, be faithful to each other. That means that you have sex only with each other and no one else.
- **Limit your number of sex partners.** Your risk of getting STIs goes up with the number of partners you have.
- **Do not douche.** Douching removes some of the normal bacteria in the vagina that protect you from infection. Douching may also raise your risk for PID by helping bacteria travel to other areas, such as your uterus, ovaries, and fallopian tubes.

- **Do not abuse alcohol or drugs.** Drinking too much alcohol or using drugs increases risky behavior and may put you at risk of sexual assault and possible exposure to STIs.

The steps work best when used together. No single step can protect you from every single type of STI.[2]

[2] Office on Women's Health (OWH), "Pelvic Inflammatory Disease," U.S. Department of Health and Human Services (HHS), December 30, 2022. Available online. URL: www.womenshealth.gov/a-z-topics/pelvic-inflammatory-disease. Accessed July 14, 2023.

Chapter 48 | Vancomycin-Resistant Enterococci Infection

Enterococci are bacteria (germs) that are normally present in the human intestines and in the female genital tract and are often found in the environment, such as in soil and water. These bacteria can cause infections.

Enterococci bacteria are constantly finding new ways to avoid the effects of the antibiotics used to treat the infections they cause. Antibiotic resistance occurs when the germs no longer respond to the antibiotics designed to kill them. If these germs develop resistance to vancomycin, an antibiotic that is used to treat some drug-resistant infections, they become vancomycin-resistant enterococci (VRE).

HOW COMMON ARE THESE INFECTIONS?

In 2017, VRE caused an estimated 54,500 infections among hospitalized patients and 5,400 estimated deaths in the United States.

WHO IS AT RISK?

Those most likely to be infected include the following:

- people who have been previously treated with antibiotics, including vancomycin, for long periods of time
- people who are hospitalized, have undergone surgical procedures, or have medical devices inserted in their bodies (such as catheters)

- people with weakened immune systems, such as patients in intensive care units or in cancer or transplant wards

HOW IS IT SPREAD?

Vancomycin-resistant enterococci can spread from one person to another through contact with contaminated surfaces or equipment or through person-to-person spread, often via contaminated hands. It is not spread through the air by coughing or sneezing.

HOW CAN YOU AVOID GETTING AN INFECTION?

If you or someone in your household has VRE, you can protect yourself by:

- keeping your hands clean to avoid getting sick and spreading germs that can cause infections:
  - Patients and their caregivers should wash their hands with soap and water or use alcohol-based hand sanitizer, particularly:
    - after using the bathroom
    - before and after handling medical devices or caring for wounds
    - before preparing food
- frequently cleaning areas of the home, such as bathrooms, that may become contaminated with VRE
- wearing gloves if hands may come in contact with body fluids that may contain VRE, such as stool (poop) or bandages from infected wounds:
  - Always wash your hands after removing gloves.
- informing health-care providers if you or someone you care for has VRE so that appropriate precautions can be taken to prevent the spread

HOW ARE THESE INFECTIONS TREATED?

When VRE infections do develop, they are generally treated with antibiotics other than vancomycin. In order to identify the best antibiotic to treat a specific infection, health-care providers will send a specimen (often called a "culture") to the laboratory and test any bacteria that grow against a set of antibiotics to determine which are active against the germ. The provider will then select an antibiotic based on the activity of the antibiotic and other factors, such as potential side effects or interactions with other drugs.

Some people will carry VRE on their body without it causing symptoms, which is called being colonized. People who are colonized do not require antibiotics.

WHAT IS THE CDC DOING TO ADDRESS VANCOMYCIN-RESISTANT ENTEROCOCCI INFECTIONS?

The Centers for Disease Control and Prevention (CDC) tracks VRE infections using data from several sources, including the National Healthcare Safety Network Patient Safety Component. This surveillance system collects reports of VRE from device-associated infections, such as central-line-associated bloodstream infections.

The CDC works with health-care facilities and state and local health departments to control outbreaks of resistant germs such as VRE and to help devise and implement prevention strategies for facilities with high numbers of VRE infections.[1]

[1] "Vancomycin-Resistant Enterococci (VRE) in Healthcare Settings," Centers for Disease Control and Prevention (CDC), November 13, 2019. Available online. URL: www.cdc.gov/hai/organisms/vre/vre.html. Accessed July 13, 2023.

Chapter 49 | Whooping Cough

Whooping cough (pertussis) can cause serious illness in people of all ages but is most dangerous for babies. Getting vaccinated is the best way to protect against pertussis. Make sure you and your loved ones are up-to-date with your whooping cough vaccines.

CAUSES AND HOW WHOOPING COUGH SPREADS

Whooping cough is a very contagious respiratory illness that spreads from person to person.

Causes of Whooping Cough

Whooping cough, also known as "pertussis," is a very contagious respiratory illness caused by a type of bacteria called "*Bordetella pertussis*." The disease is only found in humans.

Whooping cough bacteria attach to the cilia (tiny, hair-like extensions) that line part of the upper respiratory system. The bacteria release toxins (poisons), which damage the cilia and cause airways to swell.

How It Spreads

The bacteria that cause whooping cough spread easily from person to person through the air. When a person who has whooping cough sneezes or coughs, they can release small particles with the bacteria in them. Other people then breathe in the bacteria. It also spreads when people spend a lot of time together or share breathing space, such as when you hold a newborn on your chest.

PEOPLE CAN BE CONTAGIOUS FOR WEEKS

People can spread the bacteria from the start of the very first symptoms and for at least two weeks after coughing begins. Taking antibiotics early in the illness may shorten the amount of time someone is contagious.

PEOPLE CAN SPREAD THE DISEASE EVEN IF THEY DO NOT KNOW THEY HAVE IT

Some people have mild symptoms and do not know they have whooping cough, but they can still spread the bacteria to others. Many babies who get whooping cough are infected by older siblings, parents, or caregivers who do not know they have it.

SIGNS AND SYMPTOMS

Whooping cough may begin like a common cold, but unlike a cold, the coughing can last for weeks or months.

Symptoms of whooping cough usually develop within 5–10 days after you come into contact with the bacteria that cause it. Sometimes, symptoms do not develop for as long as three weeks.

Early Symptoms: Stage 1

Early symptoms can last for one to two weeks and usually include the following:

- runny or stuffed-up nose
- low-grade fever (less than 100.4 °F (38 °C))
- mild, occasional cough (Babies do not do this.)
- apnea (life-threatening pauses in breathing) and cyanosis (turning blue or purple) in babies and young children

In its early stages, whooping cough appears to be nothing more than the common cold. Therefore, doctors often do not suspect or diagnose it until more severe symptoms appear.

Later Symptoms: Stage 2

One to two weeks after the first symptoms start, people with whooping cough may develop paroxysms—rapid, violent, and uncontrolled coughing fits. These coughing fits usually last one to six weeks but can last for up to 10 weeks. Coughing fits generally get worse and become more common as the illness continues.

Coughing fits can cause people to:

- make a high-pitched "whoop" sound when they are finally able to inhale at the end of a coughing fit
- vomit during or after coughing fits
- feel very tired after the fit but usually seem well in between fits
- struggle to breathe

Babies may struggle to breathe, while teens and adults usually have mild symptoms. Many babies with whooping cough do not cough at all. Instead, it may cause them to turn blue or struggle to breathe. It may seem like a common cold for the entire illness, not just the beginning.

The infection is generally milder in teens and adults than in babies and children, especially those who have gotten vaccinated against whooping cough. It may seem like a common cold. The "whoop" is often not there for people who have a milder illness.

However, teens and adults can have serious cases of whooping cough. Teens and adults, especially those who did not get whooping cough vaccines, may have lengthy coughing fits that keep them up at night. Those who get these coughing fits say it is the worst cough of their lives. It can also cause major disruptions to daily life and serious complications.

VACCINATED PEOPLE MAY NOT GET AS SICK

Whooping cough vaccines are effective, but not perfect. The infection is usually not as bad for people who have gotten vaccinated against whooping cough but still get sick. In vaccinated people who get whooping cough:

- the cough usually will not last as many days
- coughing fits, whooping, and vomiting after coughing fits are less common
- apnea and cyanosis are less common (in vaccinated babies and children)

The Centers for Disease Control and Prevention (CDC) recommends whooping cough vaccines for people of all ages.

Recovery: Stage 3

Recovery from whooping cough can be slow. The cough becomes milder and less common as you get better. Coughing fits may stop for a while but can return if you get other respiratory infections. Coughing fits can return many months after the whooping cough illness starts. Figure 49.1 shows the progression of whooping cough disease.

COMPLICATIONS OF WHOOPING COUGH

Whooping cough (pertussis) can cause complications in people of all ages. Some people will get serious complications and need care in the hospital. Serious and sometimes deadly complications are more likely in babies under a year old.

Babies and Children

Whooping cough can cause serious and sometimes deadly complications in babies and young children. Babies and children who

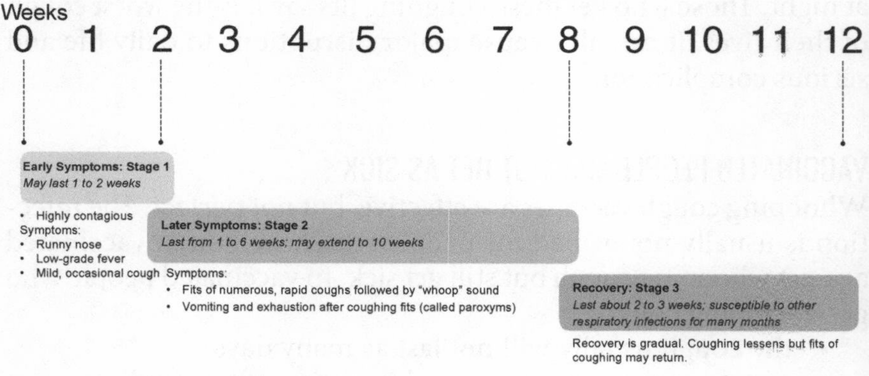

Figure 49.1. Whooping Cough Disease Progression

Centers for Disease Control and Prevention (CDC)

have not had all recommended whooping cough vaccines are more likely to get serious complications.

About one-third of babies younger than one year who get whooping cough need care in the hospital. The younger the baby, the more likely they will need treatment in the hospital. Of those babies younger than one year old who are treated in the hospital with whooping cough, about:

- 2 in 3 (68%) will have apnea (life-threatening pauses in breathing)
- 1 in 5 (22%) will get pneumonia (lung infection)
- 1 in 50 (2%) will have convulsions (violent, uncontrolled shaking)
- 1 in 150 (0.6%) will have encephalopathy (disease of the brain)
- 1 in 100 (1%) will die

Teens and Adults

Teens and adults can also get complications, such as pneumonia, from whooping cough. If they have a severe cough, teens and adults can:

- pass out
- fracture (break) a rib
- lose bladder control
- lose weight

Complications are usually less serious in this older age group, especially in those who have been vaccinated against whooping cough. However, if complications are serious, some people may need care in the hospital.

DIAGNOSIS AND TREATMENT OF WHOOPING COUGH

Treating whooping cough (pertussis) early with antibiotics may make the infection less serious and help prevent the spread of the bacteria that cause it to others.

See a doctor if you think you or your child may have whooping cough.

Diagnosis of Whooping Cough

Doctors diagnose whooping cough by considering if you have been in contact with someone who has whooping cough and by doing a:

- history of typical signs and symptoms
- physical exam
- laboratory test of a mucus sample from the back of the throat
- blood test

Treatment of Whooping Cough

Doctors generally treat whooping cough with antibiotics. There are several antibiotics available to treat whooping cough. It is very important to treat whooping cough early before coughing fits begin. Treating whooping cough early can:

- make the illness less serious
- help prevent the spreading of the bacteria that cause it to others

Starting treatment after three weeks of illness is unlikely to help even though most people will still have symptoms. By then, your body has gotten rid of the bacteria, but the symptoms are still there due to the damage already done to your body.

MANAGING SYMPTOMS AT HOME

Manage whooping cough symptoms and reduce the risk of spreading the bacteria to others.

- Take antibiotics exactly as prescribed by the doctor.
- Keep your home free from irritants—as much as possible—that can trigger coughing, such as smoke, dust, and chemical fumes.
- Use a clean, cool mist humidifier to help loosen mucus and soothe the cough.
- Wash hands often with soap and water for at least 20 seconds.
- Eat small meals every few hours to help prevent vomiting.

- Get plenty of fluids, including water, juices, and soups, and fruits to prevent dehydration (lack of fluids).
- Do not take cough medicine unless your doctor recommends them. Giving cough medicine probably will not help and is often not recommended for children younger than four years.

Report signs of dehydration to your doctor immediately. Signs of dehydration include the following:

- dry, sticky mouth
- sleepiness or tiredness
- thirst
- decreased urination or fewer wet diapers
- few or no tears when crying
- muscle weakness
- headache
- dizziness or light-headedness

GETTING TREATMENT IN A HOSPITAL

Whooping cough can sometimes be very serious and can cause complications, especially for babies. People with serious illnesses or complications need care in the hospital. About a third of babies younger than one year who get whooping cough need care in the hospital. Hospital treatment of whooping cough usually focuses on:

- keeping breathing passages clear, which may require suctioning (drawing out) mucus
- monitoring breathing and giving oxygen, if needed
- preventing or treating dehydration (People might need intravenous (IV, through the vein) fluids if they show signs of dehydration or have difficulty eating.)

PREVENTION OF WHOOPING COUGH

Whooping cough (pertussis) is a highly contagious respiratory illness that is making a comeback in the United States.

Vaccines

The best way to prevent whooping cough is to get vaccinated. Two vaccines in the United States help prevent whooping cough: diphtheria, tetanus, and pertussis (DTaP) and tetanus, diphtheria, and pertussis (Tdap). These vaccines also provide protection against tetanus and diphtheria. These vaccines cannot give you whooping cough, tetanus, or diphtheria.

Preventive Antibiotics

Preventive antibiotics, also known as "postexposure antimicrobial prophylaxis" (PEP), are medicines given to someone who has been exposed to a harmful bacterium in order to help prevent them from getting sick.

Doctors and local health departments generally determine who should get preventive antibiotics. For people exposed to whooping cough, the CDC recommends preventive antibiotics only if they:

- live with a person who has been diagnosed with whooping cough
- are at increased risk for serious disease (e.g., babies, people with certain medical conditions) or will have close contact with someone who is at increased risk for serious disease (e.g., women in their third trimester of pregnancy, people who work with or care for high-risk individuals)

If you have been exposed to the bacteria that cause whooping cough, talk to your doctor about whether you need preventive antibiotics. This is especially important if there is a baby or pregnant woman in your household or if you plan to have contact with a baby or pregnant woman.

Good Hygiene

The CDC recommends practicing good hygiene to prevent the spread of the bacteria that cause whooping cough and other respiratory illnesses.

COVER YOUR COUGH OR SNEEZE

- Cover your mouth and nose with a tissue when you cough or sneeze.
- Throw away used tissues in the wastebasket right away.
- Cough or sneeze into your upper sleeve or elbow if you do not have a tissue. Never cough into your hands because you can spread germs this way.

WASH YOUR HANDS OFTEN

- Wash your hands often with soap and water for at least 20 seconds.
- Use an alcohol-based hand sanitizer if soap and water are not available.

Temporary Immunity after Getting Sick

People who have had whooping cough have some natural immunity (protection) to future whooping cough infections. Getting sick with whooping cough does not provide lifelong protection.

The CDC recommends whooping cough vaccination even if you have had the disease before since natural immunity fades and does not offer lifelong protection.[1]

[1] "Pertussis (Whooping Cough)," Centers for Disease Control and Prevention (CDC), August 8, 2022. Available online. URL: www.cdc.gov/pertussis/index.html. Accessed July 13, 2023.

Part 4 | Parasitic and Fungal Contagious Diseases

Chapter 50 | Amebiasis

WHAT IS AMEBIASIS?

Amebiasis is a disease caused by a one-celled parasite called "*Entamoeba histolytica*."

WHO IS AT RISK FOR AMEBIASIS?

Although anyone can have this disease, it is more common in people who live in tropical areas with poor sanitary conditions. In the United States, amebiasis is most common in:

- people who have traveled to tropical places that have poor sanitary conditions
- immigrants from tropical countries that have poor sanitary conditions
- people who live in institutions that have poor sanitary conditions
- men who have sex with men (MSM)

HOW CAN YOU BECOME INFECTED WITH *ENTAMOEBA* HISTOLYTICA?

Entamoeba histolytica infection can occur when a person:

- puts anything into their mouth that has touched the feces (poop) of a person who is infected with *E. histolytica*
- swallows something, such as water or food, that is contaminated with *E. histolytica*
- swallows *E. histolytica* cysts (eggs) picked up from contaminated surfaces or fingers

WHAT ARE THE SYMPTOMS OF AMEBIASIS?

Only about 10–20 percent of people who are infected with *E. histolytica* become sick from the infection. The symptoms are often quite mild and can include loose feces (poop), stomach pain, and stomach cramping. An amebic dysentery is a severe form of amebiasis associated with stomach pain, bloody stools (poop), and fever. Rarely, *E. histolytica* invades the liver and forms an abscess (a collection of pus). In a small number of instances, it has been shown to spread to other parts of the body, such as the lungs or brain, but this is very uncommon.

IF YOU SWALLOWED *ENTAMOEBA HISTOLYTICA*, HOW QUICKLY WOULD YOU BECOME SICK?

Only about 10–20 percent of people who are infected with *E. histolytica* become sick from the infection. Those people who do become sick usually develop symptoms within two to four weeks though it can sometimes take longer.

HOW IS AMEBIASIS DIAGNOSED?

Your health-care provider will ask you to submit fecal (poop) samples. Because *E. histolytica* is not always found in every stool sample, you may be asked to submit several stool samples from several different days. Diagnosis of amebiasis can be very difficult. One problem is that other parasites and cells can look very similar to *E. histolytica* when seen under a microscope. Therefore, sometimes, people are told that they are infected with *E. histolytica* even though they are not. *E. histolytica* and another ameba, *Entamoeba dispar*, which is about 10 times more common, look the same when seen under a microscope. Unlike infection with *E. histolytica*, which sometimes makes people sick, infection with *E. dispar* does not make people sick and therefore does not need to be treated. If you have been told that you are infected with *E. histolytica*, but you are feeling fine, you might be infected with *E. dispar* instead. Unfortunately, most laboratories do not yet have the tests that can tell whether a person is infected with *E. histolytica* or with *E. dispar*.

Until these tests become more widely available, it is usually best to assume that the parasite is *E. histolytica.*

A blood test is also available but is only recommended when your health-care provider thinks that your infection may have spread beyond the intestine (gut) to some other organ of your body, such as the liver. However, this blood test may not be helpful in diagnosing your current illness because the test can be positive if you had amebiasis in the past, even if you are not infected now.

HOW IS AMEBIASIS TREATED?

Several antibiotics are available to treat amebiasis. Treatment must be prescribed by a physician. You will be treated with only one antibiotic if your *E. histolytica* infection has not made you sick. You probably will be treated with two antibiotics (first one and then the other) if your infection has made you sick.

WHAT CAN YOU CONSUME IN PLACES WITH POOR SANITATION?

You are going to travel to a country that has poor sanitary conditions. What should you eat and drink there, so you will not become infected with *E. histolytica* or other such germs?

The following items are safe to drink:

- bottled water with an unbroken seal
- tap water that has been boiled for at least 1 minute
- carbonated (bubbly) water from sealed cans or bottles
- carbonated (bubbly) drinks (such as soda) from sealed cans or bottles

You can also make tap water safe for drinking by filtering it through an "absolute 1 micron or less" filter and dissolving chlorine, chlorine dioxide, or iodine tablets in the filtered water. "Absolute 1-micron" filters can be found in camping/outdoor supply stores. The following items may not be safe to drink or eat:

- fountain drinks or any drinks with ice cubes
- fresh fruit or vegetables that you did not peel yourself

- milk, cheese, or dairy products that may not have been pasteurized
- food or drinks sold by street vendors

SHOULD YOU BE CONCERNED ABOUT SPREADING THE INFECTION TO OTHERS?

Yes, but the risk of spreading infection is low if the infected person is treated with antibiotics and practices good personal hygiene. This includes thorough handwashing with soap and water after using the toilet, after changing diapers, and before handling or preparing food.[1]

[1] "Parasites—Amebiasis—*Entamoeba histolytica* Infection," Centers for Disease Control and Prevention (CDC), December 29, 2021. Available online. URL: www.cdc.gov/parasites/amebiasis/index.html. Accessed July 11, 2023.

Chapter 51 | Cryptosporidiosis

WHAT IS CRYPTOSPORIDIOSIS?

Cryptosporidiosis is a disease that causes watery diarrhea. It is caused by microscopic germs—parasites called "*Cryptosporidium*." *Cryptosporidium*, or "Crypto" for short, can be found in water, food, or soil or on surfaces or dirty hands that have been contaminated with the feces of humans or animals infected with the parasite.

During 2001–2010, Crypto was the leading cause of waterborne disease outbreaks, linked to recreational water in the United States. The parasite is found in every region of the United States and throughout the world.

WHAT ARE THE SYMPTOMS OF CRYPTOSPORIDIOSIS?

Symptoms of Crypto generally begin 2–10 days (average 7 days) after becoming infected with the parasite. Symptoms include the following:

- watery diarrhea
- stomach cramps or pain
- dehydration
- nausea
- vomiting
- fever
- weight loss

Symptoms usually last about one to two weeks (with a range of a few days to four or more weeks) in people with healthy immune systems. The most common symptom of cryptosporidiosis is watery diarrhea. Some people with Crypto will have no symptoms at all.

WHO IS MOST AT RISK FOR CRYPTOSPORIDIOSIS?

People who are most likely to become infected with *Cryptosporidium* include the following:

- children who attend childcare centers, including diaper-aged children
- childcare workers
- parents of infected children
- older adults (aged 75 and older)
- people who take care of other people with Crypto
- international travelers
- backpackers, hikers, and campers who drink unfiltered, untreated water
- people who drink from untreated shallow, unprotected wells
- people, including swimmers, who swallow water from contaminated sources
- people who handle infected calves or other ruminants, such as sheep
- people exposed to human poop through sexual contact

Contaminated water might include water that has not been boiled or filtered, as well as contaminated recreational water sources (e.g., swimming pools, lakes, rivers, ponds, and streams). Several community-wide outbreaks have been linked to drinking tap water or recreational water contaminated with *Cryptosporidium*. Crypto's high tolerance to chlorine enables the parasite to survive for long periods of time in chlorinated drinking and swimming pool water. This means anyone swallowing contaminated water could get ill.

Note: Although Crypto can infect all people, some groups are likely to develop more serious illnesses:

- **Young children and pregnant women**. They may be more likely to get dehydrated because of their diarrhea, so they should drink plenty of fluids while ill.
- **People with severely weakened immune systems.** These people are at risk for more serious diseases.

Symptoms may be more severe and could lead to serious or life-threatening illness. Examples of people with weakened immune systems include those with human immunodeficiency virus (HIV)/acquired immunodeficiency syndrome (AIDS), those with inherited diseases that affect the immune system, and cancer and transplant patients who are taking certain immunosuppressive drugs.

HOW IS CRYPTOSPORIDIOSIS DIAGNOSED?

Cryptosporidiosis is a diarrheal disease that is spread through contact with the stool of an infected person or animal. The disease is diagnosed by examining stool samples. People infected with Crypto can shed the parasite irregularly in their poop (e.g., one day they shed the parasite, the next day they do not, the third day they do), so patients may need to give three samples collected on three different days to help make sure that a negative test result is accurate and really means they do not have Crypto. Health-care providers should specifically request testing for Crypto. Routine ova and parasite testing do not normally include Crypto testing.

WHAT IS THE TREATMENT FOR CRYPTOSPORIDIOSIS?

Most people with healthy immune systems will recover from cryptosporidiosis without treatment. The following actions may help relieve symptoms:

- Drink plenty of fluids to remain well-hydrated and avoid dehydration. Serious health problems can occur if the body does not maintain proper fluid levels. For some people, diarrhea can be severe, resulting in hospitalization due to dehydration.
- Maintain a well-balanced diet. Doing so may help speed recovery.
- Avoid beverages that contain caffeine, such as tea, coffee, and many soft drinks.
- Avoid alcohol, as it can lead to dehydration.

Over-the-counter (OTC) antidiarrheal medicine might help slow down diarrhea, but a health-care provider should be consulted before such medicine is taken.

A drug called "nitazoxanide" has been approved by the Centers for Disease Control and Prevention (CDC) for the treatment of diarrhea caused by *Cryptosporidium* in people with healthy immune systems and is available by prescription.

WHAT SHOULD YOU DO IF YOU THINK YOU MIGHT HAVE CRYPTOSPORIDIOSIS?

For diarrhea whose cause has not been determined, the following actions may help relieve symptoms:

- Drink plenty of fluids to remain well-hydrated and avoid dehydration. Serious health problems can occur if the body does not maintain proper fluid levels. For some people, diarrhea can be severe, resulting in hospitalization due to dehydration.
- Maintain a well-balanced diet. Doing so may help speed recovery.
- Avoid beverages that contain caffeine, such as tea, coffee, and many soft drinks.
- Avoid alcohol, as it can lead to dehydration.

HOW IS CRYPTOSPORIDIOSIS SPREAD?

Crypto lives in the gut of infected humans or animals. An infected person or animal sheds Crypto parasites in their poop. An infected person can shed 10,000,000–100,000,000 Crypto germs in a single bowel movement. Shedding of Crypto in poop begins when symptoms such as diarrhea begin and can last for weeks after symptoms stop. Swallowing as few as 10 Crypto germs can cause infection. Crypto can be spread by:

- swallowing recreational water (e.g., the water in swimming pools, fountains, lakes, and rivers) contaminated with Crypto
- Crypto's high tolerance to chlorine enables the parasite to survive for long periods of time in chlorinated drinking and swimming pool water

- drinking untreated water from a lake or river that is contaminated with Crypto
- swallowing water, ice, or beverages contaminated with poop from infected humans or animals
- eating undercooked food or drinking unpasteurized/raw apple cider or milk that gets contaminated with Crypto
- touching your mouth with contaminated hands
- hands that can become contaminated through a variety of activities, such as touching surfaces or objects (e.g., toys, bathroom fixtures, changing tables, diaper pails) that have been contaminated by poop from an infected person, changing diapers, caring for an infected person, and touching an infected animal
- exposure to poop from an infected person through oral–anal sexual contact

Crypto is not spread through contact with blood.

HOW TO PREVENT THE SPREAD OF CRYPTOSPORIDIOSIS

No cleaning method is guaranteed to be completely effective against Crypto. However, you can lower the chance of spreading Crypto by taking the following precautions:

- Wash linens, clothing, dishwasher- or dryer-safe soft toys, and so on soiled with poop or vomit as soon as possible.
  - Flush excess vomit or poop on clothes or objects down the toilet.
  - Use laundry detergent and wash in hot water at 113 °F (45 °C) or hotter for at least 20 minutes or at 122 °F (50 °C) or hotter for at least 5 minutes.
  - Machine dry on the highest heat setting.
- For other household objects and surfaces (e.g., diaper-change areas), do the following:
  - Remove all visible poop.
  - Clean with soap and water.

    - Let dry completely for at least four hours.
    - If possible, expose to direct sunlight for 4 hours.
- Wash your hands with soap and water after cleaning objects or surfaces that could be contaminated with Crypto.[1]

[1] "Cryptosporidiosis—General Information for the Public," Centers for Disease Control and Prevention (CDC), February 8, 2021. Available online. URL: www.cdc.gov/parasites/crypto/general-info.html. Accessed July 11, 2023.

Chapter 52 | Giardiasis

WHAT IS GIARDIASIS?

Giardiasis is a diarrheal disease caused by the microscopic parasite *Giardia duodenalis* (or "*Giardia*" for short). Once a person or animal has been infected with *Giardia*, the parasite lives in the intestines and is passed in stool (poop). Once outside the body, *Giardia* can sometimes survive for weeks or even months. *Giardia* can be found in every region of the United States and around the world.

HOW IS GIARDIASIS SPREAD?

You can get giardiasis if you swallow the *Giardia* parasite (germ). *Giardia*—or poop from people or animals infected with *Giardia*—can contaminate anything it touches. *Giardia* spreads very easily; even getting tiny amounts of poop in your mouth could make you sick.

Giardiasis can be spread by:

- swallowing unsafe food or water contaminated with *Giardia* germs
- having close contact with someone who has giardiasis, particularly in childcare settings
- traveling within areas that have poor sanitation
- exposure to poop through sexual contact from someone who is sick or recently sick with *Giardia*
- transferring *Giardia* germs picked up from contaminated surfaces (such as bathroom handles, changing tables, diaper pails, or toys) into your mouth
- having contact with infected animals or animal environments contaminated with poop

WHAT ARE THE SYMPTOMS OF GIARDIASIS?

Giardia infection (giardiasis) can cause a variety of intestinal symptoms, which include the following:

- diarrhea
- gas
- foul-smelling, greasy poop that can float
- stomach cramps or pain
- upset stomach or nausea
- dehydration

Symptoms of giardiasis generally begin by having two to five loose stools (poop) per day and progressively increasing fatigue. Other less common symptoms include fever, itchy skin, hives, and swelling of the eyes and joints. Over time, giardiasis can also cause weight loss and keep the body from absorbing nutrients it needs, such as fat, lactose, vitamin A, and vitamin B_{12}. Some people with *Giardia* infections have no symptoms at all.

HOW LONG AFTER INFECTION DO SYMPTOMS APPEAR?

Symptoms of giardiasis normally begin one to two weeks after becoming infected.

HOW LONG WILL SYMPTOMS LAST?

Symptoms generally last anywhere from two to six weeks. In people with weakened immune systems (e.g., due to illness such as human immunodeficiency virus (HIV)), symptoms may last longer. Health-care providers can prescribe the appropriate antiparasitic medications to help reduce the amount of time symptoms last.

WHO IS MOST AT RISK OF GETTING GIARDIASIS?

Anyone can become infected with *Giardia*. However, those at greatest risk are:

- people in childcare settings
- people who are in close contact with someone who has the disease

- travelers within areas that have poor sanitation
- people who have contact with poop during sexual activity
- backpackers or campers who drink untreated water from springs, lakes, or rivers
- swimmers who swallow water from swimming pools, hot tubs, splash pads, or untreated recreational water from springs, lakes, or rivers
- people who get their household water from a shallow well
- people with weakened immune systems
- people who have contact with infected animals or animal environments contaminated with poop

HOW IS GIARDIASIS DIAGNOSED?

Contact your health-care provider if you think you may have giardiasis. Your health-care provider will ask you to submit stool (poop) samples to see if you are infected. Because it can be difficult to detect *Giardia*, you may be asked to submit several stool specimens collected over several days to see if you are infected.

WHAT IS THE TREATMENT FOR GIARDIASIS?

Many prescription drugs are available to treat giardiasis. Although *Giardia* can infect all people, infants and pregnant women may be more likely to experience dehydration from diarrhea caused by giardiasis. To prevent dehydration, infants and pregnant women should drink a lot of fluids while sick. Dehydration can be life-threatening for infants, so it is especially important that parents talk to their health-care providers about treatment options for their infants.

TREATMENT FOR CHILDREN DIAGNOSED WITH GIARDIASIS WITHOUT DIARRHEA

Your child may not need treatment if they have no symptoms though it is important to consider that their poop may remain a source of infection for other household members for an uncertain period of time. However, if your child does not have diarrhea but does have other symptoms, such as nausea or upset stomach, tiredness, weight loss, or a lack of hunger, you and your health-care provider may need to consider treatment. The same is true if many family members are sick or if a family member is pregnant and unable to take the most effective medications to treat *Giardia*. Contact your health-care provider for specific treatment recommendations.

CAN YOU GET GIARDIASIS FROM YOUR PRIVATE WELL?

Giardia-contaminated poop can enter groundwater in different ways, including sewage overflows, sewage systems that are not working properly, and polluted stormwater. Wells may be more likely to be contaminated by poop after flooding, particularly if the wells are shallow, have been dug or bored, or have been covered by floodwater for long periods of time. Overused, leaky, or poorly maintained septic systems could contaminate nearby wells with germs from poop, including *Giardia*.

WHAT CAN YOU DO TO PREVENT AND CONTROL GIARDIASIS?

To prevent and control *Giardia* infection, it is important to:

- wash your hands with soap and water during key times, especially:
    - before preparing food or eating
    - after using the bathroom or changing diapers
- avoid eating food and drinking water that might be contaminated with *Giardia* germs:
    - Properly treat water from springs, lakes, or rivers (surface water) while backpacking or camping if no other source of safe water is available.
    - Avoid swallowing water from swimming pools, hot tubs, splash pads, and untreated water from springs, lakes, or rivers (surface water) while swimming.
    - Store, clean, and prepare fruits and vegetables properly.

- practice safe sex by reducing your contact with poop during sex or avoid having sex several weeks after you or your partner has recovered from giardiasis.

CAN YOU GET GIARDIASIS FROM YOUR PET?

The chances of people getting a *Giardia* infection from dogs or cats are small. The type of *Giardia* that infects humans is usually not the same type that infects dogs and cats.[1]

[1] "Parasites—Giardia," Centers for Disease Control and Prevention (CDC), February 26, 2021. Available online. URL: www.cdc.gov/parasites/giardia/general-info.html#anchor_1614258721435. Accessed July 12, 2023.

Chapter 53 | Lice Infestation

Chapter Contents

Section 53.1 | Body Lice

Adult body lice are 2.3–3.6 mm in length. Body lice live and lay eggs on clothing and only move to the skin to feed. Body lice are known to spread disease.

Body lice infestations (pediculosis) are spread most commonly by close person-to-person contact but are generally limited to persons who live under conditions of crowding and poor hygiene (e.g., the homeless, refugees, etc.). Dogs, cats, and other pets do not play a role in the transmission of human lice. Improved hygiene and access to regular changes of clean clothes is the only treatment needed for body lice infestations.

WHAT ARE BODY LICE?

Body lice are parasitic insects that live on clothing and bedding used by infested persons. Body lice frequently lay their eggs on or near the seams of clothing. Body lice must feed on blood and usually only move to the skin to feed. Body lice exist worldwide and infest people of all races. In the United States, actual infestation with body lice tends to occur only in people who do not have access to regular (at least weekly) bathing and changes of clean clothes, including people experiencing homelessness or people residing in shelters.

WHAT DO BODY LICE LOOK LIKE?

Body lice have three forms: the egg (also called a "nit"), the nymph, and the adult.

- **Nit**. Nits are lice eggs. They are generally easy to see in the seams of an infested person's clothing, particularly around the waistline and under the armpits. Body lice nits occasionally may also be attached to body hair. They are oval and usually yellow to white in color. Body lice nits may take one to two weeks to hatch.
- **Nymph**. A nymph is an immature louse that hatches from the nit (egg). A nymph looks like an adult body

louse but is smaller. Nymphs mature into adults about 9–12 days after hatching. To live, the nymph must feed on blood.

- **Adult**. The adult body louse is about the size of a sesame seed, has six legs, and is tan to grayish-white. Females lay eggs. To live, lice must feed on blood. If a louse falls off of a person, it dies within about five to seven days at room temperature.

WHERE ARE BODY LICE FOUND?

Body lice generally are found on clothing and bedding used by infested people. Sometimes, body lice are seen on the body when they feed. Body lice eggs usually are seen in the seams of clothing or on bedding. Occasionally, eggs are attached to body hair. Lice found on the head and scalp are not body lice; they are head lice.

WHAT ARE THE SIGNS AND SYMPTOMS OF BODY LICE?

Intense itching ("pruritus") and rash caused by an allergic reaction to the louse bites are common symptoms of body lice infestation. When body lice infestation has been present for a long time, heavily bitten areas of the skin can become thickened and discolored, particularly around the midsection of the body (waist, groin, or upper thighs).

As with other lice infestations, intense itching can lead to scratching, which can cause sores on the body; these sores sometimes can become infected with bacteria or fungi.

CAN BODY LICE TRANSMIT DISEASE?

Yes. Body lice can spread epidemic typhus, trench fever, and louse-borne relapsing fever. Although louse-borne (epidemic) typhus is no longer widespread, outbreaks of this disease still occur during times of war, civil unrest, and natural or human-made disasters and in prisons where people live together in unsanitary conditions. Louse-borne typhus still exists in places where climate, chronic poverty, and social customs or war and social upheaval prevent regular changes and laundering of clothing.

HOW ARE BODY LICE SPREAD?

Body lice are spread through direct physical contact with a person who has body lice or through contact with articles such as clothing, beds, bed linens, or towels that have been in contact with an infested person. In the United States, actual infestation with body lice tends to occur only in people who do not have access to regular (at least weekly) bathing and changes of clean clothes, including people experiencing homelessness or people residing in shelters.

HOW ARE BODY LICE INFESTATIONS DIAGNOSED?

Body lice infestation is diagnosed by finding eggs and crawling lice in the seams of clothing. Sometimes, a body louse can be seen crawling or feeding on the skin. Although body lice and nits can be large enough to be seen with the naked eye, a magnifying lens may be necessary to find crawling lice or eggs.

HOW ARE BODY LICE TREATED?

A body lice infestation is treated by improving the personal hygiene of the infested person, including assuring a regular (at least weekly) change of clean clothes. Clothing, bedding, and towels used by the infested person should be laundered using hot water (at least 130 °F (54.44 °C)) and machine dried using the hot cycle.

Sometimes, the infested person is also treated with a pediculicide, a medicine that can kill lice; however, a pediculicide is generally not necessary if hygiene is maintained and items are laundered appropriately at least once a week. A pediculicide should be applied exactly as directed on the bottle or by your physician.

PREVENTION AND CONTROL OF BODY LICE

Body lice are spread most commonly by direct contact with an infested person or an infested person's clothing or bedding. Body lice usually infest persons who do not launder and change their clothes regularly.

The following are steps that can be taken to help prevent and control the spread of body lice:

- Bathe regularly and change into properly laundered clothes at least once a week; launder infested clothing at least once a week.
- Machine wash and dry infested clothing and bedding using the hot water (at least 130 °F (54.44 °C)) laundry cycle and the high heat drying cycle. Clothing and items that are not washable can be dry-cleaned or sealed in a plastic bag and stored for two weeks.
- Do not share clothing, beds, bedding, and towels used by an infested person.
- Fumigation or dusting with chemical insecticides sometimes is necessary to control and prevent the spread of body lice for certain diseases (epidemic typhus).[1]

Section 53.2 | **Head Lice**

Adult head lice are roughly 2–3 mm long. Head lice infest the head and neck and attach their eggs to the base of the hair shaft. Lice move by crawling; they cannot hop or fly.

Head lice infestation, or pediculosis, is spread most commonly by close person-to-person contact. Dogs, cats, and other pets do not play a role in the transmission of human lice. Both over-the-counter (OTC) and prescription medications are available for the treatment of head lice infestations.

WHAT ARE HEAD LICE?

The head louse, or *Pediculus humanus capitis*, is a parasitic insect that can be found on the head, eyebrows, and eyelashes of people. Head lice feed on human blood several times a day and live close to the human scalp. Head lice are not known to spread disease.

[1] "Body Lice," Centers for Disease Control and Prevention (CDC), September 12, 2019. Available online. URL: www.cdc.gov/parasites/lice/body/index.html. Accessed July 12, 2023.

WHO IS AT RISK FOR GETTING HEAD LICE?

Head lice are found worldwide. In the United States, infestation with head lice is most common among preschool children attending childcare, elementary schoolchildren, and the household members of infested children. Although reliable data on how many people in the United States get head lice each year are not available, an estimated 6–12 million infestations occur each year in the United States among children 3–11 years of age. In the United States, infestation with head lice is much less common among African Americans than among persons of other races, possibly because the claws of the head louse found most frequently in the United States are better adapted for grasping the shape and width of the hair shaft of other races.

Head lice move by crawling; they cannot hop or fly. Head lice are spread by direct contact with the hair of an infested person. Anyone who comes in head-to-head contact with someone who already has head lice is at greatest risk. Spread by contact with clothing (such as hats, scarves, and coats) or other personal items (such as combs, brushes, or towels) used by an infested person is uncommon. Personal hygiene or cleanliness in the home or school has nothing to do with getting head lice.

WHAT DO HEAD LICE LOOK LIKE?

Head lice have three forms: the egg (also called a "nit"), the nymph, and the adult.

- **Egg/Nit.** Nits are lice eggs laid by the adult female head louse at the base of the hair shaft nearest the scalp. Nits are firmly attached to the hair shaft and are oval-shaped and very small (about the size of a knot in thread) and hard to see. Nits often appear yellow or white although live nits sometimes appear to be the same color as the hair of the infested person. Nits are often confused with dandruff, scabs, or hair spray droplets. Head lice nits usually take about 8–9 days to hatch. Eggs that are likely to hatch are usually located no more than ¼ inch from the base of the hair shaft. Nits located further than ¼ inch from the base of the hair shaft may very well be already hatched, nonviable nits, or empty nits or casings. This is difficult to distinguish with the naked eye.

- **Nymph**. A nymph is an immature louse that hatches from the nit. A nymph looks like an adult head louse but is smaller. To live, a nymph must feed on blood. Nymphs mature into adults about 9–12 days after hatching from the nit.
- **Adult**. The fully grown and developed adult louse is about the size of a sesame seed, has six legs, and is tan to grayish-white in color. Adult head lice may look darker in persons with dark hair than in persons with light hair. To survive, adult head lice must feed on blood. An adult head louse can live about 30 days on a person's head but will die within one or two days if it falls off a person. Adult female head lice are usually larger than males and can lay about six eggs each day.

WHERE ARE HEAD LICE MOST COMMONLY FOUND?

Head lice and head lice nits are found almost exclusively on the scalp, particularly around and behind the ears and near the neckline at the back of the head. Head lice or head lice nits sometimes are found on the eyelashes or eyebrows, but this is uncommon. Head lice hold tightly to hair with hook-like claws at the end of each of their six legs. Head lice nits are cemented firmly to the hair shaft and can be difficult to remove even after the nymphs hatch and empty casings remain.

WHAT ARE THE SIGNS AND SYMPTOMS OF HEAD LICE INFESTATION?

- tickling feeling of something moving in the hair
- itching that is caused by an allergic reaction to the bites of the head louse
- irritability and difficulty sleeping (Head lice are most active in the dark.)
- sores on the head caused by scratching, which can sometimes become infected with bacteria found on the person's skin

DIAGNOSIS OF HEAD LICE INFESTATION

Misdiagnosis of head lice infestation is common. The diagnosis of head lice infestation is best made by finding a live nymph or adult louse on the scalp or hair of a person. Because adult and nymph lice are very small, move quickly, and avoid light, they may be difficult to find. The use of a fine-toothed louse comb may facilitate the identification of live lice.

If crawling lice are not seen, finding nits attached firmly within ¼ inch of the base of hair shafts suggests, but does not confirm, the person is infested. Nits are frequently seen on hair behind the ears and near the back of the neck. Nits that are attached more than ¼ inch from the base of the hair shaft are almost always nonviable (hatched or dead). Head lice and nits can be visible with the naked eye although the use of a magnifying lens may be necessary to find crawling lice or to identify a developing nymph inside a viable nit. Nits are often confused with other particles found in hair, such as dandruff, hair spray droplets, and dirt particles.

If no nymphs or adults are seen and the only nits found are more than ¼ inch from the scalp, then the infestation is probably old and no longer active—and does not need to be treated.

TREATMENT FOR HEAD LICE INFESTATION

Treatment for head lice is recommended for persons diagnosed with an active infestation. All household members and other close contacts should be checked; those persons with evidence of an active infestation should be treated. Some experts believe prophylactic treatment is prudent for persons who share the same bed with actively infested individuals. All infested persons (household members and close contacts) and their bedmates should be treated at the same time.

Some pediculicides (medicines that kill lice) have an ovicidal effect (kill eggs). For pediculicides that are only weakly ovicidal or not ovicidal, routine retreatment is recommended. For those that are more strongly ovicidal, retreatment is recommended only if live (crawling) lice are still present several days after treatment. To be most effective, retreatment should occur after all eggs have hatched but before new eggs are produced.

When treating head lice, supplemental measures can be combined with recommended medicine (pharmacologic treatment); however, such additional (nonpharmacologic) measures generally are not required to eliminate a head lice infestation. For example, hats, scarves, pillowcases, bedding, clothing, and towels worn or used by the infested person in the two-day period just before treatment is started can be machine washed and dried using hot water and hot air cycles because lice and eggs are killed by exposure for five minutes to temperatures greater than 128.3 °F (53.5 °C). Items that cannot be laundered may be dry-cleaned or sealed in a plastic bag for two weeks. Items such as hats, grooming aids, and towels that come in contact with the hair of an infested person should not be shared. Vacuuming furniture and floors can remove an infested person's hair that might have viable nits attached.

The infested person(s) can be treated using an OTC or prescription medication. Follow these treatment steps:

- Before applying treatment, it may be helpful to remove clothing that can become wet or stained during treatment.
- Apply lice medicine, also called "pediculicide," according to the instructions contained in the box or printed on the label. If the infested person has very long hair (longer than shoulder-length), it may be necessary to use a second bottle. Pay special attention to instructions on the label or in the box regarding how long the medication should be left on the hair and how it should be washed out.

  Warning. Do not use a combination shampoo/conditioner or conditioner before using lice medicine. Do not rewash the hair for one to two days after the lice medicine is removed.
- Have the infested person put on clean clothing after treatment.
- If a few live lice are still found 8–12 hours after treatment but are moving more slowly than before, do not retreat. The medicine may take longer to kill all the lice. Comb dead and any remaining live lice out of the hair using a fine-toothed nit comb.

- If, after 8–12 hours of treatment, no dead lice are found and lice seem as active as before, the medicine may not be working. Do not retreat until speaking with your health-care provider; a different pediculicide may be necessary. If your health-care provider recommends a different pediculicide, carefully follow the treatment instructions contained in the box or printed on the label.
- Nit (head lice egg) combs, often found in lice medicine packages, should be used to comb nits and lice from the hair shaft. Many flea combs made for cats and dogs are also effective.
- After each treatment, checking the hair and combing with a nit comb to remove nits and lice every two to three days may decrease the chance of self-reinfestation. Continue to check for two to three weeks to be sure all lice and nits are gone. Nit removal is not needed when treated with spinosad topical suspension.
- Retreatment is meant to kill any surviving hatched lice before they produce new eggs. For some drugs, retreatment is recommended routinely about a week after the first treatment (seven to nine days, depending on the drug), and for others, only if crawling lice are seen during this period. Retreatment with lindane shampoo is not recommended.

Supplemental Measures. Head lice do not survive long if they fall off a person and cannot feed. You do not need to spend a lot of time or money on housecleaning activities. Follow these steps to help avoid reinfestation by lice that have recently fallen off the hair or crawled onto clothing or furniture.

- Machine wash and dry clothing, bed linens, and other items that the infested person wore or used during the two days before treatment using the hot water (130 °F (54.44 °C)) laundry cycle and the high heat drying cycle. Clothing and items that are not washable can be dry-cleaned or sealed in a plastic bag and stored for two weeks.

- Soak combs and brushes in hot water (at least 130 °F (54.44 °C)) for 5–10 minutes.
- Vacuum the floor and furniture, particularly where the infested person sat or lay. However, the risk of getting infested by a louse that has fallen onto a rug or carpet or furniture is very small. Head lice survive less than one to two days if they fall off a person and cannot feed; nits cannot hatch and usually die within a week if they are not kept at the same temperature as that found close to the human scalp. Spending much time and money on housecleaning activities is not necessary to avoid reinfestation by lice or nits that may have fallen off the head or crawled onto furniture or clothing.
- Do not use fumigant sprays; they can be toxic if inhaled or absorbed through the skin.

Over-the-Counter Medications

Many head lice medications are available "OTC" without a prescription at a local drug store or pharmacy. Each OTC product approved by the U.S. Food and Drug Administration (FDA) for the treatment of head lice contains one of the following active ingredients. Always follow the label instructions when administering these medications. If crawling lice are still seen after a full course of treatment, contact your health-care provider.

PYRETHRINS COMBINED WITH PIPERONYL BUTOXIDE

- **Brand name products:** A–200*, Pronto*, R&C*, Rid*, and Triple X*. Pyrethrins are naturally occurring pyrethroid extracts from the chrysanthemum flower. Pyrethrins are safe and effective when used as directed. Pyrethrins can only kill live lice, not unhatched eggs (nits). A second treatment is recommended 9–10 days after the first treatment to kill any newly hatched lice before they can produce new eggs. Pyrethrins generally should not be used by persons who are allergic to chrysanthemums or ragweed. Pyrethrin is approved for use on children aged two and older. The efficacy of pyrethrins may be reduced because of the development of resistance, but the prevalence of resistance has not been well studied and is unknown. If crawling lice are still seen after a full course of treatment, contact your health-care provider.

PERMETHRIN LOTION, 1 PERCENT

- **Brand name product:** Nix*. Permethrin is a synthetic pyrethroid similar to naturally occurring pyrethrins. Permethrin lotion 1 percent is approved by the FDA for the treatment of head lice. Permethrin is safe and effective when used as directed. Permethrin kills live lice but not unhatched eggs. Permethrin may continue to kill newly hatched lice for several days after treatment. A second treatment often is necessary on day nine to kill any newly hatched lice before they can produce new eggs. Permethrin is approved for use on children two months of age and older. Resistance to 1 percent permethrin has been reported, but its prevalence is unknown. If crawling lice are still seen after a full course of treatment, contact your health-care provider.

Prescription Medications

The following medications, in alphabetical order, approved by the FDA for the treatment of head lice, are available only by prescription. Always follow the instructions of your health-care provider when administering these medications. If crawling lice are still seen after a full course of treatment, contact your health-care provider.

BENZYL ALCOHOL LOTION, 5 PERCENT: BRAND NAME PRODUCT: ULESFIA LOTION

Benzyl alcohol is an aromatic alcohol. Benzyl alcohol lotion, 5 percent, has been approved by the FDA for the treatment of head lice and is considered safe and effective when used as directed. It kills lice, but it is not ovicidal. A second treatment is needed seven days after the first treatment to kill any newly hatched lice before they can produce new eggs. Benzyl alcohol lotion is intended for use on persons who are six months of age and older, and its safety in persons aged more than 60 years has not been established. It can be irritating to the skin.

IVERMECTIN LOTION, 0.5 PERCENT: BRAND NAME PRODUCT: SKLICE

Ivermectin lotion, 0.5 percent was approved by the FDA in 2012 for treatment of head lice in persons aged six months and older. It is not ovicidal but appears to prevent nymphs (newly hatched lice) from surviving. It is effective in most patients when given as a single application on dry hair without nit combing. It should not be used for retreatment without talking to a health-care provider. Given as a tablet in mass drug administrations, oral ivermectin has been used extensively and safely for over two decades in many countries to treat filarial worm infections. Although not FDA-approved for the treatment of lice, ivermectin tablets given in a single oral dose of 200 mcg/kg or 400 mcg/kg repeated in 9–10 days have been shown effective against head lice. It should not be used in children weighing less than 15 kg or in pregnant women.

MALATHION LOTION, 0.5 PERCENT: BRAND NAME PRODUCT: OVIDE

Malathion is an organophosphate. The formulation of malathion approved in the United States for the treatment of head lice is a lotion that is safe and effective when used as directed. Malathion is pediculicidal (that kills live lice) and partially ovicidal (that kills some lice eggs). A second treatment is recommended if live lice still are present seven to nine days after treatment. Malathion is intended for use on persons six years of age and older. Malathion can be irritating to the skin. Malathion lotion is flammable; do not smoke or use electrical heat sources, including hair dryers, curlers, and curling or flat irons when applying malathion lotion and while the hair is wet.

SPINOSAD 0.9 PERCENT TOPICAL SUSPENSION: BRAND NAME PRODUCT: NATROBA

Spinosad is derived from soil bacteria. Spinosad topical suspension, 0.9 percent, was approved by the FDA in 2011. Since it kills live lice as well as unhatched eggs, retreatment is usually not needed. Nit combing is not required. Spinosad topical suspension is approved for the treatment of children aged six months and older. It is safe and effective when used as directed. Repeat treatment should be given only if live (crawling) lice are seen seven days after the first treatment.

LINDANE SHAMPOO, 1 PERCENT: BRAND NAME PRODUCTS: NONE AVAILABLE (FOR SECOND-LINE TREATMENT ONLY)

Lindane is an organochloride. The American Academy of Pediatrics (AAP) no longer recommends it as a pediculicide. Although lindane shampoo 1 percent is approved by the FDA for the treatment of head lice, it is not recommended as a first-line treatment. Overuse, misuse, or accidentally swallowing lindane can be toxic to the brain and other parts of the nervous system; its use should be restricted to patients for whom prior treatments have failed or who cannot tolerate other medications that pose less risk. Lindane should not be used to treat premature infants, persons with human immunodeficiency virus (HIV) or a seizure disorder, women who are pregnant or breastfeeding, persons who have very irritated skin or sores where the lindane will be applied, infants, children, the elderly, and persons who weigh less than 110 pounds. Retreatment should be avoided.

When treating head lice:

- Do not use extra amounts of any lice medication unless instructed to do so by your physician and pharmacist. The drugs used to treat lice are insecticides and can be dangerous if they are misused or overused.
- All the medications listed above should be kept out of the eyes. If they get into the eyes, they should be immediately flushed away.
- Do not treat an infested person more than two to three times with the same medication if it does not seem to be working. This may be caused by using the medicine

incorrectly or by resistance to the medicine. Always seek the advice of your health-care provider if this should happen. He/she may recommend an alternative medication.

- Do not use different head lice drugs at the same time unless instructed to do so by your physician and pharmacist.
- The AAP recommends rinsing all topical pediculicides from the hair over a sink, rather than in the shower or bath to limit skin exposure and to use warm water rather than hot water to minimize absorption.

PREVENTION AND CONTROL

Head lice are spread most commonly by direct head-to-head (hair-to-hair) contact. However, much less frequently, they are spread by sharing clothing or belongings onto which lice have crawled or nits attached to shed hairs may have fallen. The risk of getting infested by a louse that has fallen onto a carpet or furniture is very small. Head lice survive less than one to two days if they fall off a person and cannot feed; nits cannot hatch and usually die within a week if they are not kept at the same temperature as that found close to the scalp.

The following are steps that can be taken to help prevent and control the spread of head lice:

- Avoid head-to-head (hair-to-hair) contact during play and other activities at home, school, and elsewhere (sports activities, playground, slumber parties, camp).
- Do not share clothing such as hats, scarves, coats, sports uniforms, hair ribbons, or barrettes.
- Do not share combs, brushes, or towels. Disinfect combs and brushes used by an infested person by soaking them in hot water (at least 130 °F (54.44 °C)) for 5–10 minutes.
- Do not lie on beds, couches, pillows, carpets, or stuffed animals that have recently been in contact with an infected person.

- Machine wash and dry clothing, bed linens, and other items that an infested person wore or used during the two days before treatment using the hot water (130 °F (54.44 °C)) laundry cycle and the high heat drying cycle. Clothing and items that are not washable can be dry-cleaned or sealed in a plastic bag and stored for two weeks.
- Vacuum the floor and furniture, particularly where the infested person sat or lay. However, spending much time and money on housecleaning activities is not necessary to avoid reinfestation by lice or nits that may have fallen off the head or crawled onto furniture or clothing.
- Do not use fumigant sprays or fog; they are not necessary to control head lice and can be toxic if inhaled or absorbed through the skin.

To help control a head lice outbreak in a community, school, or camp, children can be taught to avoid activities that may spread head lice.

**Use of trade names is for identification purposes only and does not imply endorsement by the Public Health Service or by the U.S. Department of Health and Human Services (HHS).*[2]

[2] "Head Lice," Centers for Disease Control and Prevention (CDC), June 15, 2023. Available online. URL: www.cdc.gov/parasites/lice/head/index.html. Accessed July 12, 2023.

Section 53.3 | Pubic Lice

WHAT ARE PUBIC LICE?

Also called "crab lice" or "crabs," pubic lice are parasitic insects found primarily in the pubic or genital area of humans. Pubic lice infestation is found worldwide and occurs in all races, ethnic groups, and levels of society.

WHAT DO PUBIC LICE LOOK LIKE?

Pubic lice have three forms: the egg (also called a "nit"), the nymph, and the adult.

- **Nit.** Nits are lice eggs. They can be hard to see and are found firmly attached to the hair shaft. They are oval and usually yellow to white. Pubic lice nits take about 6–10 days to hatch.
- **Nymph.** The nymph is an immature louse that hatches from the nit (egg). A nymph looks like an adult pubic louse, but it is smaller. Pubic lice nymphs take about two to three weeks after hatching to mature into adults capable of reproducing. To live, a nymph must feed on blood.
- **Adult.** The adult pubic louse resembles a miniature crab when viewed through a strong magnifying glass. Pubic lice have six legs; their two front legs are very large and look like the pincher claws of a crab. This is how they got the nickname "crabs." Pubic lice are tan to grayish-white in color. Females lay nits and are usually larger than males. To live, lice must feed on blood. If the louse falls off a person, it dies within one to two days.

WHERE ARE PUBIC LICE FOUND?

Pubic lice are usually found in the genital area on pubic hair; but they may occasionally be found on other coarse body hair, such as hair on the legs, armpits, mustache, beard, eyebrows, or eyelashes. Pubic lice on the eyebrows or eyelashes of children may be a sign of sexual exposure or abuse. Lice found on the head generally are head lice, not pubic lice. Animals do not get or spread pubic lice.

WHAT ARE THE SIGNS AND SYMPTOMS OF PUBIC LICE?

Signs and symptoms of pubic lice include the following:

- itching in the genital area
- visible nits (lice eggs) or crawling lice

HOW DO YOU GET PUBIC LICE?

Pubic lice are usually spread through sexual contact and are most common in adults. Pubic lice found on children may be a sign of sexual exposure or abuse. Occasionally, pubic lice may be spread by close personal contact or contact with articles such as clothing, bed linens, or towels that have been used by an infested person. A common misconception is that pubic lice are spread easily by sitting on a toilet seat. This would be extremely rare because lice cannot live long away from a warm human body, and they do not have feet designed to hold onto or walk on smooth surfaces, such as toilet seats. Persons infested with pubic lice should be examined for the presence of other sexually transmitted diseases (STDs).

HOW IS A PUBIC LICE INFESTATION DIAGNOSED?

Pubic lice are short and crab-like and appear very different from head and body lice. Pubic lice infestation is diagnosed by finding a "crab" louse or eggs on hair in the pubic region or, less commonly, elsewhere on the body (eyebrows, eyelashes, beard, mustache, armpit, perianal area, groin, trunk, and scalp). Although pubic lice and nits can be large enough to be seen with the naked eye, a magnifying lens may be necessary to find lice or eggs.

HOW IS A PUBIC LICE INFESTATION TREATED?

A lice-killing lotion containing 1 percent permethrin or a mousse containing pyrethrins and piperonyl butoxide can be used to treat pubic ("crab") lice. These products are available over the counter without a prescription at a local drug store or pharmacy. These medications are safe and effective when used exactly according to the instructions in the package or on the label.

Lindane shampoo is a prescription medication that can kill lice and lice eggs. However, lindane is not recommended as a first-line therapy. Lindane can be toxic to the brain and other parts of the nervous system; its use should be restricted to patients who have failed treatment with or cannot tolerate other medications that pose less risk. Lindane should not be used to treat premature infants, persons with a seizure disorder, women who are pregnant or breastfeeding, persons who have very irritated skin or sores where the lindane will be applied, infants, children, the elderly, and persons who weigh less than 110 pounds.

Malathion* lotion 0.5 percent (Ovide*) is a prescription medication that can kill lice and some lice eggs; however, malathion lotion (Ovide*) currently has not been approved by the U.S. Food and Drug Administration (FDA) for treatment of pubic ("crab") lice.

Both topical and oral ivermectin have been used successfully to treat lice; however, only topical ivermectin lotion currently is approved by the FDA for the treatment of lice. Oral ivermectin is not FDA-approved for the treatment of lice.

How to Treat Pubic Lice Infestations

(Warning: See special instructions for treatment of lice and nits on eyebrows or eyelashes. The lice medications described here should not be used near the eyes.)

- Wash the infested area and towel dry.
- Carefully follow the instructions in the package or on the label. Thoroughly saturate the pubic hair and other infested areas with lice medication. Leave medication on hair for the time recommended in the instructions. After waiting for the recommended time, remove the medication by carefully following the instructions on the label or in the box.
- Following treatment, most nits will still be attached to hair shafts. Nits may be removed with fingernails or by using a fine-toothed comb.
- Put on clean underwear and clothing after treatment.
- To kill any lice or nits remaining on clothing, towels, or bedding, machine wash and machine dry those items that the infested person used during the two to three

days before treatment. Use hot water (at least 130 °F (54.44 °C)) and the hot dryer cycle.
- Items that cannot be laundered can be dry-cleaned or stored in a sealed plastic bag for two weeks.
- All sex partners from within the previous month should be informed that they are at risk for infestation and should be treated.
- Persons should avoid sexual contact with their sex partner(s) until both they and their partners have been successfully treated and reevaluated to rule out persistent infestation.
- Repeat treatment in 9–10 days if live lice are still found.
- Persons with pubic lice should be evaluated for other STDs.

Special Instructions for Treatment of Lice and Nits Found on Eyebrows or Eyelashes

- If only a few live lice and nits are present, it may be possible to remove these with fingernails or a nit comb.
- If additional treatment is needed for lice or nits on the eyelashes, careful application of ophthalmic-grade petrolatum ointment (only available by prescription) to the eyelid margins two to four times a day for 10 days is effective. Regular petrolatum (e.g., Vaseline)* should not be used because it can irritate the eyes if applied.

PREVENTION AND CONTROL OF PUBIC LICE INFESTATION

Pubic ("crab") lice most commonly are spread directly from person to person by sexual contact. Pubic lice very rarely may be spread by clothing, bedding, or a toilet seat.

The following are steps that can be taken to help prevent and control the spread of pubic ("crab") lice:

- All sexual contacts of the infested person should be examined. All those who are infested should be treated.
- Sexual contact between the infested person(s) and their sexual partner(s) should be avoided until all have been

examined, treated as necessary, and reevaluated to rule out persistent infestation.
- Machine wash and dry clothing worn and bedding used by the infested person in the hot water (at least 130 °F (54.44 °C)) laundry cycle and the high heat drying cycle. Clothing and items that are not washable can be dry-cleaned or sealed in a plastic bag and stored for two weeks.
- Do not share clothing, bedding, and towels used by an infested person.
- Do not use fumigant sprays or fogs; they are not necessary to control pubic ("crab") lice and can be toxic if inhaled or absorbed through the skin.

Persons with pubic lice should be examined and treated for any other STDs that may be present.

**Use of trade names is for identification purposes only and does not imply endorsement by the Public Health Service or by the U.S. Department of Health and Human Services.*[3]

[3] "Pubic 'Crab' Lice," Centers for Disease Control and Prevention (CDC), June 15, 2023. Available online. URL: www.cdc.gov/parasites/lice/pubic/index.html. Accessed July 12, 2023.

Chapter 54 | Pinworm Infections

WHAT IS A PINWORM?

A pinworm ("threadworm") is a small, thin, white roundworm (nematode) called "*Enterobius vermicularis*" that sometimes lives in the colon and rectum of humans. Pinworms are about the length of a staple. While an infected person sleeps, female pinworms leave the intestine through the anus and deposit their eggs on the surrounding skin.

WHAT ARE THE SYMPTOMS OF PINWORM INFECTION?

Pinworm infection (called "enterobiasis" or "oxyuriasis") causes itching around the anus that can lead to difficulty sleeping and restlessness. Symptoms are caused by the female pinworm laying her eggs. Symptoms of pinworm infection are usually mild, and some infected people have no symptoms.

WHO IS AT RISK FOR PINWORM INFECTION?

Pinworm infection occurs worldwide and affects persons of all ages and socioeconomic levels. It is the most common worm infection in the United States. Pinworm infection occurs most commonly among:

- school- and preschool-aged children
- institutionalized persons
- household members and caretakers of persons with pinworm infection

Pinworm infection often occurs in more than one person in household and institutional settings. Childcare centers are often the sites of cases of pinworm infection.

HOW IS PINWORM INFECTION SPREAD?

Pinworm infection is spread by the fecal–oral route, that is, by the transfer of infective pinworm eggs from the anus to someone's mouth, either directly by hand or indirectly through contaminated clothing, bedding, food, or other articles.

Pinworm eggs become infective within a few hours after being deposited on the skin around the anus and can survive for two to three weeks on clothing, bedding, or other objects. People become infected, usually unknowingly, by swallowing (ingesting) infective pinworm eggs that are on fingers, under fingernails, or on clothing, bedding, and other contaminated objects and surfaces. Because of their small size, pinworm eggs sometimes can become airborne and ingested while breathing.

DIAGNOSIS OF PINWORM INFECTIONS

A person infected with pinworm is often asymptomatic, but itching around the anus is a common symptom. Diagnosis of pinworm can be reached from three simple techniques. The first option is to look for the worms in the perianal region two to three hours after the infected person is asleep. The second option is to touch the perianal skin with transparent tape to collect possible pinworm eggs around the anus first thing in the morning. If a person is infected, the eggs on the tape will be visible under a microscope. The tape method should be conducted on three consecutive mornings right after the infected person wakes up and before he/she does any washing. Since anal itching is a common symptom of pinworm, the third option for diagnosis is analyzing samples from under fingernails under a microscope. An infected person who has scratched the anal area may have picked up some pinworm eggs under the nails that could be used for diagnosis.

Since pinworm eggs and worms are often sparse in stool, examining stool samples is not recommended. Serologic tests are not available for diagnosing pinworm infections.

TREATMENT OF PINWORM INFECTIONS

The medications used for the treatment of pinworm are either mebendazole, pyrantel pamoate, or albendazole. Any of these drugs are given in one dose initially and then another single dose of the same drug two weeks later. Pyrantel pamoate is available without a prescription. The medication does not reliably kill pinworm eggs. Therefore, the second dose is to prevent reinfection by adult worms that hatch from any eggs not killed by the first treatment. Health practitioners and parents should weigh the health risks and benefits of these drugs for patients under two years of age.

Repeated infections should be treated by the same method as the first infection. In households where more than one member is infected or where repeated symptomatic infections occur, it is recommended that all household members be treated at the same time. In institutions, mass and simultaneous treatment, repeated in two weeks, can be effective.

PREVENTION AND CONTROL OF PINWORM INFECTIONS

Washing your hands with soap and warm water after using the toilet, after changing diapers, and before handling food is the most successful way to prevent pinworm infection. In order to stop the spread of pinworm and possible reinfection, people who are infected should shower every morning to help remove a large amount of the eggs on the skin. Showering is a better method than taking a bath because showering avoids potentially contaminating the bath water with pinworm eggs. Infected people should not cobathe with others during their time of infection.

Also, infected people should comply with good hygiene practices such as washing their hands with soap and warm water after using the toilet, after changing diapers, and before handling food. They should also cut fingernails regularly and avoid biting the nails and scratching around the anus. Frequent changing of underclothes and bed linens first thing in the morning is a great way to prevent possible transmission of eggs into the environment and risk of reinfection. These items should not be shaken and carefully placed into a washer and laundered in hot water followed by a hot dryer to kill any eggs that may be there.

In institutions, daycare centers, and schools, control of pinworm can be difficult, but mass drug administration during an outbreak can be successful. Teach children the importance of washing hands to prevent infection.[1]

[1] "Parasites—Enterobiasis (Also Known as Pinworm Infection)," Centers for Disease Control and Prevention (CDC), June 5, 2023. Available online. URL: www.cdc.gov/parasites/pinworm. Accessed July 10, 2023.

Chapter 55 | Scabies

WHAT IS SCABIES?

Scabies is an infestation of the skin by the human itch mite (*Sarcoptes scabiei* var. *hominis*). The microscopic scabies mite burrows into the upper layer of the skin where it lives and lays its eggs. The most common symptoms of scabies are intense itching and a pimple-like skin rash. The scabies mite is usually spread by direct, prolonged, skin-to-skin contact with a person who has scabies.

Scabies is found worldwide and affects people of all races and social classes. Scabies can spread rapidly under crowded conditions where close body and skin contact is frequent. Institutions such as nursing homes, extended-care facilities, and prisons are often sites of scabies outbreaks. Childcare facilities are also common sites of scabies infestations.

WHAT IS CRUSTED SCABIES?

Crusted scabies is a severe form of scabies that can occur in some persons who are immunocompromised (have a weak immune system), elderly, disabled, or debilitated. It is also called "Norwegian scabies." Persons with crusted scabies have thick crusts of skin that contain large numbers of scabies mites and eggs. Persons with crusted scabies are very contagious to other persons and can spread the infestation easily both by direct skin-to-skin contact and by contamination of items such as their clothing, bedding, and furniture. Persons with crusted scabies may not show the usual signs and symptoms of scabies, such as the characteristic rash or itching (pruritus). Persons with crusted scabies should receive quick and aggressive medical treatment for their infestation to prevent outbreaks of scabies.

HOW SOON AFTER INFESTATION DO SYMPTOMS OF SCABIES BEGIN?

If a person has never had scabies before, symptoms may take four to eight weeks to develop. It is important to remember that an infested person can spread scabies during this time, even if he/she does not have symptoms yet. In a person who has had scabies before, symptoms usually appear much sooner (one to four days) after exposure.

WHAT ARE THE SIGNS AND SYMPTOMS OF SCABIES INFESTATION?

The most common signs and symptoms of scabies are intense itching (pruritus), especially at night, and a pimple-like (papular) itchy rash. The itching and rash each may affect much of the body or be limited to common sites such as the wrist, elbow, armpit, webbing between the fingers, nipple, penis, waist, beltline, and buttocks. The rash can also include tiny blisters (vesicles) and scales. Scratching the rash can cause skin sores; sometimes, these sores become infected by bacteria.

Tiny burrows sometimes are seen on the skin; these are caused by the female scabies mite tunneling just beneath the surface of the skin. These burrows appear as tiny raised and crooked (serpiginous) grayish-white or skin-colored lines on the skin surface. Because mites are often few in number (only 10–15 mites per person), these burrows may be difficult to find. They are found most often in the webbing between the fingers, in the skin folds on the wrist, elbow, or knee, and on the penis, breast, or shoulder blades.

The head, face, neck, palms, and soles often are involved in infants and very young children, but usually not in adults and older children. Persons with crusted scabies may not show the usual signs and symptoms of scabies, such as the characteristic rash or itching (pruritus).

HOW DO YOU GET SCABIES?

Scabies is usually spread by direct, prolonged, skin-to-skin contact with a person who has scabies. Contact generally must be prolonged; a quick handshake or hug usually will not spread scabies. Scabies is spread easily to sexual partners and household members. Scabies in adults frequently is sexually acquired. Scabies is sometimes spread indirectly by sharing articles such as clothing, towels, or bedding used by an infested person; however, such indirect spread can occur much more easily when the infested person has crusted scabies.

HOW IS SCABIES INFESTATION DIAGNOSED?

Diagnosis of a scabies infestation is usually made based on the customary appearance and distribution of the rash and the presence of burrows. Whenever possible, the diagnosis of scabies should be confirmed by identifying the mite, mite eggs, or mite fecal matter (scybala). This can be done by carefully removing a mite from the end of its burrow using the tip of a needle or by obtaining skin scraping to examine under a microscope for mites, eggs, or mite fecal matter. It is important to remember that a person can still be infested even if mites, eggs, or fecal matter cannot be found; typically fewer than 10–15 mites can be present on the entire body of an infested person who is otherwise healthy. However, persons with crusted scabies can be infested with thousands of mites and should be considered highly contagious.

HOW LONG CAN SCABIES MITES LIVE?

On a person, scabies mites can live for as long as one to two months. Off a person, scabies mites usually do not survive more than 48–72 hours. Scabies mites will die if exposed to a temperature of 122 °F (50 °C) for 10 minutes.

CAN SCABIES BE TREATED?

Yes. Products used to treat scabies are called "scabicides" because they kill scabies mites; some also kill eggs. Scabicides to treat human scabies are available only with a doctor's prescription; no "over-the-counter" (OTC) (nonprescription) products have been tested and approved for humans.

Always follow carefully the instructions provided by the doctor and pharmacist, as well as those contained in the box or printed on the label. When treating adults and older children, scabicide cream or lotion is applied to all areas of the body from the neck down to the feet and toes; when treating infants and young children, the cream or lotion also is applied to the head and neck. The medication should be left on the body for the recommended time before it is washed off. Clean clothes should be worn after treatment.

WHO SHOULD BE TREATED FOR SCABIES?

Anyone who is diagnosed with scabies, as well as his or her sexual partners and other contacts who have had prolonged skin-to-skin contact with the infested person, should be treated. Treatment is recommended for members of the same household as the person with scabies, particularly those persons who have had prolonged skin-to-skin contact with the infested person. All persons should be treated at the same time to prevent reinfestation.

HOW SOON AFTER TREATMENT WILL YOU FEEL BETTER?

If itching continues more than two to four weeks after initial treatment or if new burrows or rashes continue to appear (if initial treatment includes more than one application or dose, then the two to four time period begins after the last application or dose), retreatment with scabicide may be necessary; seek the advice of a physician.

DID YOU GET SCABIES FROM YOUR PET?

No. Animals do not spread human scabies. Pets can become infested with a different kind of scabies mite that does not survive or reproduce on humans but causes "mange" in animals. If an animal with "mange" has close contact with a person, the animal mite can get under the person's skin and cause temporary itching and skin irritation. However, the animal mite cannot reproduce on a person and will die on its own in a couple of days. Although the person does not need to be treated, the animal should be treated because its mites can continue to burrow into the person's skin and cause symptoms until the animal has been treated successfully.

CAN SCABIES BE SPREAD BY SWIMMING IN A PUBLIC POOL?

Scabies is spread by prolonged skin-to-skin contact with a person who has scabies. Scabies sometimes can also be spread by contact with items such as clothing, bedding, or towels that have been used by a person with scabies, but such spread is very uncommon unless the infested person has crusted scabies.

Scabies is very unlikely to be spread by water in a swimming pool. Except for a person with crusted scabies, only about 10–15 scabies mites are present on an infested person; it is extremely unlikely that any would emerge from under wet skin. Although uncommon, scabies can be spread by sharing a towel or item of clothing that has been used by a person with scabies.

HOW CAN YOU REMOVE SCABIES MITES FROM YOUR HOUSE, CARPET, AND CLOTHES?

Scabies mites do not survive more than two to three days away from human skin. Items such as bedding, clothing, and towels used by a person with scabies can be decontaminated by machine washing in hot water and drying using the hot cycle or by dry-cleaning. Items that cannot be washed or dry-cleaned can be decontaminated by removing from any body contact for at least 72 hours.

Because persons with crusted scabies are considered very infectious, careful vacuuming of furniture and carpets in rooms used by these persons is recommended. Fumigation of living areas is unnecessary.

YOUR SPOUSE STILL HAS SYMPTOMS AFTER TREATMENT WHILE YOU ARE CURED. WHY?

The rash and itching of scabies can persist for several weeks to a month after treatment, even if the treatment was successful and all the mites and eggs have been killed. Your health-care provider may prescribe additional medication to relieve itching if it is severe. Symptoms that persist for longer than two weeks after treatment can be due to a number of reasons, including:

- **Incorrect diagnosis of scabies**. Many drug reactions can mimic the symptoms of scabies and cause a skin rash and itching; the diagnosis of scabies should be confirmed by skin scraping that includes observing the mite, eggs, or mite feces (scybala) under a microscope. If you are sleeping in the same bed with your spouse and have not become reinfested and you have not retreated yourself for at least 30 days, then it is unlikely that your spouse has scabies.

- **Reinfestation**. Reinfestation with scabies from a family member or other infested person if all patients and their contacts are not treated at the same time; infested persons and their contacts must be treated at the same time to prevent reinfestation.
- **Treatment failure**. It may be caused by resistance to medication, by faulty application of topical scabicides, or by failure to do a second application when necessary; no new burrows should appear 24–48 hours after effective treatment.
- **Treatment failure of crusted scabies**. This is because of poor penetration of scabicide into thick scaly skin containing large numbers of scabies mites; repeated treatment with a combination of both topical and oral medication may be necessary to treat crusted scabies successfully.
- **Reinfestation from items (fomites)**. Items include clothing, bedding, or towels that were not appropriately washed or dry-cleaned (this is mainly of concern for items used by persons with crusted scabies); potentially contaminated items (fomites) should be machine washed in hot water and dried using the hot temperature cycle, dry-cleaned, or removed from skin contact for at least 72 hours.
- **An allergic skin rash (dermatitis)**. This may also be one of the reasons.
- **Exposure to household mites**. This exposure causes symptoms to persist because of cross-reactivity between mite antigens.

If itching continues for more than two to four weeks or if new burrows or rash continue to appear, seek the advice of a physician; retreatment with the same or a different scabicide may be necessary.

IF YOU COME IN CONTACT WITH A PERSON WHO HAS SCABIES, SHOULD YOU TREAT YOURSELF?

No. If a person thinks he or she might have scabies, he/she should contact a doctor. The doctor can examine the person, confirm the diagnosis of scabies, and prescribe an appropriate treatment. Products used to treat scabies in humans are available only with a doctor's prescription.

Sleeping with or having sex with any scabies-infested person presents a high risk for transmission. The longer a person has skin-to-skin exposure, the greater the likelihood for transmission to occur. Although briefly shaking hands with a person who has non-crusted scabies could be considered as presenting a relatively low risk, holding the hand of a person with scabies for 5–10 minutes could be considered to present a relatively high risk of transmission. However, transmission can occur even after brief skin-to-skin contact, such as a handshake, with a person who has crusted scabies. In general, a person who has skin-to-skin contact with a person who has crusted scabies would be considered a good candidate for treatment.

To determine when prophylactic treatment should be given to reduce the risk of transmission, early consultation should be sought with a health-care provider who understands:

- the type of scabies (i.e., non-crusted versus crusted) to which a person has been exposed
- the degree and duration of skin exposure that a person has had to the infested patient
- whether the exposure occurred before or after the patient was treated for scabies
- whether the exposed person works in an environment where he/she would be likely to be exposed to other people during the asymptomatic incubation period

(For example, a nurse or caretaker who works in a nursing home or hospital often would be treated prophylactically to reduce the risk of further scabies transmission in the facility.)[1]

[1] "Scabies Frequently Asked Questions (FAQs)," Centers for Disease Control and Prevention (CDC), September 1, 2020. Available online. URL: www.cdc.gov/parasites/scabies/gen_info/faqs.html. Accessed July 12, 2023.

Chapter 56 | Trichomoniasis

WHAT IS TRICHOMONIASIS?

Trichomoniasis, or trich, is a sexually transmitted infection (STI) caused by a parasite. The parasite is spread most often through vaginal, oral, or anal sex. It is one of the most common STIs in the United States and affects more women than men. It is treated easily with antibiotics, but many women do not have symptoms. If left untreated, trichomoniasis can raise your risk of getting human immunodeficiency virus (HIV).

WHO GETS TRICHOMONIASIS?

Trichomoniasis is more common in women than men. It affects more than two million women aged 14–49 in the United States.

Trichomoniasis affects more African-American women than White and Hispanic women. The risk for African-American women goes up with age and lifetime number of sex partners.

HOW DO YOU GET TRICHOMONIASIS?

Trichomoniasis is spread through the following ways:

- **Vaginal, oral, or anal sex**. Trichomoniasis can be spread even if there are no symptoms. This means you can get trichomoniasis from someone who has no signs or symptoms.
- **Genital touching**. A man does not need to ejaculate (come) for trichomoniasis to spread. Trichomoniasis can also be passed between women who have sex with women.

WHAT ARE THE SYMPTOMS OF TRICHOMONIASIS?

Most infected women have no symptoms. If you do get symptoms, they might appear 5–28 days after exposure and can include the following:

- irritation and itching in the genital area
- thin or frothy discharge with an unusual foul odor that can be clear, white, yellowish, or greenish
- discomfort during sex and when urinating
- lower abdominal pain (which is rare)

If you think you may have trichomoniasis, you and your sex partner(s) need to see a doctor or nurse as soon as possible.

HOW IS TRICHOMONIASIS DIAGNOSED?

To find out whether you have trichomoniasis, your doctor or nurse may:

- do a pelvic exam
- use a cotton swab to take a fluid sample from your vagina to look for the parasite under a microscope
- do a lab test, such as a deoxyribonucleic acid (DNA) test or a fluid culture (A culture test uses urine or a swab from your vagina. The parasite then grows in a lab. It takes up to a week for the parasite to grow enough to be seen.)

A Papanicolaou (Pap) test is not used to detect trichomoniasis. If you have trichomoniasis, you need to be tested for other STIs, too.

HOW IS TRICHOMONIASIS TREATED?

Trichomoniasis is easily cured with one of the following two antibiotics:

- metronidazole
- tinidazole

These antibiotics are usually a pill you swallow in a single dose. If you are treated for trichomoniasis, your sex partner(s) needs to be treated, too. Do not have sex until you and your sex partner(s) finish taking all of the antibiotics and have no symptoms.

WHAT CAN HAPPEN IF TRICHOMONIASIS IS NOT TREATED?

Most people with trichomoniasis have no symptoms and never know they have it. Even without symptoms, it can be passed to others.

If you have trichomoniasis, you are at higher risk of getting HIV (the virus that causes acquired immunodeficiency syndrome (AIDS)) if you are exposed to HIV. If you are HIV-positive, having trichomoniasis also raises your risk of passing HIV to your sex partner(s). The Centers for Disease Control and Prevention (CDC) recommends that women with HIV get screened for trichomoniasis at least once a year.

WHAT SHOULD YOU DO IF YOU HAVE TRICHOMONIASIS?

Trichomoniasis is easy to treat. But you need to be tested and treated as soon as possible. If you have trichomoniasis, do the following:

- See a doctor or nurse as soon as possible. Antibiotics will treat trichomoniasis.
- Take all of your medicine. Even if symptoms go away, you need to finish all of the antibiotics.
- Tell your sex partner(s), so they can be tested and treated.
- Avoid sexual contact until you and your partner(s) have been treated and cured. Even after you finish your antibiotics, you can get trichomoniasis again if you have sex with someone who has trichomoniasis.
- See your doctor or nurse again if you have symptoms that do not go away within a few days after finishing the antibiotics.

HOW DOES TRICHOMONIASIS AFFECT PREGNANCY?

Pregnant women with trichomoniasis are at higher risk of premature birth (babies born before 37 weeks of pregnancy) or a low-birth-weight baby (less than 5½ pounds). Premature birth and a low birth weight raise the risk of health and developmental problems at birth and later in life.

The antibiotic metronidazole can be used to treat trichomoniasis during any stage of pregnancy. Talk to your doctor about the benefits and risks of taking any medicine during pregnancy.

CAN YOU TAKE MEDICINE FOR TRICHOMONIASIS IF YOU ARE BREASTFEEDING?

You can take the antibiotic metronidazole if you are breastfeeding. Your doctor may suggest waiting 12–24 hours after taking metronidazole before breastfeeding. Do not take tinidazole if you are breastfeeding.

HOW CAN YOU PREVENT TRICHOMONIASIS?

The best way to prevent trichomoniasis or any STI is to not have vaginal, oral, or anal sex. If you do have sex, lower your risk of getting an STI with the following steps:

- **Use condoms**. Condoms are the best way to prevent STIs when you have sex. Because a man does not need to ejaculate (come) to give or get trichomoniasis, make sure to put the condom on before the penis touches the vagina, mouth, or anus. Other methods of birth control, such as birth control pills, shots, implants, or diaphragms, will not protect you from STIs.
- **Get tested**. Be sure you and your partner are tested for STIs. Talk to each other about the test results before you have sex.
- **Be monogamous**. Having sex with just one partner can lower your risk for STIs. After being tested for STIs, be faithful to each other. That means that you have sex only with each other and no one else.
- **Limit your number of sex partners**. Your risk of getting STIs goes up with the number of partners you have.
- **Do not douche**. Douching removes some of the normal bacteria in the vagina that protects you from infection. This may increase your risk of getting STIs.

- **Do not abuse alcohol or drugs.** Drinking too much alcohol or using drugs increases risky behavior and may put you at risk of sexual assault and possible exposure to STIs.

The steps work best when used together. No single step can protect you from every single type of STI.[1]

[1] Office on Women's Health (OWH), "Trichomoniasis," U.S. Department of Health and Human Services (HHS), December 30, 2022. Available online. URL: www.womenshealth.gov/a-z-topics/trichomoniasis. Accessed July 12, 2023.

Chapter 57 | **Fungal Infections**

Chapter Contents

Section 57.1 | *Pneumocystis* Pneumonia

WHAT IS *PNEUMOCYSTIS* PNEUMONIA?

Pneumocystis pneumonia (PCP) is a serious infection caused by the fungus *Pneumocystis jirovecii*. Most people who get PCP have a medical condition that weakens their immune system, such as human immunodeficiency virus (HIV)/acquired immunodeficiency syndrome (AIDS), or take medicines (such as corticosteroids) that lower the body's ability to fight germs and sickness. In the United States, people with HIV/AIDS are less likely to get PCP today than before the availability of antiretroviral therapy (ART). However, PCP is still a substantial public health problem. Much of the information we have about PCP and its treatment comes from caring for patients with HIV/AIDS.

Scientists have changed both the classification and the name of this organism since it first appeared in patients with HIV in the 1980s. *P. jirovecii* used to be classified as a protozoan but is now considered a fungus. *P. jirovecii* used to be called "*Pneumocystis carinii*." When scientists renamed *P. carinii* to *P. jirovecii*, some people considered using the abbreviation "PJP," but to avoid confusion, *P. jirovecii* pneumonia is still abbreviated as "PCP."

SYMPTOMS OF *PNEUMOCYSTIS* PNEUMONIA

The symptoms of PCP can develop over several days or weeks and include the following:

- fever
- cough
- difficulty breathing
- chest pain
- chills
- fatigue (tiredness)

Contact your health-care provider if you have symptoms that you think are related to PCP.

WHO GETS *PNEUMOCYSTIS* PNEUMONIA?

Pneumocystis pneumonia is extremely rare in healthy people, but the fungus that causes this disease can live in their lungs without causing symptoms. In fact, up to 20 percent of adults might carry this fungus at any given time, and the immune system removes the fungus after several months.

Most people who get PCP have weakened immune systems, meaning that their bodies do not fight infections well. About 30–40 percent of people who get PCP have HIV/AIDS. The other people who get PCP are usually taking medicine (such as corticosteroids) that lowers the body's ability to fight germs or sickness or have other medical conditions, such as:

- chronic lung diseases
- cancer
- inflammatory diseases or autoimmune diseases (e.g., lupus or rheumatoid arthritis (RA))
- solid organ or stem cell transplant

HOW *PNEUMOCYSTIS* PNEUMONIA SPREADS

Pneumocystis pneumonia spreads from person to person through the air. Some healthy adults can carry the *Pneumocystis* fungus in their lungs without having symptoms, and it can spread to other people, including those with weakened immune systems.

Many people are exposed to *Pneumocystis* as children, but they likely do not get sick because their immune systems prevent the fungus from causing an infection. In the past, scientists believed that people who had been exposed to *Pneumocystis* as children could later develop PCP from that childhood infection if their immune systems became weakened. However, it is more likely that people get PCP after being exposed to someone else who has PCP or who is carrying the fungus in their lungs without having symptoms.

DIAGNOSIS AND TESTING FOR *PNEUMOCYSTIS* PNEUMONIA

Pneumocystis pneumonia is diagnosed using a sample from a patient's lungs. The sample is usually mucus that is either coughed up by the patient (called "sputum") or collected by a procedure called "bronchoalveolar lavage." Sometimes, a small sample of lung tissue (a biopsy) is used to diagnose PCP. The patient's sample is sent to a laboratory, usually to be examined under a microscope. Polymerase chain reaction (PCR) can also be used to detect *Pneumocystis* deoxyribonucleic acid (DNA) in different types of samples. A blood test to detect β-D-glucan (a part of the cell wall of many different types of fungi) can also help diagnose PCP.

TREATMENT AND OUTCOMES OF *PNEUMOCYSTIS* PNEUMONIA

Pneumocystis pneumonia must be treated with prescription medicine. Without treatment, PCP can cause death. The most common form of treatment is trimethoprim/sulfamethoxazole (TMP/SMX), which is also known as "co-trimoxazole" and by several different brand names, including Bactrim, Septra, and Cotrim. This medicine is given by mouth or through a vein for three weeks. TMP/SMX can cause side effects such as rash and fever. Other medicines are available for patients who cannot take TMP/SMX.

PREVENTION OF *PNEUMOCYSTIS* PNEUMONIA

There is no vaccine to prevent PCP. A health-care provider might prescribe medicine to prevent PCP for people who are more likely to develop the disease. The medicine most commonly used to prevent PCP is called "TMP/SMX."

Medicine to prevent PCP is recommended for some people infected with HIV, stem cell transplant patients, and some solid organ transplant patients. Health-care providers might also prescribe medicine to prevent PCP in other patients, such as people who are taking long-term, high-dose corticosteroids.[1]

[1] "*Pneumocystis* Pneumonia," Centers for Disease Control and Prevention (CDC), October 13, 2021. Available online. URL: www.cdc.gov/fungal/diseases/pneumocystis-pneumonia/index.html. Accessed July 13, 2023.

Section 57.2 | Tinea Infections

WHAT IS RINGWORM?

Ringworm is a common infection of the skin and nails that is caused by fungus. The infection is called "ringworm" because it can cause an itchy, red, circular rash. Ringworm is also called "tinea" or "dermatophytosis." The different types of ringworm are usually named for the location of the infection on the body. Areas of the body that can be affected by ringworm include the following:

- feet (tinea pedis, commonly called "athlete's foot")
- groin, inner thighs, or buttocks (tinea cruris, commonly called "jock itch")
- scalp (tinea capitis)
- beard (tinea barbae)
- hands (tinea manuum)
- toenails or fingernails (tinea unguium, also called "onychomycosis")
- other parts of the body such as arms or legs (tinea corporis)

Approximately 40 different species of fungi can cause ringworm; the scientific names for the types of fungi that cause ringworm are *Trichophyton*, *Microsporum*, and *Epidermophyton*.

Symptoms of Ringworm Infections

Ringworm can affect the skin on almost any part of the body as well as fingernails and toenails. The symptoms of ringworm often depend on which part of the body is infected, but they generally include the following:

- itchy skin
- ring-shaped rash
- red, scaly, cracked skin
- hair loss

Symptoms typically appear between 4 and 14 days after the skin comes in contact with the fungi that cause ringworm. Symptoms of ringworm by location on the body include the following:

- **Feet (tinea pedis or "athlete's foot")**. The symptoms of ringworm on the feet include red, swollen, peeling, itchy skin between the toes (especially between the pinky toe and the one next to it). The sole and heel of the foot may also be affected. In severe cases, the skin on the feet can blister.
- **Scalp (tinea capitis)**. Ringworm on the scalp usually looks like a scaly, itchy, red, circular bald spot. The bald spot can grow in size, and multiple spots might develop if the infection spreads. Ringworm on the scalp is more common in children than it is in adults.
- **Groin (tinea cruris or "jock itch")**. Ringworm on the groin looks like scaly, itchy, red spots, usually on the inner sides of the skin folds of the thigh.
- **Beard (tinea barbae)**. Symptoms of ringworm on the beard include scaly, itchy, red spots on the cheeks, chin, and upper neck. The spots might become crusted over or filled with pus, and the affected hair might fall out.

Ringworm Risk

Ringworm is very common. Anyone can get ringworm, but people who have weakened immune systems may be especially at risk for infection and may have problems fighting off a ringworm infection. People who use public showers or locker rooms, athletes (particularly those who are involved in contact sports such as wrestling), people who wear tight shoes and have excessive sweating, and people who have close contact with animals may also be more likely to come in contact with the fungi that cause ringworm.

How Does Ringworm Spread?

The fungi that cause ringworm can live on the skin and in the environment. The following are the three main ways that ringworm can spread:

- **From a person who has ringworm**. People can get ringworm after contact with someone who has the infection. To avoid spreading the infection, people with ringworms should not share clothing, towels, combs, or other personal items with other people.
- **From an animal that has ringworm**. People can get ringworm after touching an animal that has ringworm. Many different kinds of animals can spread ringworm to people, including dogs and cats, especially kittens and puppies. Other animals, such as cows, goats, pigs, and horses, can also spread ringworm to people.
- **From the environment**. The fungi that cause ringworm can live on surfaces, particularly in damp areas such as locker rooms and public showers. For that reason, it is a good idea not to walk barefoot in these places.

Diagnosis and Testing for Ringworm

Your health-care provider might suspect you have ringworm by looking at the affected skin and asking questions about your symptoms. Your health-care provider will generally take a small skin scraping or nail sample to examine under a microscope or send it to a laboratory for further testing.

Treatment for Ringworm

The treatment for ringworm depends on its location on the body and how serious the infection is. Some forms of ringworm can be treated with nonprescription (over-the-counter (OTC)) medications, but other forms of ringworm need treatment with prescription antifungal medication.

- Ringworm on the skin, such as athlete's foot (tinea pedis) and jock itch (tinea cruris), can usually be treated with nonprescription antifungal creams, lotions, or powders applied to the skin for two to four weeks. There are many nonprescription products available to treat ringworm, including the following:

- clotrimazole (Lotrimin and Mycelex)
- miconazole (Aloe Vesta Antifungal, Azolen, Baza Antifungal, Carrington Antifungal, Critic Aid Clear, Cruex Prescription Strength, DermaFungal, Desenex, Fungoid Tincture, Micaderm, Micatin, Micro-Guard, Miranel, Mitrazol, Podactin, Remedy Antifungal, and Secura Antifungal)
- terbinafine (Lamisil)
- ketoconazole (Xolegel)

For nonprescription creams, lotions, or powders, follow the directions on the package label. Contact your health-care provider if your infection does not go away or gets worse.

- Ringworm on the scalp (tinea capitis) usually needs to be treated with prescription antifungal medication taken by mouth for one to three months. Creams, lotions, or powders do not work for ringworms on the scalp. Prescription antifungal medications used to treat ringworm on the scalp include the following:
    - griseofulvin (Grifulvin V and Gris-PEG)
    - terbinafine
    - itraconazole (Onmel and Sporanox)
    - fluconazole (Diflucan)

You should contact your health-care provider if:

- your infection gets worse or does not go away after using nonprescription medications
- you or your child has ringworm on the scalp

Prevention of Ringworm Infections

- Keep your skin clean and dry.
- Wear shoes that allow air to circulate freely around your feet.

- Do not walk barefoot in areas such as locker rooms or public showers.
- Clip your fingernails and toenails short and keep them clean.
- Change your socks and underwear at least once a day.
- Do not share clothing, towels, sheets, or other personal items with someone who has ringworm.
- Wash your hands with soap and running water after playing with pets. If you suspect that your pet has ringworm, take it to see a veterinarian.
- If you are an athlete involved in close contact sports, shower immediately after your practice session or match and keep all of your sports gear and uniform clean. Do not share sports gear (helmet, etc.) with other players.[2]

ATHLETE'S FOOT (TINEA PEDIS)

Athlete's foot, or tinea pedis, is an infection of the skin and feet that can be caused by a variety of different fungi. Although tinea pedis can affect any portion of the foot, the infection most often affects the space between the toes. Athlete's foot is typically characterized by skin fissures or scales that can be red and itchy.

Tinea pedis is spread through contact with infected skin scales or contact with fungi in damp areas (e.g., showers, locker rooms, and swimming pools). Tinea pedis can be a chronic infection that recurs frequently. Treatment may include topical creams (applied to the surface of the skin) or oral medications. Appropriate hygiene techniques may help prevent or control tinea pedis. The following hygiene techniques can be helpful:

- Athlete's foot can be prevented in the following ways:
  - Nails should be clipped short and kept clean. Nails can house and spread the infection.

[2] "About Ringworm," Centers for Disease Control and Prevention (CDC), February 26, 2021. Available online. URL: www.cdc.gov/fungal/diseases/ringworm/definition.html. Accessed July 13, 2023.

    - Avoid walking barefoot in locker rooms or public showers (wear sandals).
- To control athlete's foot infection, persons with active tinea pedis infection should:
    - keep feet clean, dry, and cool
    - avoid using swimming pools, public showers, or foot baths
    - wear sandals when possible or air shoes out by alternating them every two to three days
    - avoid wearing closed shoes and wearing socks made from fabric that does not dry easily (e.g., nylon)
    - treat the infection with recommended medication[3]

Section 57.3 | **Vaginal Yeast Infections**

WHAT IS A VAGINAL YEAST INFECTION?

A vaginal yeast infection is an infection of the vagina that causes itching and burning of the vulva, the area around the vagina. Vaginal yeast infections are caused by an overgrowth of the fungus *Candida*.

WHO GETS VAGINAL YEAST INFECTIONS?

Women and girls of all ages can get vaginal yeast infections. Three out of four women will have a yeast infection at some point in their life. Almost half of women have two or more infections. Vaginal yeast infections are rare before puberty and after menopause.

ARE SOME WOMEN MORE AT RISK FOR YEAST INFECTIONS?

Yes. Your risk for yeast infections is higher if:

- you are pregnant

[3] "Hygiene-Related Diseases," Centers for Disease Control and Prevention (CDC), February 6, 2017. Available online. URL: www.cdc.gov/healthywater/hygiene/disease/athletes_foot.html. Accessed July 13, 2023.

- you have diabetes and your blood sugar is not under control
- you use a type of hormonal birth control that has higher doses of estrogen
- you douche or use vaginal sprays
- you recently took antibiotics such as amoxicillin or steroid medicines
- you have a weakened immune system, such as from human immunodeficiency virus (HIV)

WHAT ARE THE SYMPTOMS OF VAGINAL YEAST INFECTIONS?

The most common symptom of a vaginal yeast infection is extreme itchiness in and around the vagina. Other signs and symptoms include the following:

- burning, redness, and swelling of the vagina and the vulva
- pain when urinating
- pain during sex
- soreness
- a thick, white vaginal discharge that looks like cottage cheese and does not have a bad smell

You may have only a few of these symptoms. They may be mild or severe.

WHAT CAUSES YEAST INFECTIONS?

Yeast infections are caused by overgrowth of the microscopic fungus *Candida*. Your vagina may have small amounts of yeast at any given time without causing any symptoms. But, when too much yeast grows, you can get an infection.

CAN YOU GET A YEAST INFECTION FROM HAVING SEX?

Yes. A yeast infection is not considered a sexually transmitted infection (STI) because you can get a yeast infection without having sex. But you can get a yeast infection from your sexual partner.

Condoms and dental dams may help prevent getting or passing yeast infections through vaginal, oral, or anal sex.

SHOULD YOU CALL YOUR DOCTOR OR NURSE IF YOU THINK YOU HAVE A YEAST INFECTION?

Yes. Seeing your doctor or nurse is the only way to know for sure if you have a yeast infection and not a more serious type of infection. The signs and symptoms of a yeast infection are a lot like symptoms of other more serious infections, such as STIs and bacterial vaginosis (BV). If left untreated, STIs and BV raise your risk of getting other STIs, including HIV, and can lead to problems getting pregnant. BV can also lead to problems during pregnancy, such as premature delivery.

HOW IS A YEAST INFECTION DIAGNOSED?

Your doctor will do a pelvic exam to look for swelling and discharge. Your doctor may also use a cotton swab to take a sample of the discharge from your vagina. A lab technician will look at the sample under a microscope to see whether there is an overgrowth of the fungus *Candida* that causes a yeast infection.

HOW IS A YEAST INFECTION TREATED?

Yeast infections are usually treated with antifungal medicine. See your doctor or nurse to make sure that you have a vaginal yeast infection and not another type of infection.

You can then buy antifungal medicine for yeast infections at a store, without a prescription. Antifungal medicines come in the form of creams, tablets, ointments, or suppositories that you insert into your vagina. You can apply treatment in one dose or daily for up to seven days, depending on the brand you choose.

Your doctor or nurse can also give you a single dose of antifungal medicine taken by mouth, such as fluconazole. If you get more than four vaginal yeast infections a year or if your yeast infection does not go away after using over-the-counter (OTC) treatment, you may need to take regular doses of antifungal medicine for up to six months.

IS IT SAFE TO USE OVER-THE-COUNTER MEDICINES FOR YEAST INFECTIONS?

Yes, but always talk with your doctor or nurse before treating yourself for a vaginal yeast infection. This is for the following reasons:

- You may be trying to treat an infection that is not a yeast infection. Studies show that two out of three women who buy yeast infection medicine do not really have a yeast infection. Instead, they may have an STI or BV. STIs and BV require different treatments than yeast infections and, if left untreated, can cause serious health problems.
- Using treatment when you do not actually have a yeast infection can cause your body to become resistant to the yeast infection medicine. This can make actual yeast infections harder to treat in the future.
- Some yeast infection medicines may weaken condoms and diaphragms, increasing your chance of getting pregnant or an STI when you have sex. Talk to your doctor or nurse about what is best for you and always read and follow the directions on the medicine carefully.

HOW DO YOU TREAT A YEAST INFECTION IF YOU ARE PREGNANT?

During pregnancy, it is safe to treat a yeast infection with vaginal creams or suppositories that contain miconazole or clotrimazole. Do not take the oral fluconazole tablet to treat a yeast infection during pregnancy. It may cause birth defects.

CAN YOU GET A YEAST INFECTION FROM BREASTFEEDING?

Yes. Yeast infections can happen on your nipples or in your breast (commonly called "thrush") from breastfeeding. Yeast thrive on milk and moisture. A yeast infection you get while breastfeeding is different from a vaginal yeast infection. However, it is caused by an overgrowth of the same fungus.

Symptoms of thrush during breastfeeding include the following:

- sore nipples that last more than a few days, especially after several weeks of pain-free breastfeeding
- flaky, shiny, itchy, or cracked nipples
- deep pink and blistered nipples
- achy breast
- shooting pain in the breast during or after feedings

If you have any of these signs or symptoms or think your baby might have thrush in his or her mouth, call your doctor.

IF YOU HAVE A YEAST INFECTION, DOES YOUR SEXUAL PARTNER NEED TO BE TREATED?

Maybe. Yeast infections are not STIs. But it is possible to pass yeast infections to your partner during vaginal, oral, or anal sex.

- If your partner is a man, the risk of infection is low. About 15 percent of men get an itchy rash on the penis if they have unprotected sex with a woman who has a yeast infection. If this happens to your partner, he should see a doctor. Men who have not been circumcised and men with diabetes are at higher risk.
- If your partner is a woman, she may be at risk. She should be tested and treated if she has any symptoms.

HOW CAN YOU PREVENT A YEAST INFECTION?

You can take steps to lower your risk of getting yeast infections:

- Do not douche. Douching removes some of the normal bacteria in the vagina that protects you from infection.
- Do not use scented feminine products, including bubble bath, sprays, pads, and tampons.
- Change tampons, pads, and panty liners often.
- Do not wear tight underwear, pantyhose, pants, or jeans. These can increase body heat and moisture in your genital area.

- Wear underwear with a cotton crotch. Cotton underwear helps keep you dry and does not hold in warmth and moisture.
- Change out of wet swimsuits and workout clothes as soon as you can.
- After using the bathroom, always wipe from front to back.
- Avoid hot tubs and very hot baths.
- If you have diabetes, be sure your blood sugar is under control.

DOES YOGURT PREVENT OR TREAT YEAST INFECTIONS?

Maybe. Studies suggest that eating eight ounces of yogurt with "live cultures" daily or taking *Lactobacillus acidophilus* capsules can help prevent infection.

But more research still needs to be done to say for sure if yogurt with *Lactobacillus* or other probiotics can prevent or treat vaginal yeast infections. If you think you have a yeast infection, see your doctor or nurse to make sure before taking any OTC medicine.

WHAT SHOULD YOU DO IF YOU GET REPEAT YEAST INFECTIONS?

If you get four or more yeast infections in a year, talk to your doctor or nurse. About 5 percent of women get four or more vaginal yeast infections in one year. This is called "recurrent vulvovaginal candidiasis" (RVVC). RVVC is more common in women with diabetes or weak immune systems, such as with HIV, but it can also happen in otherwise healthy women. Doctors most often treat RVVC with antifungal medicine for up to six months. Researchers are also studying the effects of a vaccine to help prevent RVVC.[4]

---

[4] Office on Women's Health (OWH), "Vaginal Yeast Infections," U.S. Department of Health and Human Services (HHS), February 22, 2021. Available online. URL: www.womenshealth.gov/a-z-topics/vaginal-yeast-infections. Accessed July 13, 2023.

Part 5 | Self-Care and Treatment for Contagious Diseases

Chapter 58 | **Self-Care for Colds or Flu**

Chapter Contents

Section 58.1 | Managing Colds and Coughs

WHAT ARE COLD AND COUGH MEDICINES?

Cold and cough medicines can help relieve symptoms of a common cold. The symptoms of a cold can include a sore throat, stuffy or runny nose, sneezing, and coughing.

You do not usually need to treat a cold or cough. You cannot cure a cold, and antibiotics will not help you get better. But, sometimes, the symptoms can keep you awake or cause a lot of discomfort. In that case, cold and cough medicines can sometimes be helpful.

WHAT ARE THE DIFFERENT TYPES OF COLD AND COUGH MEDICINES?

There are lots of different cold and cough medicines, and they do different things:

- **Nasal decongestants.** Unclog a stuffy nose.
- **Cough suppressants.** Quiet a cough.
- **Expectorants.** Loosen mucus in your lungs, so you can cough it up.
- **Antihistamines.** Stop runny noses and sneezing.
- **Pain relievers.** Ease fever, headaches, and minor aches and pains.

WHAT DO YOU NEED TO KNOW ABOUT TAKING COLD AND COUGH MEDICINES?

Before taking these medicines, read the labels and follow the instructions carefully. Many cold and cough medicines contain the same active ingredients. For example, some of them include pain relievers. If you are taking these medicines and are also taking a separate pain reliever, you could be getting a dangerous amount of the pain reliever.

Do not give cold or cough medicines to children under two and do not give aspirin to children.

WHAT ELSE CAN YOU DO TO FEEL BETTER FOR A COLD OR COUGH?

If you decide that you do not want to take cold and cough medicines, there are other ways to feel better:

- Drink lots of fluids.
- Get plenty of rest.
- Use a cool mist humidifier.
- Use saline nose drops or sprays.
- Use nasal suctioning with a bulb syringe, which can be very helpful in children under a year old.[1]

Section 58.2 | Differentiating Cold, COVID-19, Flu, or Allergy

Feeling sick can be especially concerning these days. Could your sniffles be caused by COVID-19? Or the flu? Or a cold? Or maybe allergies?

Determining the cause of an illness can be tricky because many share some symptoms. They can leave you sniffling, coughing, and feeling tired. But there are important differences. Figuring out what is making you sick can help you recover and prevent spreading sickness to others.

FLU VERSUS COVID-19

"Distinguishing COVID from flu can be difficult because the symptoms overlap so much," explains Dr. Brooke Bozick, program officer in the Respiratory Diseases Branch in the Division of Microbiology and Infectious Diseases (DMID) at the National Institute of Allergy and Infectious Diseases (NIAID) within the National Institutes of Health (NIH).

Flu and COVID-19 are caused by different viruses that can be spread among people. Flu is caused by the influenza virus. COVID-19 is caused by severe acute respiratory syndrome coronavirus 2 (SARS-CoV-2). Both can give you a fever, cough, headaches, and body aches.

[1] MedlinePlus, "Cold and Cough Medicines," National Institutes of Health (NIH), February 8, 2022. Available online. URL: https://medlineplus.gov/coldandcoughmedicines.html.htm. Accessed July 4, 2023.

Flu and COVID-19 also spread similarly. They are transmitted by small particles that come from your nose and mouth when you sneeze, cough, sing, or talk, raising the possibility of infecting people who are nearby. Infected people may not have symptoms but can still pass along either virus. "Both influenza and COVID can be spread to other people before individuals develop symptoms," notes Dr. Aubree Gordon, associate professor in the Department of Epidemiology in the School of Public Health at the University of Michigan.

COVID-19 symptoms can take longer than flu symptoms to develop, she explains. Someone with flu usually has symptoms one to four days after being infected. A person with COVID-19 typically shows symptoms about five days after infection although this can range from 2 to 14 days. One telling sign of COVID-19 in some cases is loss of smell or taste. But, because of other similar symptoms, there is really only one way to be certain if you have COVID-19 or flu: Get tested. "You can go and get a COVID test at many pharmacies, and your doctor can administer tests for flu," Dr. Bozick says. COVID-19 tests are also available at many health centers. And you can buy testing kits approved for use at home.

COULD IT BE A COLD? OR ALLERGIES?

Like flu and COVID-19, colds are also caused by viruses and can be passed to others. Symptoms of a cold tend to be mild. You may have a runny nose, cough, congestion, and sore throat. But you would not usually have the aches and fever that are common with COVID-19 and flu. Often, you will feel better in a couple of days.

There is no cure for the common cold. Typical treatments include rest, fluids, and over-the-counter (OTC) medicines. Some complementary treatments may help with cold symptoms, too. Taking honey may help with nighttime cough for children over one year old. Rinsing your nose and sinuses can help with congestion. You can use a neti pot or other nasal rinsing device. Be sure to only use water that has been properly processed, such as distilled or boiled water, not tap water. Nasal rinses can bring relief for both colds and allergies.

Allergies can cause a runny nose and sneezing. But they are not contagious. If your eyes, nose, or ears itch, that could also be an allergy. Exposure to things such as dust, pets, and tree or grass pollen can trigger allergies, which are caused by the immune system overreacting.

Allergy symptoms tend to stop when you are no longer exposed to the cause. Unless you have asthma, allergies typically do not cause breathing problems. Allergies can be treated with drugs such as antihistamines, decongestants, and nasal steroids.

WINTERY MIX OF VIRUSES

Winter is the prime cold and flu season. You are more likely to be indoors and closer to others when it is colder outside. Weather also plays a role in the spread of viruses. "Cold and flu viruses survive better and are more transmissible if it is cooler and if there is lower humidity," Dr. Gordon explains.

Experts are concerned that flu and COVID-19 cases may increase and overlap in the winter. Flu cases usually start to increase around October and peak between December and February. Being infected with flu and SARS-CoV-2 at the same time is possible, as is showing symptoms of both.

If you are sick with the flu, your doctor may prescribe antiviral drugs. Such drugs can make your flu milder and shorten the time you are sick. They work best if they are used early in your illness.

The U.S. Food and Drug Administration (FDA) has also approved one antiviral drug, called "remdesivir," to treat COVID-19. Other treatments are in development and under review. No complementary approaches have been shown to be helpful for fighting off flu or COVID-19.

Fortunately, strategies to prevent the spread of COVID-19 also prevent the spread of flu and colds. "Measures such as masking and social distancing work for other respiratory viruses, as well as COVID-19," says Dr. Chip Walter, pediatrician and chief medical officer at the Duke Human Vaccine Institute.[2]

---

[2] *NIH News in Health*, "Is It Flu, COVID-19, Allergies, or a Cold?" National Institutes of Health (NIH), January 1, 2022. Available online. URL: https://newsinhealth.nih.gov/2022/01/it-flu-covid-19-allergies-or-cold. Accessed July 4, 2023.

Section 58.3 | Healthy Habits to Prevent Flu

The single best way to reduce the risk of seasonal flu and its potentially serious complications is to get vaccinated each year, but good health habits such as avoiding people who are sick, covering your cough, and washing your hands can often help stop the spread of germs and prevent respiratory illnesses, such as flu. There are also flu antiviral drugs that can be used to treat and prevent flu. The following tips and resources will help you learn about actions you can take to protect yourself and others from flu and help stop the spread of germs:

- **Avoid close contact**. Avoid close contact with people who are sick. When you are sick, keep your distance from others to protect them from getting sick too.
- **Stay home when you are sick**. If possible, stay home from work, school, and errands when you are sick. This will help prevent the spread of your illness to others.
- **Cover your mouth and nose**. When coughing or sneezing, cover your mouth and nose with a tissue. It may prevent those around you from getting sick. Flu viruses spread mainly by droplets made when people with flu cough, sneeze, or talk.
- **Clean your hands**. Washing your hands often will help protect you from germs. If soap and water are not available, use an alcohol-based hand rub.
- **Avoid touching your eyes, nose, or mouth**. Germs can be spread when a person touches something that is contaminated with germs and then touches his or her eyes, nose, or mouth.
- **Practice other good health habits**. Clean and disinfect frequently touched surfaces at home, work, or school, especially when someone is ill. Get plenty of sleep, be physically active, manage your stress, drink plenty of fluids, and eat nutritious food.

PREVENTING FLU AT WORK AND SCHOOL

At School

- Find out about plans your child's school, childcare program, and/or college has if an outbreak of flu or another illness occurs and whether flu vaccinations are offered on-site.
- Make sure your child's school, childcare program, and/or college routinely cleans frequently touched objects and surfaces and that they have a good supply of tissues, soap, paper towels, alcohol-based hand rubs, and disposable wipes on-site.
- Ask how sick students and staff are separated from others and who will care for them until they can go home and about the absentee policy for sick students and staff.

At Work

- Find out about your employer's plans if an outbreak of flu or another illness occurs and whether flu vaccinations are offered on-site.
- Routinely clean frequently touched objects and surfaces, including doorknobs, keyboards, and phones, to help remove germs.
- Make sure your workplace has an adequate supply of tissues, soap, paper towels, alcohol-based hand rubs, and disposable wipes.
- Train others on how to do your job, so they can cover for you in case you or a family member gets sick and you have to stay home.
- If you begin to feel sick while at work, go home as soon as possible.[3]

[3] "Healthy Habits to Help Protect against Flu," Centers for Disease Control and Prevention (CDC), August 26, 2021. Available online. URL: www.cdc.gov/flu/prevent/actions-prevent-flu.htm. Accessed July 4, 2023.

Section 58.4 | Taking Care of Yourself When You Have Seasonal Flu

WHAT SHOULD YOU DO IF YOU GET SICK?

Most people with flu have mild illness and do not need medical care or antiviral drugs. If you get sick with flu symptoms, in most cases, you should stay home and avoid contact with other people except to get medical care.

If, however, you have symptoms of flu and are in a higher-risk group or are very sick or worried about your illness, contact your health-care provider (doctor, physician assistant, etc.).

Certain people are at increased risk of serious flu-related complications (including young children, people aged 65 and older, pregnant women, and people with certain medical conditions). For a full list of people at increased risk of flu-related complications, visit www.cdc.gov/flu/highrisk/index.htm. If you are in a higher-risk group and develop flu symptoms, it is best for you to contact your doctor early in your illness. Remind them about your higher-risk status for flu. The Centers for Disease Control and Prevention (CDC) recommends that people at higher risk for complications should get antiviral treatment as early as possible because the benefit is greatest if treatment is started within two days after illness onset.

DO YOU NEED TO GO TO THE EMERGENCY ROOM IF YOU ARE ONLY A LITTLE SICK?

No. The emergency room should be used for people who are very sick. You should not go to the emergency room if you are only mildly ill.

If you have emergency warning signs of flu sickness, you should go to the emergency room. If you get sick with flu symptoms and are at higher risk of flu complications or you are concerned about your illness, call your health-care provider for advice.

WHAT ARE EMERGENCY WARNING SIGNS OF FLU?

People experiencing any of these warning signs should obtain medical care right away.

Warning Signs in Children

- fast breathing or trouble breathing
- bluish lips or face
- ribs pulling in with each breath
- chest pain
- severe muscle pain (child refusing to walk)
- dehydration (no urine for eight hours, dry mouth, and/or no tears when crying)
- not alert or interacting when awake
- seizures
- fever above 104 °F (40 °C)
- any fever in children less than 12 weeks
- fever or cough that improves but then returns or worsens
- worsening of chronic medical conditions

Warning Signs in Adults

- difficulty breathing or shortness of breath
- persistent pain or pressure in the chest or abdomen
- persistent dizziness, confusion, inability to arouse
- seizures
- not urinating
- severe muscle pain
- severe weakness or unsteadiness
- fever or cough that improves but then returns or worsens
- worsening of chronic medical conditions

These lists are not all-inclusive. Please consult your medical provider for any other symptom that is severe or concerning.

ARE THERE MEDICINES TO TREAT FLU?

Yes. There are drugs your doctor may prescribe for treating flu called "antivirals." These drugs can make you better faster and may also prevent serious complications.

HOW LONG SHOULD YOU STAY HOME IF YOU ARE SICK?

The CDC recommends that you stay home for at least 24 hours after your fever is gone except to get medical care or other necessities.

Your fever should be gone without the need to use a fever-reducing medicine, such as Tylenol®. Until then, you should stay home from work, school, travel, shopping, social events, and public gatherings.

The CDC also recommends that children and teenagers (anyone aged 18 and younger) who have flu or are suspected to have flu should not be given aspirin (acetylsalicylic acid) or any salicylate-containing products (e.g., Pepto-Bismol); this can cause a rare, very serious complication called "Reye syndrome."

WHAT SHOULD YOU DO WHILE YOU ARE SICK?

Stay away from others as much as possible to keep from infecting them. If you must leave home, for example, to get medical care, wear a face mask if you have one or cover coughs and sneezes with a tissue. Wash your hands often to keep from spreading the flu to others.[4]

[4] "Flu: What to Do If You Get Sick," Centers for Disease Control and Prevention (CDC), December 15, 2022. Available online. URL: www.cdc.gov/flu/treatment/takingcare.htm. Accessed July 4, 2023.

Chapter 59 | Sore Throat Care

Is it painful to swallow? Or is your throat scratchy? A virus may be causing your sore throat (refer to Figure 59.1).

CAUSES OF SORE THROAT

Causes of sore throat include the following:

- viruses, such as those that cause colds or flu
- bacteria group A strep, which causes strep throat (also called "streptococcal pharyngitis")
- allergies
- smoking or exposure to secondhand smoke

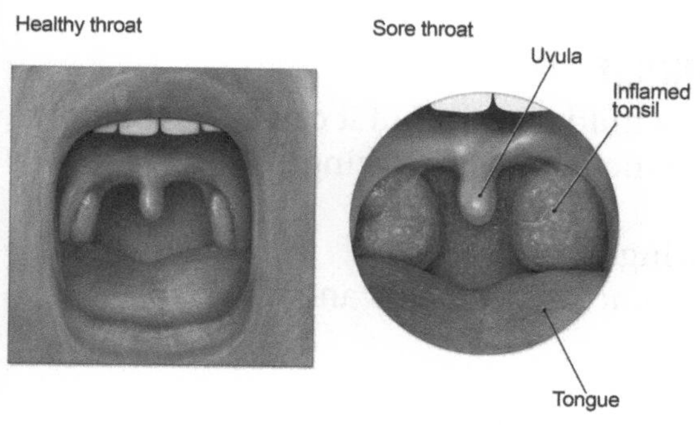

Figure 59.1. Sore Throat

Centers for Disease Control and Prevention (CDC)

Of these, infections from viruses are the most common cause of sore throats. Strep throat is an infection in the throat and tonsils caused by bacteria. These bacteria are called "group A *Streptococcus*" (also called "*Streptococcus pyogenes*"). A virus causes the most common type of sore throat and is not strep throat.

- Only 3 in 10 children with a sore throat have strep throat.
- Only about 1 in 10 adults with a sore throat has strep throat.

SYMPTOMS OF SORE THROAT

A sore throat can make it painful to swallow. A sore throat can also feel dry and scratchy. A sore throat can be a symptom of strep throat, the common cold, allergies, or other upper respiratory tract illnesses. Sore throat caused by a virus or the bacteria called "group A *Streptococcus*" can have similar symptoms. Sometimes, the following symptoms suggest a virus is causing the illness instead of strep throat:

- cough
- runny nose
- hoarseness (changes in your voice that make it sound breathy, raspy, or strained)
- conjunctivitis (also called "pink eye")

SYMPTOMS OF STREP THROAT

In general, strep throat is a mild disease, but it can be very painful. Common symptoms may include the following:

- fever
- pain when swallowing
- sore throat that can start very quickly and may look red
- red and swollen tonsils
- white patches or streaks of pus on the tonsils
- tiny, red spots on the roof of the mouth, called "petechiae"
- swollen lymph nodes in the front of the neck

The following symptoms suggest a virus is causing the illness instead of strep throat:

- cough
- runny nose
- hoarseness (changes in your voice that make it sound breathy, raspy, or strained)
- conjunctivitis (also called "pink eye")

WHEN TO SEEK MEDICAL CARE

Talk to your doctor if you or your child have symptoms of sore throat. They may need to test you or your child for strep throat. Also, see a doctor if you or your child have any of the following:

- difficulty breathing
- difficulty swallowing
- blood in saliva or phlegm
- excessive drooling (in young children)
- dehydration
- joint swelling and pain
- rash

This list is not all-inclusive. Please see your doctor for any symptom that is severe or concerning. See a doctor if symptoms do not improve within a few days or get worse. Tell your doctor if you or your child have recurrent sore throats.

TREATMENT FOR SORE THROAT

A doctor will determine what type of illness you have by asking about symptoms and doing a physical examination. Sometimes, they will also swab your throat.

Since bacteria cause strep throat, antibiotics are needed to treat the infection and prevent rheumatic fever and other complications. A doctor cannot tell if someone has strep throat just by looking in the throat. If your doctor thinks you might have strep throat, they can test you to determine if it is causing your illness.

Anyone with strep throat should stay home from work, school, or daycare until they no longer have a fever and have taken antibiotics for at least 12 hours.

If a virus causes a sore throat, antibiotics will not help. Most sore throats will get better on their own within one week. Your doctor may prescribe other medicine or give you tips to help you feel better.

When antibiotics are not needed, they will not help you, and their side effects could still cause harm. Side effects can range from mild reactions, such as a rash, to more serious health problems. These problems can include severe allergic reactions, antibiotic-resistant infections, and *Clostridium difficile* (*C. difficile*) infections. *Clostridium difficile* causes diarrhea that can lead to severe colon damage and death.

HOW TO FEEL BETTER

Some ways you can feel better when you have a sore throat are as follows:

- Suck on ice chips, Popsicles, or lozenges (do not give lozenges to children younger than two years).
- Use a clean humidifier or cool mist vaporizer.
- Gargle with salt water.
- Drink warm beverages and plenty of fluids.
- Use honey to relieve cough for adults and children at least one year of age or older.
- Ask your doctor or pharmacist about over-the-counter (OTC) medicines that can help you feel better. Always use OTC medicines as directed.[1]

[1] "Sore Throat," Centers for Disease Control and Prevention (CDC), October 6, 2021. Available online. URL: www.cdc.gov/antibiotic-use/sore-throat.html. Accessed July 3, 2023.

Chapter 60 | Fever: What You Can Do

A fever—also called "high temperature" or "pyrexia"—is a temporary rise in the body's temperature. It is not an illness itself but a natural defense against bacteria or viruses that thrives best at normal body temperature, around 98.6 °F (37 °C).

Hyperthermia is a form of fever in which the body's temperature rises far above normal and can be caused, for example, by side effects of illicit drugs or certain medications, stroke, or temperature-related conditions, such as heat stroke. Usually, a fever is not considered life-threatening, but hyperthermia can lead to a critical elevation of the body's temperature.

An adult is considered to have a fever if the body temperature is above 99–99.5 °F (37.2–37.5 °C), depending on the time of the day. (Body temperature is usually highest in late afternoon.) A child is considered to have a fever if the temperature is at or above:

- 100.4 °F (38 °C) rectally
- 99.5 °F (37.5 °C) orally
- 99 °F (37.2 °C) axillary (measured under the arm)

WHAT CAUSES FEVER?

The hypothalamus, a region in the brain that helps the body maintain its normal temperature, may cause temperature to fluctuate in response to a number of factors, such as eating, heavy clothing, high humidity, medications, physical activity, room temperature, strong emotions, and menstrual cycles in women. The hypothalamus may also cause an increase in the body temperature as a response to an infection or illness.

Although the most frequent causes of fever are common infections, such as colds, other possibilities include:

- appendicitis
- autoimmune or inflammatory conditions
- blood clots or thrombophlebitis
- bone infections (osteomyelitis)
- cancer, particularly leukemia, Hodgkin disease, and non-Hodgkin lymphoma
- reaction to medications, such as certain antibiotics, antihistamines, and seizure medicines
- hormone disorders, such as hyperthyroidism
- immunization, in some children
- infections of the bladder or kidney
- meningitis
- respiratory infections, such as flu, sinus infections, mononucleosis, bronchitis, pneumonia, and tuberculosis
- side effects of drugs such as amphetamines and cocaine
- skin infections or cellulitis
- teething

SIGNS AND SYMPTOMS OF FEVER

In addition to an elevated body temperature, other symptoms of fever, depending on its underlying cause, can include headache, sweating, chills, muscle aches, weakness, and dehydration.

In children, symptoms may also include fussiness, lethargy, poor appetite, stiff neck, rashes, earache, sore throat, cough, vomiting, diarrhea, and a weakened immune system.

HOW IS A FEVER DIAGNOSED?

Once a fever is measured with a thermometer, a physician will attempt to determine its cause by a physical examination (including a thorough examination of the skin, eyes, ears, nose, throat, neck, chest, and abdomen) and by asking about recent behavior and interactions, including travel to regions that are known to be sources of infections. For instance, conditions such as Lyme disease and Rocky Mountain spotted fever (RMSF) are endemic to certain parts of the United States, while conditions such as malaria are more common in sub-Saharan Africa and southern Asia. In certain cases, a person might be diagnosed with a "fever of unknown origin," one in which the cause is not attributable to an obvious condition.

To diagnose fever, the doctor may order tests that include:

- blood tests (such as a complete blood count or blood differential)
- chest x-ray
- urinalysis

HOW IS A FEVER TREATED?

A fever is treated based on its duration and cause, along with other symptoms that may accompany the elevated temperature. Typically, medications for fever include over-the-counter drugs, such as acetaminophen (Tylenol), and nonsteroidal anti-inflammatory medicines, such as naproxen (Aleve) and ibuprofen (Advil and Motrin). If the fever is the result of a bacterial infection, such as strep throat, antibiotics would be prescribed. Aspirin may be taken by adults but is not recommended for children and teens, as it is associated with Reye syndrome, which can cause damage to the brain and liver.

HOME CARE

Fever is not necessarily a symptom of a serious problem. While a simple cold can lead to body temperatures as high as 104 °F (40 °C), some serious conditions may cause no fever at all.

A mild fever does not generally require treatment; enough rest and proper fluid consumption will usually suffice. The condition is most likely not serious if the patient:

- is alert and active
- continues to eat and drink well
- has a normal skin color
- looks well when the body temperature returns to normal

If a person with a high body temperature is uncomfortable and experiences vomiting, dehydration, or inadequate sleep, follow these steps to reduce the fever:

- Make the room comfortable. It should neither be too hot nor too cool.
- Remove excess clothing from the person. A single layer of lightweight clothing will be sufficient. If the patient has chills, do not bundle him/her up excessively.
- Cool the person with a lukewarm bath or sponge bath. This may be particularly effective after medication is given.
- Avoid cold baths, ice, or alcohol rubs, as they worsen the situation by making the person shiver, which can increase the core body temperature.

When taking medicine to lower a fever, do the following:

- Always consult a doctor before giving medicines to a child aged three months or younger.
- In adults and children, acetaminophen and ibuprofen help reduce fever. A doctor may recommend the use of either type of medicine although ibuprofen is not generally recommended for children under the age of six months.
- Aspirin is highly effective for treating fever but is recommended only for adults unless prescribed for a child by a doctor.
- The correct dose of medicine should be given to a child based on the child's weight and per the instructions on the package.

It is important for adults, and even more so for children, to drink plenty of fluids to keep the body hydrated. Water, soup, Popsicles, and gelatin are good choices. Consumption of fruit juice should be limited, and sports drinks should be avoided in young children. Eating is fine; however, food should not be forced.

WHEN TO CONTACT A MEDICAL PROFESSIONAL

Call a doctor immediately if the fever:

- is 100.4 °F (38 °C) or higher in a child aged three months or younger
- is 102.2 °F (39 °C) or higher in children between the ages of 3 and 12 months
- is 105 °F (40.5 °C) or higher and does not come down readily when treated and the person is not comfortable
- lasts longer than 24–48 hours in children aged two years or younger
- lasts longer than 48–72 hours in those older than two years

Medical assistance will also be required if the patient:

- has a fever that stays at 103 °F (37 °C) or keeps rising
- has symptoms (such as a sore throat, cough, or earache) that are usually associated with other illnesses
- has had recurrent mild fevers for a week or more
- has bruises or a new rash
- has been vaccinated recently
- has pain when urinating
- traveled to another region or country recently
- is suffering from a serious medical condition, such as diabetes, heart disease, sickle cell anemia, chronic obstructive pulmonary disease (COPD), other chronic lung problems, or cystic fibrosis
- has problems with the immune system (such as one caused by a bone marrow or organ transplant, cancer treatment, chronic steroid therapy, human immunodeficiency virus (HIV), or spleen removal)

If an infant aged three months or younger has a temperature above 100.4 °F (38 °C) or any child has a temperature above 104 °F (38 °C), you should call a doctor or visit an emergency room immediately since this could be a sign of the potentially life-threatening condition. Febrile seizures can occur in some children with such high body temperatures although this generally does not cause any permanent damage. But brain damage can occur if the fever is above 107.6 °F (42 °C).

References

Blahd, William. "Fever Facts," WebMD, LLC, April 16, 2015. Available online. URL: www.webmd.com/first-aid/fevers-causes-symptoms-treatments. Accessed August 18, 2023.

Kaneshiro, Neil K. "Fever," MedlinePlus, U.S. National Library of Medicine, August 30, 2014. Available online. URL: https://medlineplus.gov/ency/article/003090.htm. Accessed August 18, 2023.

Chapter 61 | Mouth Sores: Causes and Care

Mouth sores are common ailments that appear on the soft tissues of your mouth, including the cheeks, lips, tongue, gums, roof, and floor of the mouth. There is also a possibility of developing mouth sores in your esophagus. There are many types of mouth sores; however, the most common types are cold sores and canker sores. Cold sores, sometimes called "fever blisters," form around your lips. Canker sores, also called "aphthous ulcers," are shallow, small lesions that develop on the soft tissues in the mouth or at the base of your gums.

CAUSES OF MOUTH SORES

Mostly, mouth sores occur as a result of irritation from:

- biting your cheek, tongue, or lip
- burning your mouth from hot drinks or foods
- chewing tobacco
- a sharp or broken tooth
- braces

In other cases, mouth sores can develop due to the following reasons:

- high acidic foods
- stress
- hormonal changes during pregnancy
- vitamin and folate deficiencies

The sores can spread from person to person through close contact (such as kissing). Cold sores are caused by the herpes simplex virus (HSV) and are contagious. Unlike cold sores, canker sores do not occur on the surface of the lips and are not contagious. The cause of the canker sores remains unclear, but it may be related to:

- virus
- irritation
- minor injury during dental operations
- overzealous brushing
- mouth rinses and toothpaste containing lauryl sulfate
- a diet lacking in vitamin B_{12}, zinc, folate, or iron
- hormonal changes during menstruation

Rarely, mouth sores can be a sign of a tumor or illness. In such cases, they may form in response to:

- mouth cancer
- infection (such as hand-foot-and-mouth syndrome)
- bleeding disorders
- weakened immune system
- autoimmune disorders

Certain drugs and medications, such as aspirin, penicillin, phenytoin, streptomycin, chemotherapeutic agents, and sulfa drugs, tend to cause mouth sores.

SIGNS AND SYMPTOMS OF MOUTH SORES

Cold Sores

Cold sores are tiny, fluid-filled blisters that occur around your lips. These blisters are often grouped together in patches. The symptoms of cold sores are:

- blisters, lesions, or ulcers in the mouth
- pain in the mouth or tongue
- lip swelling
- sore throat
- difficulty swallowing
- swollen glands

- fever
- headache

The signs and symptoms may vary depending on whether it is a recurrence or the first outbreak.

Canker Sores

Canker sores appear either as a single pale or yellow ulcer with a red outer ring or as a cluster of sores. The major symptoms of canker sores are:

- severe pain
- fever
- extreme difficulty eating and drinking

HOW TO TAKE CARE OF YOUR MOUTH SORES

Mouth sores can last for 10–14 days. Usually, mouth sores do not need any treatment, but persistent, large, and painful sores often do need medical attention. Follow these steps to make yourself feel better:

- Gargle with salt or cold water.
- Apply cool compression.
- Avoid hot beverages.
- Avoid eating spicy and salty foods.
- Avoid citrus fruits.
- Avoid alcohol.
- Take pain relievers, such as acetaminophen.

For canker sores, follow these steps:

- Apply a thin paste of water and baking soda to the sore.
- For severe cases, anti-inflammatory amlexanox paste (Aphthasol®) or fluocinonide gel (Lidex®) is recommended.

Over-the-counter (OTC) medicines (such as creams, pastes, gels, or liquids) can help relieve the pain caused by mouth sores and to speed up the healing process.

WHEN TO SEE THE DOCTOR

You must consult the doctor if:

- you have large patches on the tongue or roof of the mouth
- the sore begins after starting a new medication
- the sore lasts more than two weeks
- you have other symptoms, such as a skin rash, drooling, fever, or difficulty swallowing

WHAT TO EXPECT DURING A DOCTOR'S VISIT

The doctor will perform a physical examination of your tongue and mouth and review your medical history and symptoms. The treatment will consist of the following:

- antiviral medication to treat the sores that are caused by the herpes simplex virus (HSV)
- medicine to numb the area that is causing extreme pain, which may be prescribed as an ointment, such as lidocaine (which must not be used for children)
- steroid gel to apply to the mouth sore
- a paste that stops swelling and inflammation (Aphthasol)

The doctor will prescribe a mouthwash, such as chlorhexidine gluconate (Peridex), or a solution to use to rinse the mouth. This will help you heal and prevent further infections. The doctor may recommend a nutritional supplement, such as folate, zinc, or vitamin B_{12}, if you are low on nutrients.

PREVENTION OF MOUTH SORES

Mouth sores are common and can be prevented from spreading. Follow these steps to prevent mouth sores from spreading:

- Avoid close contact with people who have sores. The virus spreads more quickly when the sores secrete moisture from blisters.
- Avoid sharing personal items. Towels, utensils, and lip balms can spread the virus when blisters are present.
- Keep your hands clean.

References

"Canker Sore," Mayo Foundation for Medical Education and Research (MFMER), April 3, 2018. Available online. URL: www.mayoclinic.org/diseases-conditions/canker-sore/diagnosis-treatment/drc-20370620. Accessed August 18, 2023.

"Cold Sore," Mayo Foundation for Medical Education and Research (MFMER), January 24, 2023. Available online. URL: www.mayoclinic.org/diseases-conditions/cold-sore/symptoms-causes/syc-20371017. Accessed August 18, 2023.

Felman, Adam. "Everything You Need to Know about Cold Sores," Medical News Today, September 25, 2020. Available online. URL: www.medicalnewstoday.com/articles/172389.php. Accessed August 18, 2023.

Fletcher, Jenna. "Mouth Sores: Everything You Need to Know," Medical News Today, March 12, 2019. Available online. URL: www.medicalnewstoday.com/articles/324680. Accessed August 18, 2023.

Chapter 62 | **Over-the-Counter Medications for Contagious Diseases**

Chapter Contents

Section 62.1 | Understanding Over-the-Counter Medicines

WHAT ARE OVER-THE-COUNTER MEDICINES?

Over-the-counter (OTC) medicines are those that can be sold directly to people without a prescription. OTC medicines treat a variety of illnesses and their symptoms, including pain, coughs and colds, diarrhea, constipation, acne, and others. Some OTC medicines have active ingredients with the potential for misuse at higher-than-recommended dosages.

HOW DO PEOPLE USE AND MISUSE OVER-THE-COUNTER MEDICINES?

Misuse of an OTC medicine means:

- taking medicine in a way or dose other than directed on the package
- taking medicine for the effect it causes, for example, to get high
- mixing OTC medicines together to create new products

WHAT ARE SOME OF THE COMMONLY MISUSED OVER-THE-COUNTER MEDICINES?

There are two OTC medicines that are most commonly misused:

- **Dextromethorphan (DXM).** DXM is a cough suppressant found in many OTC cold medicines. The most common sources of abused DXM are "extra-strength" cough syrup, tablets, and gel capsules. OTC medications that contain DXM often also contain antihistamines and decongestants. DXM may be swallowed in its original form or may be mixed with soda for flavor, called "robotripping" or "skittling." Users sometimes inject it. These medicines are often misused in combination with other drugs, such as alcohol and marijuana.
- **Loperamide.** This is an antidiarrheal that is available in tablet, capsule, or liquid form. When misusing loperamide, people swallow large quantities of the medicine. It is unclear how often this drug is misused.

HOW DO THESE OVER-THE-COUNTER MEDICINES AFFECT THE BRAIN?

- **DXM**. DXM is an opioid without effects on pain reduction and does not act on the opioid receptors. When taken in large doses, DXM causes a depressant effect and sometimes a hallucinogenic effect, similar to phencyclidine (PCP) and ketamine. Repeatedly seeking to experience that feeling can lead to addiction—a chronic relapsing brain condition characterized by the inability to stop using a drug despite damaging consequences to a person's life and health.
- **Loperamide**. Loperamide is an opioid designed not to enter the brain. However, when taken in large amounts and combined with other substances, it may cause the drug to act in a similar way to other opioids. Other opioids, such as certain prescription pain relievers and heroin, bind to and activate opioid receptors in many areas of the brain, especially those involved in feelings of pain and pleasure. Opioid receptors are also located in the brain stem, which controls important processes, such as blood pressure, arousal, and breathing.

WHAT ARE THE HEALTH EFFECTS OF THESE OVER-THE-COUNTER MEDICINES?

Dextromethorphan

Short-term effects of DXM misuse can range from mild stimulation to alcohol- or marijuana-like intoxication. At high doses, a person may have hallucinations or feelings of physical distortion, extreme panic, paranoia, anxiety, and aggression.

Other health effects from DXM misuse can include the following:

- hyperexcitability
- poor motor control
- lack of energy
- stomach pain
- vision changes
- slurred speech

- increased blood pressure
- sweating

Misuse of DXM products containing acetaminophen can cause liver damage.

Loperamide

In the short term, loperamide is sometimes misused to lessen cravings and withdrawal symptoms; however, it can cause euphoria, similar to other opioids.

Loperamide misuse can also lead to fainting, stomach pain, constipation, eye changes, and loss of consciousness. It can cause the heart to beat erratically or rapidly or cause kidney problems. These effects may increase if taken with other medicines that interact with loperamide. Other effects have not been well studied, and reports are mixed, but the physical consequences of loperamide misuse can be severe.

CAN A PERSON OVERDOSE ON THESE OVER-THE-COUNTER MEDICINES?

Yes, a person can overdose on cold medicines containing DXM or loperamide. An overdose occurs when a person uses enough of the drug to produce a life-threatening reaction or death.

As with other opioids, when people overdose on DXM or loperamide, their breathing often slows or stops. This can decrease the amount of oxygen that reaches the brain, a condition called "hypoxia." Hypoxia can have short- and long-term mental effects and effects on the nervous system, including coma, permanent brain damage, and death.

HOW CAN THESE OVER-THE-COUNTER MEDICINE OVERDOSES BE TREATED?

A person who has overdosed needs immediate medical attention. Call 911. If the person has stopped breathing or if breathing is weak, begin cardiopulmonary resuscitation (CPR). DXM overdoses can also be treated with naloxone.

Certain medications can be used to treat heart rhythm problems caused by loperamide overdose. If the heart stops, health-care providers will perform CPR and other cardiac support therapies.

CAN MISUSE OF THESE OVER-THE-COUNTER MEDICINES LEAD TO ADDICTION?

Yes, misuse of DXM or loperamide can lead to addiction. An addiction develops when continued use of the drug causes issues, such as health problems and failure to meet responsibilities at work, school, or home. The symptoms of withdrawal from DXM and loperamide have not been well studied.

HOW CAN PEOPLE GET TREATMENT FOR ADDICTION TO THESE OVER-THE-COUNTER MEDICINES?

There are no medications approved specifically to treat DXM or loperamide addiction. Behavioral therapies, such as cognitive-behavioral therapy (CBT) and contingency management, may be helpful. CBT helps modify the patient's drug-use expectations and behaviors and effectively manage triggers and stress. Contingency management provides vouchers or small cash rewards for positive behaviors such as staying drug-free.[1]

[1] National Institute on Drug Abuse (NIDA), "Over-the-Counter Medicines DrugFacts," National Institutes of Health (NIH), December 17, 2017. Available online. URL: https://nida.nih.gov/publications/drugfacts/over-counter-medicines. Accessed July 3, 2023.

Section 62.2 | Over-the-Counter Medicines for Children

Use care when giving any medicine to an infant or a child. Even over-the-counter (OTC) medicines that you buy are serious medicines. The following is advice for giving OTC medicine to your child, from the U.S. Food and Drug Administration (FDA) and the makers of OTC medicines:

- **Always read and follow the Drug Facts label on your OTC medicine.** This is important for choosing and safely using all OTC medicines. Read the label every time before you give the medicine. Be sure you clearly understand how much medicine to give and when the medicine can be taken again.
- **Know the "active ingredient" in your child's medicine.** This is what makes the medicine work and is always listed at the top of the Drug Facts label. Sometimes, an active ingredient can treat more than one medical condition. For that reason, the same active ingredient can be found in many different medicines that are used to treat different symptoms. For example, a medicine for a cold and a medicine for a headache could each contain the same active ingredient. So, if you are treating a cold and a headache with two medicines and both have the same active ingredient, you could be giving two times the normal dose. If you are confused about your child's medicines, check with a doctor, nurse, or pharmacist.
- **Give the right medicine, in the right amount, to your child. Not all medicines are right for an infant or a child.** Medicines with the same brand name can be sold in many different strengths, such as infant, child, and adult formulas. The amount and directions are also different for children of different ages or weights. Always use the right medicine and follow the directions exactly. Never use more medicine than directed, even if your child seems sicker than the last time.

- **Talk to your doctor, pharmacist, or nurse to find out what mixes well and what does not.** Medicines, vitamins, supplements, foods, and beverages do not always mix well with each other. Your health-care professional can help.
- **Use the dosing tool that comes with the medicine, such as a dropper or a dosing cup.** A different dosing tool, or a kitchen spoon, could hold the wrong amount of medicine.
- **Know the difference between a tablespoon (tbsp.) and a teaspoon (tsp.).** Do not confuse them! A tablespoon holds three times as much medicine as a teaspoon. On measuring tools, a teaspoon (tsp) is equal to "5 cc" or "5 mL."
- **Know your child's weight.** Directions on some OTC medicines are based on weight. Never guess the amount of medicine to give to your child or try to figure it out from the adult dose instructions. If a dose is not listed for your child's age or weight, call your doctor or other members of your health-care team.
- **Prevent a poison emergency by always using a child-resistant cap.** Relock the cap after each use. Be especially careful with any products that contain iron; they are the leading cause of poisoning deaths in young children.
- **Store all medicines in a safe place.** Today's medicines are tasty and colorful, and many can be chewed. Kids may think that these products are candy. To prevent an overdose or poisoning emergency, store all medicines and vitamins in a safe place out of your child's (and even your pet's) sight and reach. If your child takes too much, call the Poison Center Hotline at 800-222-1222 (open 24 hours every day, seven days a week) or call 911.
- **Check the medicine three times.** First, check the outside packaging for such things as cuts, slices, or tears. Second, once you are at home, check the label on the inside package to be sure you have the

right medicine. Make sure the lid and seal are not broken. Third, check the color, shape, size, and smell of the medicine. If you notice anything different or unusual, talk to a pharmacist or another health-care professional.[2]

[2] "Kids Aren't Just Small Adults—Medicines, Children, and the Care Every Child Deserves," U.S. Food and Drug Administration (FDA), December 17, 2017. Available online. URL: www.fda.gov/drugs/resourcesforyou/consumers/ucm312776.htm. Accessed July 3, 2023.

Chapter 63 | **Prescription Medicines for Contagious Diseases**

Although evidence suggests that the use of medicines to treat infections, also known as "antimicrobial chemotherapy," may date back to ancient times, the modern use of this treatment began in the early 20th century when researchers in the lab of Paul Ehrlich, a German physician and scientist, synthesized an arsenical compound called "arsphenamine." This drug, manufactured under the trade name Salvarsan, went on to become the first chemotherapeutic agent proven effective against human parasitic disease and was widely used in the treatment of syphilis.

This was followed by the discovery of penicillin in 1928 by Alexander Fleming, a Scottish scientist, who noticed that the accidental growth of Penicillium mold in a petri dish inhibited the growth of *Staphylococcus aureus* bacteria. By the forties, this wonder drug was being used to treat a number of infections—some life-threatening—of skin, blood, bone, and vital organs caused by *Staphylococcus*. During World War II, penicillin saved millions of lives and prevented the debilitating effects of wounds from dangerous infections. These early discoveries set the stage for the development of numerous anti-infective agents capable of preventing and treating a wide range of microbial infections.

Infections are generally caused when infective agents, such as bacteria, viruses, or fungi, invade the tissues of an organism, sometimes called the "host." These organisms multiply inside the host and produce toxins, provoking a reaction in the host tissues that could either result in an acute infection (short term) or a chronic infection (long term). There are a number of anti-infective agents that are used to treat infections. These agents work either by killing the infectious agent or pathogen or by inhibiting its growth. While antimicrobial chemotherapy refers to the treatment of infections caused by infective agents, antimicrobial prophylaxis is used to prevent the spread of infection caused by pathogens. Anti-infective agents are classified on the basis of the infective agents they fight. For example, antibacterials are pharmacologic agents generally used to treat infections caused by bacteria. Antifungals are primarily effective against fungi and include fungistats (which inhibit fungal growth and proliferation) and fungicides (which kill fungal cells and spores). Antivirals and antiprotozoals act against viruses and protozoa, respectively.

ANTIBIOTICS

The discovery of antimicrobial agents, particularly antibiotics, is often regarded as one of the greatest achievements of modern medicine since it led to a significant decline in mortality rates from infectious diseases. The term "antibiotic" was first suggested by Selman Waksman, a Russian-born American biochemist and microbiologist credited with the discovery of several antibiotics, including streptomycin and neomycin, which have found extensive use in the treatment of many infectious diseases. The term is used to define the activity or application of a chemical compound, and it includes any molecule that kills or inhibits the growth of bacteria.

Classes of Antibiotics

Antibiotics may be derived from certain classes of microorganisms or living systems and are used to fight against one or more types of disease-causing microorganisms. They may also be derived from nonorganic sources, as in the case of sulfonamides and quinolones. Some antibiotics are effective against a number of bacteria, both gram-positive and gram-negative; these are termed broad-spectrum antibiotics. Other antibiotics, called "narrow-spectrum," are used to treat infections caused by specific families of bacteria.

Mode of Action

Most antibiotics work by disrupting the bacteria's metabolic processes. Although the exact mechanism of how this is brought about is still under study, it is believed that most antibacterial action targets enzymes that regulate the biosynthesis of the cell wall or cell proteins, while others target enzymes that regulate nucleic acid metabolism of the bacterial cell. Some, like ionophores, work by interfering with cell membrane integrity. Antibiotics such as penicillin and cephalosporins act on the bacterial cell wall, while quinolones and sulfonamides target the bacterial enzymes. Lincosamides and tetracyclines are examples of antibiotics that interfere with protein synthesis in bacterial cells.

Although the discovery of antibiotics was thought to herald the end of infectious diseases, their rampant misuse and overuse in humans, as well as in food-producing animals, in the last few decades have led to the emergence of antibiotic-resistant strains of bacteria. Antibiotics that were used successfully in the treatment of many infections in the past have now become inefficient against the same infection, and the dire need for new antibiotics—along with a slowdown in antibiotic discovery programs in the pharmaceutical industry—poses a serious challenge to public health worldwide.

ANTIVIRALS

Drugs used to treat infections caused by viruses are called "antiviral drugs." Unlike bacteria, viruses are difficult to treat because they are obligate parasites, meaning they can grow and multiply only within living hosts. This makes it impossible to use prophylactic measures to contain viral infections. Contrary to popular belief, antibiotics do not treat viral infections, such as influenza, bronchitis, ear infections, or chest colds in otherwise healthy people. Most of the antiviral remedies currently in use include vaccines, which have successfully controlled—and in some cases eradicated—such serious viral infections as smallpox and poliomyelitis. The last few decades have seen growing interest in developing antiviral drugs to prevent the multiplication of the virus and cause the illness to run its course rapidly. Unfortunately, these drugs are only partially effective and work only on a very few specific viruses. The most difficult aspect of developing antiviral agents is the astounding diversity in the structural characteristics of viruses, of which there can be more than 50 different types for any given virus. In addition, the viral antigen, a protein coded by the viral genome that provokes an immune response in the host cell, periodically mutates making it particularly difficult to contain the infection with specific therapy.

Select Classes of Antiviral Drugs

ANTI-HEPATITIS

Viral hepatitis can be treated with several antiviral medications, most of which work by preventing viral replication in infected cells. Ribavirin is commonly used to treat hepatitis C, while lamivudine and adefovir are used to treat chronic hepatitis B infections. In addition to treating viral hepatitis, these drugs are also used to treat human immunodeficiency virus (HIV) infections. Interferons are another important class of drugs used in the treatment regimen for hepatitis, and they are commonly used in combination with other antiviral agents, such as ribavirin.

ANTI-HERPES

Anti-herpes medications such as acyclovir, penciclovir, and their respective prodrugs (an inactive form of medication that is metabolized into a pharmacologically active drug inside the body) interfere with viral deoxyribonucleic acid (DNA) replication and help control their spread to new cells. While anti-herpes drugs cannot eradicate the virus, they can help control symptoms and reduce the course of infections.

ANTI-INFLUENZA

Anti-influenza medications are not substitutes for vaccination but are used in conjunction with vaccines. Some strains of the influenza virus have become resistant to older antiviral drugs, such as amantadine and rimantadine, and are no longer used although their potential use against new strains of virus that may be susceptible to these drugs cannot be ruled out. Some of the FDA-approved anti-influenza drugs include oseltamivir (Tamiflu), zanamivir

(Relenza), and peramivir (Rapivab). These drugs can ease the severity of symptoms and reduce the course of infection. The government maintains a stockpile of anti-influenza medications in preparation for a pandemic emergency.

ANTIRETROVIRAL (ART)

Antiretroviral drugs work by suppressing a virus and retarding the progression of the disease. Although the antiretroviral drugs do not kill the virus or cure the disease, they slow down viral replication and substantially reduce the amount of virus in the body. This helps the immune system stay healthy and also reduces the risk of transmission to other people. More often than not, a cocktail of drugs from three or more classes of antiretroviral drugs is used for maximum effect. Referred to as highly active antiretroviral therapy (HAART), this treatment regimen has substantially reduced HIV-related morbidity and mortality around the world.

ANTIPROTOZOALS

These are drugs that are used to treat infections caused by single-celled protozoans, such as *Entamoeba histolytica*, which causes amoebiasis, and plasmodium, the pathogen that causes malaria. Like many other infective agents, antiprotozoals work on specific targets and inhibit their growth and reproduction. Antimalarial drugs, which include a diverse class of quinoline derivatives, act by targeting the erythrocytic (red blood cell) stage of the infection, which can be life-threatening, since blood circulates through all tissues and organs. In addition to antimalarials, there are several other classes of antiprotozoals, some of which may also be used to treat certain bacterial infections. Two of the most commonly used drugs in this group are metronidazole and tinidazole, which are used to treat a variety of parasitic and amoebic infections.

ANTIFUNGAL DRUGS

This class of medication controls a diverse range of infections caused by fungi, from simple infections such as athlete's foot to extremely dangerous infections such as cryptococcal meningitis, which affects the brain and spinal cord. Antifungal medications are based on mechanisms that inhibit vital cell processes in the organism. They work by either disrupting the integrity of the fungal cell membrane or cell wall or interfering with cell division by preventing DNA replication.

Antifungal agents are broadly classified as topical and systemic drugs. While topical antifungal agents may be directly applied to skin, nails, or hair to treat superficial fungal infections, systemic antifungal agents are used to treat invasive fungal infections that affect body tissues or internal organs. Antifungal drugs come as lotions, sprays, creams, tablets, injections, and pessaries (for vaginal use).

As in the case of antibiotics, drug resistance has become a major concern with a number of antifungal drugs as a result of their indiscriminate use in health-care settings. For example, low dosage or short-term treatments may be a common cause of antifungal resistance in candidemia—one of the most common bloodstream infections in hospital settings—which incurs substantial health-care costs. Although drug resistance in several species of *Candida* is a serious problem, studies show that drug resistance in other fungal species, such as *Aspergillus*, is also becoming a cause for concern. Some studies also show that the overuse of antibiotics could lead to resistance by inhibiting gut bacteria and favoring the growth of fungal species such as *Candida*.

References

"Antiviral Drug," Encyclopaedia Britannica, August 1, 2023. Available online. URL: www.britannica.com/science/antiviral-drug. Accessed August 18, 2023.

Coates, Anthony RM; Halls, Gerry; and Hu, Yanmin. "Novel Classes of Antibiotics or More of the Same?" *British Journal of Pharmacology*, 163, no. 1 (2011): 184–194. 10.1111/j.1476-5381.2011.01250.

Davies, Julian and Davies, Dorothy. "Origins and Evolution of Antibiotic Resistance," *Microbiology and Molecular Biology Reviews*, 74, no. 3 (2010): 417–433. 10.1128/MMBR.00016-10.

Chapter 64 | **Antiviral Drugs for Seasonal Flu**

NEURAMINIDASE INHIBITORS

Neuraminidase inhibitors are chemically related antiviral medications that block the viral neuraminidase enzyme and have activity against both influenza A and B viruses. The neuraminidase inhibitors include the following:

- **Oseltamivir.** This (available as a generic or under the trade name Tamiflu® for oral administration) is approved by the U.S. Food and Drug Administration (FDA) for early treatment of uncomplicated influenza in people aged two weeks and older and for chemoprophylaxis to prevent influenza in people aged one year and older. Although not part of the FDA-approved indications, the use of oral oseltamivir for treatment of influenza in infants younger than 14 days and for chemoprophylaxis in infants aged 3 months to 1 year is recommended by the Centers for Disease Control and Prevention (CDC) and the American Academy of Pediatrics (AAP). If a child is younger than three months, the use of oseltamivir for chemoprophylaxis is not recommended unless the situation is judged critical, due to limited data in this age group.
- **Zanamivir (trade name Relenza®) for oral inhalation.** This is FDA-approved for early treatment of uncomplicated influenza in people aged seven and older and to prevent influenza in people aged five and older. It is not recommended for use in people with

underlying respiratory disease, including people with asthma.

- **Peramivir (trade name Rapivab®) for intravenous administration**. This is FDA-approved for early treatment of uncomplicated influenza in people aged six months and older.

CAP-DEPENDENT ENDONUCLEASE INHIBITOR

An endonuclease inhibitor has a different mechanism of action than a neuraminidase inhibitor. Endonuclease inhibitors interfere with viral ribonucleic acid (RNA) transcription and block virus replication in both influenza A and B viruses. There is only one approved cap-dependent endonuclease inhibitor:

- **Baloxavir marboxil (trade name Xofluza®) for oral administration**. This is FDA-approved for early treatment of uncomplicated influenza in otherwise healthy non-high-risk people of 5 to less than 12 years of age and for all persons aged 12 and older and for post-exposure prophylaxis of influenza in people aged 5 and older. Baloxavir is not recommended for pregnant women, immunocompromised persons, breastfeeding mothers, outpatients with complicated or progressive illnesses, or hospitalized patients.

ADAMANTANES

The adamantanes target the M2 ion channel protein of influenza A viruses. (Therefore, these medications are active against influenza A viruses, but not influenza B viruses.) The adamantanes are not currently recommended for use in the United States because of widespread antiviral resistance in circulating influenza A viruses. The adamantanes include the following:

- **Amantadine (generic) for oral administration**. This is FDA-approved to treat and prevent only influenza A viruses in people older than one year.
- **Rimantadine (generic or under the trade name Flumadine®) for oral administration**. This is

FDA-approved to prevent only influenza A virus infection among people older than one year. It is approved to treat only influenza A virus infections in people aged 17 and older.[1]

[1] "Antiviral Drugs for Seasonal Influenza: Additional Links and Resources," Centers for Disease Control and Prevention (CDC), September 1, 2022. Available online. URL: www.cdc.gov/flu/professionals/antivirals/links.htm. Accessed June 13, 2023.

Chapter 65 | **Drug Resistance**

Chapter Contents

WHAT IS THE RIGHT WAY TO TAKE ANTIBIOTICS?

If you need antibiotics, take them exactly as prescribed. Never save your antibiotics for later use or share them with family or friends. Taking antibiotics only when needed helps keep us healthy now, helps fight antibiotic resistance, and ensures that these lifesaving drugs will be available for future generations. Talk with your health-care professional if you have any questions about your antibiotics, including how they could interact with other medications you are taking, or if you develop any side effects.

WHAT ARE THE SIDE EFFECTS?

Common side effects range from minor to very severe health problems and can include:

- rash
- dizziness
- nausea
- diarrhea
- yeast infections

Get immediate medical help if you experience:

- severe diarrhea, which could be a symptom of a *Clostridium difficile* (*C. diff*) infection that can lead to severe colon damage and death
- severe and life-threatening allergic reactions, such as wheezing, hives, shortness of breath, and anaphylaxis (which also includes feeling that your throat is closing or choking or your voice is changing)

WHY DOES TAKING ANTIBIOTICS LEAD TO ANTIBIOTIC RESISTANCE?

Any time you take antibiotics, they can cause side effects and contribute to the development of antibiotic resistance. Antibiotic resistance is one of the most urgent threats to the public's health. Always remember the following:

- Antibiotic resistance does not mean the body is becoming resistant to antibiotics; it means bacteria are developing the ability to defeat the antibiotics designed to kill them.
- When bacteria become resistant, antibiotics cannot fight them, and the bacteria multiply.
- Some resistant bacteria can be harder to treat and can spread to other people.
- More than 2.8 million antibiotic-resistant infections occur in the United States each year, and more than 35,000 people die as a result.

HOW CAN YOU STAY HEALTHY?

You can stay healthy and keep others healthy by:

- cleaning hands by washing with soap and water for 20 seconds or using a hand sanitizer that contains at least 60 percent alcohol
- covering your mouth and nose with a tissue when you cough or sneeze or use the inside of your elbow
- getting recommended vaccines, such as the flu vaccine

Talk to your health-care professional about steps you can take to help prevent illness.

WHAT DO ANTIBIOTICS TREAT?

Antibiotics are only needed for treating certain infections caused by bacteria. Antibiotics are critical tools for treating life-threatening conditions such as pneumonia and sepsis, which is the body's extreme response to an infection.

WHAT ANTIBIOTICS DO NOT TREAT

Antibiotics do not work on viruses, such as those that cause colds, flu, bronchitis, or runny noses, even if the mucus is thick, yellow, or green. Antibiotics also would not help some common bacterial infections, including most cases of bronchitis, many sinus infections, and some ear infections.

USE ANTIBIOTICS ONLY AS PRESCRIBED

Antibiotics are powerful, life-saving drugs. When your health-care professional prescribes antibiotics, take them as directed. Patients can experience side effects while taking antibiotics. But remember, when antibiotics are needed, their benefits outweigh the risks of side effects and antibiotic resistance. When antibiotics are not needed, they would not help you, and the side effects could still cause harm. Reactions from antibiotics cause one out of five medication-related visits to the emergency room.[1]

WHAT IS THE U.S. FOOD AND DRUG ADMINISTRATION DOING?

The U.S. Food and Drug Administration (FDA) is combating antibiotic resistance through activities that include the following:

- **Approval of certain new antibiotics**. Since 2015, the FDA approved new antibiotics that can treat certain resistant bacteria. Health-care professionals are encouraged to use the new antibiotics appropriately and, for some antibiotics, use only in patients who have limited or no other treatment options.
- **Labeling regulations addressing proper use of antibiotics**. Antibiotic labeling contains required statements in several places advising health-care professionals that these drugs should be used only to treat infections that are believed to be caused by bacteria. Labeling also encourages health-care professionals to counsel patients about proper use.
- **Partnering to promote public awareness**. The FDA is partnering with the Centers for Disease Control and Prevention (CDC) on "Get Smart: Know When Antibiotics Work" (www.cdc.gov/getsmart/community/

[1] "Antibiotics Aren't Always the Answer," Centers for Disease Control and Prevention (CDC), July 16, 2021. Available online. URL: www.cdc.gov/antibiotic-use/pdfs/AntibioticsArentAlwaystheAnswer-H.pdf. Accessed June 13, 2023.

materials-references/index.html), a campaign that offers web pages, brochures, fact sheets, and other information sources aimed at helping the public learn about preventing antibiotic-resistant infections.

- **Encouraging the development of new antibiotics.** The FDA developed guidances for the industry on the types of clinical studies that could be performed to evaluate how an antibacterial drug works for the treatment of different types of infections. The FDA organized and participated in workshops aimed at addressing the development of new antibiotics that treat resistant bacterial infections.[2]

Section 65.2 | Antimicrobial (Drug) Resistance

Bacteria, fungi, and other microbes evolve over time and can develop resistance to antimicrobial drugs. Microbes naturally develop resistance; however, using antibiotics too often in humans and animals and in cases where antibiotics are not an appropriate treatment can make resistance develop more quickly.

CAUSES OF ANTIMICROBIAL (DRUG) RESISTANCE

Microbes, such as bacteria, viruses, fungi, and parasites, are living organisms that evolve over time. Their primary function is to reproduce, thrive, and spread quickly and efficiently. Therefore, microbes adapt to their environments and change in ways that ensure their survival. If something stops their ability to grow, such as an antimicrobial, genetic changes can occur that enable the microbe to survive. There are several ways this happens.

[2] "Combating Antibiotic Resistance," U.S. Food and Drug Administration (FDA), July 16, 2021. Available online. URL: www.cdc.gov/antibiotic-use/pdfs/AntibioticsArentAlwaystheAnswer-H.pdf. Accessed June 13, 2023.

Natural (Biological) Causes

SELECTIVE PRESSURE

In the presence of an antimicrobial, microbes are either killed or, if they carry resistance genes, survive. These survivors will replicate, and their progeny will quickly become the dominant type throughout the microbial population.

Nonresistant bacteria multiply, and upon drug treatment, the bacteria die. Drug-resistant bacteria multiply as well, but upon drug treatment, the bacteria continue to spread.

MUTATION

Most microbes reproduce by dividing every few hours, allowing them to evolve rapidly and adapt quickly to new environmental conditions. During replication, mutations arise, and some of these mutations may help an individual microbe survive exposure to an antimicrobial.

Some of those mutations can make the bacteria resistant to drug treatment. In the presence of the drugs, only the resistant bacteria survive and then multiply and thrive.

GENE TRANSFER

Microbes may also get genes from each other, including genes that make the microbe drug-resistant. Bacteria multiply by the billions. Bacteria that have drug-resistant deoxyribonucleic acid (DNA) may transfer a copy of these genes to other bacteria. Nonresistant bacteria receive the new DNA and become resistant to drugs. In the presence of drugs, only drug-resistant bacteria survive. The drug-resistant bacteria multiply and thrive.

Bacteria multiply by the billions. Bacteria that have drug-resistant DNA may transfer a copy of these genes to other bacteria. Nonresistant bacteria receive the new DNA and become resistant to drugs. In the presence of drugs, only drug-resistant bacteria survive. The drug-resistant bacteria multiply and thrive.

SOCIETAL PRESSURES

The use of antimicrobials, even when used appropriately, creates a selective pressure for resistant organisms. However, there are additional societal pressures that act to accelerate the increase of antimicrobial resistance.

INAPPROPRIATE USE

The selection of resistant microorganisms is exacerbated by the inappropriate use of antimicrobials. Sometimes, health-care providers will prescribe antimicrobials inappropriately, wishing to placate an insistent patient who has a viral infection or an as-yet undiagnosed condition.

INADEQUATE DIAGNOSTICS

More often, health-care providers must use incomplete or imperfect information to diagnose an infection and thus prescribe an antimicrobial just in case or prescribe a broad-spectrum antimicrobial when a specific antibiotic might be better. These situations contribute to selective pressure and accelerate antimicrobial resistance.

HOSPITAL USE

Critically ill patients are more susceptible to infections and, thus, often require the aid of antimicrobials. However, the heavier use of antimicrobials in these patients can worsen the problem by selecting antimicrobial-resistant microorganisms. The extensive use of antimicrobials and close contact among sick patients creates a fertile environment for the spread of antimicrobial-resistant germs.

AGRICULTURAL USE

Scientists also believe that the practice of adding antibiotics to agricultural feed promotes drug resistance. More than half of the antibiotics produced in the United States are used for agricultural purposes. However, there is still much debate about whether drug-resistant microbes in animals pose a significant public health burden.

DIAGNOSIS: ANTIMICROBIAL (DRUG) RESISTANCE

Without appropriate diagnostic tests, it can be difficult to know what type of pathogen is causing an infection. Viral infections can be mistaken for bacterial infections and improperly treated with antibiotics, while bacterial infections can be treated with the wrong antibiotic, causing prolonged disease. Furthermore, standard diagnostic tests can take two to three days or longer to yield a result. The process involves culturing the infecting organism to identify the species and performing tests to see which types of antibiotics work against that particular strain. Reliable, rapid tests are urgently needed to avoid delays in appropriate treatment.

The National Institute of Allergy and Infectious Diseases (NIAID) is supporting the development of rapid, multiplexed diagnostics platforms and biomarkers. This includes tests that can identify if a pathogen will be susceptible to a particular antibiotic, tests that can distinguish colonization from infection, and tests that do not require culturing bacteria.

The NIAID scientists are studying the mechanisms of antimicrobial resistance and novel approaches for detecting resistance based on large-scale studies of proteins and other biomarkers. In addition, NIAID's Antibacterial Resistance Leadership Group (ARLG) is testing a biomarker that could distinguish bacterial viral and bacterial infections to determine if antibiotics are necessary. The ARLG also conducts studies on improving the utility of current diagnostics. An ARLG study showed that a test previously approved by the U.S. Food and Drug Administration (FDA) to detect gonorrhea and chlamydia in urine and reproductive samples could also be used to accurately detect gonorrhea and chlamydia in throat and rectum samples.

Antimicrobial Resistance Diagnostic Challenge

The National Institutes of Health (NIH) and the Biomedical Advanced Research and Development Authority (BARDA) are supporting a federal prize competition seeking to identify innovative and rapid point-of-need diagnostic tests to help inform appropriate antibiotic treatment and facilitate antimicrobial stewardship efforts.

TREATMENT: ANTIMICROBIAL (DRUG) RESISTANCE

The rise of antimicrobial-resistant microbes has led to an urgent need to preserve the efficacy of current antibiotics, develop new ones, and identify alternative treatment strategies. The NIAID has a substantial research program to spur the development of new therapeutics against drug-resistant viruses, bacteria, parasites, and fungi and to identify alternative approaches.

Novel Antibiotics

The NIAID-supported researchers are working to develop and advance promising therapeutics. Most bacteria are classified as gram-positive or gram-negative. Gram-negative bacteria, such as *Pseudomonas aeruginosa* and carbapenem-resistant Enterobacteriaceae (CRE), have a double membrane that cannot be penetrated by many antibiotics. They also have special proteins called "efflux pumps" that eject antibiotics out of the cell. These features make gram-negative bacterial infections difficult to treat.

The NIAID is funding research projects that aim to develop models and tests to predict and measure the potency of candidate therapeutics based on an understanding of how molecules enter and leave gram-negative pathogens. Researchers are also working to develop novel drugs that directly target efflux pumps or the biofilm that protects some bacteria from the immune system.

The NIAID also has supported clinical trials evaluating novel antibiotics against gram-negative infections. An NIAID-supported phase 2 clinical trial showed that the novel oral antibiotic zoliflodacin was well-tolerated and successfully cured most cases of uncomplicated gonorrhea. Researchers are also exploring combination therapies to treat gram-negative infections that target both the bacteria's essential functions and factors contributing to resistance.

In another effort to identify novel antibiotics, scientists are exploring potential antimicrobial compounds from nature, including new classes of antibiotics found in soil.

The NIAID supports the global nonprofit public–private partnership called "combating antibiotic-resistant bacteria biopharmaceutical accelerator" (CARB-X). The partnership aims to accelerate a diverse portfolio of antibacterial products toward clinical development. CARB-X prioritizes treatments for target pathogens defined by the CDC and the World Health Organization (WHO), including *Clostridium difficile* (*C. diff*) infection, methicillin-resistant *Staphylococcus aureus* (MRSA) infection, CRE, *Neisseria gonorrhoeae*, and *Acinetobacter*.

Optimizing Existing Antibiotics

The NIAID-supported clinical trials are testing optimized treatment regimens of older antibiotics to more effectively treat infections and suppress the emergence of resistance. For example, NIAID is funding a trial testing an intravenous formulation of the antibiotic fosfomycin as a treatment for bacterial lung infections. Additional trials are exploring the most effective duration of treatment for pediatric urinary tract infections and community-acquired pneumonia. Researchers are also studying combination therapy regimens. One trial is testing whether the antibiotic colistin alone or colistin combined with a carbapenem is effective in treating multidrug-resistant gram-negative bacterial infections and in reducing the emergence of resistance to colistin.

Microbiome-Based Approaches

Scientists are exploring nontraditional approaches to treating antibacterial-resistant infections, including live microbiome-based therapeutic products. The NIAID scientists collaborated with researchers in Thailand on a project that showed that *Bacillus*, a "good" bacterium commonly found in probiotic digestive supplements, helps eliminate *Staphylococcus aureus*. The NIAID is also exploring the use of fecal microbiota transplantation for the treatment of recurrent *C. diff*-associated disease (CDAD), a potentially life-threatening diarrheal illness. The process involves putting stool that has been prescreened for infectious agents and antibiotic-resistant organisms from a healthy donor in the colon of a recipient to restore a healthy and diverse gut microbiome.

Phage Therapy

Bacteriophages (phages) are viruses that selectively infect and kill bacteria. Phage therapy has been used to treat patients with severe, multidrug-resistant infections under compassionate use conditions with promising results. However, knowledge gaps hinder the development and regulation of phage therapy in the U.S. NIAID plans to support researchers who are developing novel platforms for the discovery of new phages and are working to improve our understanding of how phages interact with their bacterial host, antibiotics, and the human immune system.

PREVENTION: ANTIMICROBIAL (DRUG) RESISTANCE

The NIAID supports basic, translational, and clinical research on ways to prevent serious drug-resistant infections, including vaccines, monoclonal antibody therapies, and compounds that modulate innate immunity. The NIAID also supports research on antibacterial resistance stewardship and infection control strategies.

Vaccines and Immune-Based Interventions

Vaccines for bacterial infections are urgently needed. Vaccines could be used to mitigate symptoms and disease progression or prevent infection or reduce colonization. For example, NIAID is supporting research on vaccine targets for *N. gonorrhoeae*, how the bacteria cause disease, and how our immune systems respond to it. The NIAID is also funding the Sexually Transmitted Infections Cooperative Research Centers, which aim to develop vaccines against gonorrhea, chlamydia, and syphilis.

In 2019, the NIAID established the Infectious Diseases Clinical Research Consortium, a clinical trials network that encompasses the institute's long-standing Vaccine and Treatment Evaluation Units (VTEUs). The consortium leadership group will prioritize candidate vaccines and other interventions to test in clinical trials.

The NIAID scientists are also developing a potential immunotherapy approach for the treatment of multidrug-resistant *Klebsiella pneumoniae* infections. While antibiotics target bacterial pathogens, immunotherapy approaches enhance the immune system's ability to fight specific bacteria. The NIAID's ARLG has also evaluated investigational antibody-based therapies aimed at preventing potentially antibiotic-resistant infections.

Antimicrobial Stewardship and Infection Control Strategies

Effectively controlling the spread of antimicrobial-resistant bacteria can help prevent infections. Certain types of bacteria can spread through the food supply, animals, and the environment (e.g., water). In health-care facilities, specialized infection control procedures, including best practices for using medical devices such as central venous catheters, can help reduce the transmission of harmful bacteria. The NIAID is supporting research on further improving infection control techniques. Prior research has indicated that decolonization strategies (removing skin-surface bacteria that are normally harmless, but that may enter the bloodstream following surgery or other procedures and cause infection, including life-threatening sepsis) can benefit patients in intensive care units. An NIAID-supported study found that decolonization through daily bathing with chlorhexidine, a type of antiseptic soap, benefited patients with medical devices.[3]

Section 65.3 | Surveillance of Antimicrobial Resistance Patterns and Rates

Antimicrobial drug resistance has become such a global concern that it was the focus of the 2011 World Health Day sponsored by the World Health Organization (WHO). Although antimicrobial drug resistance is well-mapped and tightly monitored in some well-resourced countries, such processes do not exist in under-resourced countries. An increasing body of evidence reveals accelerating rates

[3] "Antimicrobial (Drug) Resistance," National Institute of Allergy and Infectious Diseases (NIAID), October 5, 2022. Available online. URL: www.niaid.nih.gov/research/antimicrobial-resistance. Accessed June 13, 2023.

of antimicrobial drug resistance in these countries. Resistance may arise in the absence of any surveillance and threatens the achievement of the Millennium Goals for Development in terms of the reduction of maternal and infant deaths. The problem is even more pressing because, in a globalized world, microorganisms and their resistance genes travel faster and farther than ever before, and the pipeline of new drugs is faltering.

Mapping antimicrobial drug resistance in under-resourced countries is urgently needed so that measures can be set up to curb it. Such mapping must rely on efficient surveillance networks, endowed with adequate laboratory capacity, and take into account up-to-date diagnostic techniques. The way forward is to assess the effects of resistance, its clinical effects, and the increase in deaths, with the ultimate objective of providing achievable guidelines for surveillance and control.

WHAT ARE THE MAIN THREATS?

Tuberculosis

Resistance of *Mycobacterium tuberculosis* to antimycobacterial drugs is a global concern. In 2010, an estimated 650,000 cases of multidrug-resistant tuberculosis (MDR TB; i.e., infections with strains resistant to, at minimum, rifampin and isoniazid) occurred worldwide. An estimated 10 percent of cases were extensively drug-resistant (XDR; i.e., MDR strains that are also resistant to second-line drugs). Almost no surveillance system is in place, and no data exist on TB resistance in sub-Saharan Africa (apart from South Africa) and Asia.

Malaria

Plasmodium falciparum strains resistant to chloroquine, fansidar, and mefloquine are widespread. Interventions using artemisinin and insecticide-treated bed nets have led to a drop of 40 percent in malaria cases since 2004 according to the WHO. An estimated 750,000 lives were saved in Africa alone. Those efforts are potentially hindered by the emergence of resistance to artemisinin, which was first reported in 2008 at the Thailand–Cambodia border and subsequently reported in neighboring countries although not in Africa so far. Resistance mechanisms to artemisinin are poorly understood although mutations in some parasite genes have been partially correlated with resistance.

Severe Acute Respiratory Infections

Severe acute respiratory infections (SARIs) kill an estimated 1.4 million children younger than five years of age every year. The emergence of resistance to neuraminidase inhibitors would potentially have dramatic consequences because they are the first-line response to pandemics caused by highly virulent influenza viruses. Resistance of *Streptococcus pneumoniae* to antimicrobial drugs is also a concern. The extent of outpatient penicillin usage correlates with the level of resistance. A prospective surveillance study of 2,184 patients hospitalized with pneumococcal pneumonia in 11 Asian countries in 2008–2009 found that high-level penicillin resistance was rare, that resistance to erythromycin was highly prevalent (72.7%), and that MDR was observed for 59.3 percent of *S. pneumoniae* isolates. Of 20,100 cases of invasive pneumococcal diseases identified in South Africa during 2003–2008, a total of 3,708 (18%) were caused by isolates resistant to at least three antimicrobial drugs.

Gram-Negative Bacteria Infections

Gram-negative bacteria resistant to β-lactams are spreading worldwide. CTX-M-15, a heterogeneous and mobile resistance gene first described in 2001 in India, has since been reported all over the world and is transmissible between different species of *Enterobacteriaceae*. New Delhi metallo-β-lactamase-1 (NDM-1) is a gene that confers resistance to all β-lactams, including carbapenems, which are the only alternative for treating severe infections such as neonatal sepsis caused by MDR strains. First identified in 2008, it is now widespread in *Escherichia coli* and *Klebsiella pneumoniae* isolates from the Indian subcontinent and is found in many countries. The spread of gram-negative resistant bacteria from the hospital to the environment by direct person-to-person contact or through unsanitized water is a concern in under-resourced countries. The worldwide increase in the number of travelers, some of whom have diarrhea, is a major cause of the spread of resistance. A study conducted in Barcelona, Spain, showed that nalidixic acid resistance in enterotoxigenic or enteroaggregative *E. coli* strains isolated from patients returning from India increased from 6 percent during 1994–1997 to 64 percent during 2001–2004. Sixty-five percent of strains isolated from patients who had traveled to India were resistant to quinolones.

Methicillin-Resistant *Staphylococcus aureus* Infections

Methicillin-resistant *Staphylococcus aureus* (MRSA) infections have become widespread even in under-resourced countries. Pakistan and India have reported MRSA percentages of 42–54.9 percent, with an increasing trend.

The above sections describing antimicrobial drug resistance in various diseases are not exhaustive. Careful attention must be given to the potential spread of antimicrobial drug resistance in the drugs used to treat highly prevalent infectious diseases, such as typhoid, meningitis, HIV, and hepatitis, in under-resourced countries.

WHO ARE THE MOST VULNERABLE POPULATIONS?

Antimicrobial drug resistance accounts for excess deaths in infants and childbearing women because of poor intrapartum and postnatal infection–control practices. In 2005, infections in hospital-born babies were estimated to account for 4–56 percent of all deaths in the neonatal period in some under-resourced countries. *K. pneumoniae, E. coli, Pseudomonas* spp., *Acinetobacter* spp., and *S. aureus* were the most frequent causative pathogens of neonatal sepsis; 70 percent of these isolates would not be eliminated by an empiric regimen of ampicillin and gentamicin. Many infections might be untreatable in resource-constrained environments. Fifty-one percent of *Klebsiella* spp. were extended-spectrum β-lactamase (ESBL) producers; 38 percent of *S. aureus* strains were methicillin-resistant; and 64 percent were resistant to co-trimoxazole. Preliminary data from Kilifi District Hospital (Kenya) also show alarming rates of ESBL positivity: 180 (39%) of 459 *Enterobacteriaceae* clinical isolates from child and adult patients (including 115 isolates of *K. pneumoniae*) collected from August 2010 to August 2012 were ESBL-positive.

The Division of Women and Child Health at the Aga Khan University Medical College in Karachi, Pakistan, has proposed a model for monitoring the development of neonatal infections and outcomes in southern Asia, on the basis of a cohort of 69,450 births. Resistance rates are constantly increasing. Antimicrobial drug resistance is estimated to result in an additional 96,000 (26%, range: 16–37%) deaths each year from neonatal sepsis in southern Asia, highlighting the toll that children pay for drug resistance.[4]

Section 65.4 | **Influenza Antiviral Drug Resistance**

WHAT ARE REDUCED SUSCEPTIBILITY AND ANTIVIRAL RESISTANCE?

When an antiviral drug is fully effective against a virus, that virus is said to be susceptible to that antiviral drug. Flu viruses are constantly changing, and some changes can make antiviral drugs work less well or not work at all against these viruses. Antiviral drugs work by targeting a specific location or site found on a flu virus. When a flu virus develops changes to the site that antiviral drugs target, that virus may show reduced or no susceptibility to that antiviral drug. Flu viruses can show reduced susceptibility to one or more flu antiviral drugs. Reduced susceptibility that is detected using laboratory methods can be a sign of potential antiviral drug resistance in clinical settings. Typically, a flu virus is called "resistant" after sufficient laboratory evidence is available to show that the antiviral drug lacks activity against the virus.

[4] "Surveillance for Antimicrobial Drug Resistance in Under-Resourced Countries," Centers for Disease Control and Prevention (CDC), February 19, 2014. Available online. URL: wwwnc.cdc.gov/eid/article/20/3/12-1157_article. Accessed June 13, 2023.

In the United States, there are four antiviral drugs approved by the U.S. Food and Drug Administration (FDA) that are recommended by the Centers for Disease Control and Prevention (CDC) in October 2022. Three are neuraminidase inhibitor antiviral drugs: oseltamivir (available as a generic version or under the trade name Tamiflu®) for oral administration, zanamivir (trade name Relenza®) for oral inhalation using an inhaler device, and peramivir (trade name Rapivab®) for intravenous administration. The fourth is a cap-dependent endonuclease inhibitor, baloxavir marboxil (trade name Xofluza®) for oral administration. Baloxavir marboxil was approved for use in the United States by the FDA in October 2018.

There is another class of FDA-approved antiviral drugs, M2 inhibitors amantadine and rimantadine, also called the "adamantanes," that in the past were active against flu A viruses (but not flu B viruses). However, the adamantane antiviral drugs have not been recommended for use to treat flu in the United States for many years because of widespread antiviral resistance to this class of antivirals among circulating flu A viruses.

HOW WIDESPREAD ARE REDUCED SUSCEPTIBILITY AND ANTIVIRAL RESISTANCE IN THE UNITED STATES?

In the United States, the majority of the recently circulating flu viruses have been fully susceptible to neuraminidase inhibitors and baloxavir. However, nearly all flu A viruses are resistant to the M2 inhibitors, which is why they are not recommended for the treatment of seasonal influenza.

HOW DOES REDUCED SUSCEPTIBILITY AND ANTIVIRAL RESISTANCE HAPPEN?

Flu viruses are constantly changing; they can change in significant ways from one season to the next and can even change within the course of one flu season. As a flu virus replicates (i.e., making copies of itself), its genetic makeup may change in a way that results in the virus becoming less susceptible to one or more of the antiviral drugs used to treat or prevent flu. Flu viruses can become less susceptible to antiviral drugs during the course of antiviral treatment or emerge spontaneously. Antiviral-resistant flu viruses vary in their ability to infect people and are not necessarily more or less transmissible than susceptible flu viruses.

HOW ARE REDUCED SUSCEPTIBILITY AND ANTIVIRAL RESISTANCE DETECTED?

The CDC routinely analyzes flu viruses collected through domestic and global surveillance to see if they have genetic changes that are associated with reduced susceptibility to any flu antiviral drugs. Such changes can potentially cause viruses to be resistant to antiviral treatment with reduced or no effectiveness for treated patients. In addition, numerous state public health laboratories participate in the screening of flu viruses for genetic changes indicative of potential resistance to neuraminidase inhibitor antivirals. The CDC is also collaborating with the Wadsworth Center public health laboratory of New York State's Department of Health (NYSDOH), a National Influenza Reference Center (NIRC), to establish additional laboratory-testing capacity for monitoring baloxavir antiviral susceptibility. This combined data informs public health policy recommendations about the use of flu antiviral medications.

The CDC is continuously improving testing algorithms and methods used for monitoring antiviral susceptibility in circulating viruses. Detection of reduced susceptibility and antiviral resistance involves several laboratory tests, including phenotypic assays (testing in the presence of an antiviral drug) and molecular techniques (next-generation sequence analysis and pyrosequencing) to look for genetic changes that have been associated with reduced antiviral susceptibility.

HOW HAS THE CDC PREPARED TO TEST FOR REDUCED SUSCEPTIBILITY AND ANTIVIRAL RESISTANCE TO THE NEW FLU ANTIVIRAL BALOXAVIR?

The CDC's Influenza Division took specific laboratory actions to incorporate the antiviral drug baloxavir into routine virologic surveillance. This included the creation and validation of new assays to determine baloxavir susceptibility and the training of laboratorians to conduct baloxavir susceptibility testing.

Seasonal flu A and B viruses in humans as well as several flu A viruses that circulate in animals were tested to establish baseline susceptibility to baloxavir. In addition, the susceptibility of other distantly related flu viruses to baloxavir was tested. The CDC also collaborated with the Association of Public Health Laboratories (APHL) and the Wadsworth Center NYSDOH, a National Influenza Reference Center (NIRC), to establish laboratory-testing capacity for baloxavir susceptibility. The CDC has trained staff within these partner organizations to use the CDC's method for assessing baloxavir susceptibility.

WHAT IS OSELTAMIVIR RESISTANCE, AND WHAT CAUSES IT?

Flu viruses are constantly changing. Changes that occur in circulating flu viruses typically involve the structures of the viruses' two primary surface proteins: hemagglutinin (HA) and neuraminidase (NA).

Oseltamivir is the most commonly prescribed antiviral drug of those recommended in the United States to treat flu illness. Oseltamivir is known as a "NA inhibitor" because this antiviral drug binds to NA proteins of a flu virus and inhibits the enzymatic activity of these proteins. By inhibiting NA activity, oseltamivir prevents flu viruses from spreading from infected cells to other healthy cells.

Changes in the NA proteins of a flu virus can reduce oseltamivir's binding to them. As a result, oseltamivir's ability to inhibit the enzyme activity of NA proteins can be diminished, and this may cause "oseltamivir resistance" (non-susceptibility). A particular genetic change known as the "H275Y" mutation in the NA is the mutation that is known to confer oseltamivir resistance in A(H1N1)pdm09 flu viruses. Flu viruses that have the "H275Y" mutation show highly reduced inhibition by oseltamivir in laboratory assays. The "H275Y" mutation makes oseltamivir ineffective in treating illnesses with that flu virus by preventing oseltamivir from inhibiting NA activity, which then allows the virus to infect healthy cells. The "H275Y" mutation also reduces the effectiveness of peramivir in treating infections caused by a flu virus with this mutation. Some other mutations in the NA proteins of circulating viruses have been shown to affect oseltamivir's ability to inhibit the enzyme activity of the viruses' NA proteins. Such viruses can show "reduced" or even "highly reduced" inhibition by oseltamivir and other NA inhibitors in laboratory tests; however, not all are considered "resistant" due to insufficient data to support their drug resistance from clinical settings.

HOW DOES THE CDC IMPROVE MONITORING OF INFLUENZA VIRUSES FOR REDUCED SUSCEPTIBILITY AND ANTIVIRAL RESISTANCE?

The CDC continually improves the ability to rapidly detect flu viruses with antiviral reduced susceptibility and antiviral resistance through improvements in laboratory methods, increasing the number of surveillance sites in the United States and worldwide, and increasing the number of laboratories that can test for reduced susceptibility and antiviral resistance. Enhanced surveillance efforts have provided the CDC with the capability to detect antiviral-resistant flu viruses more quickly and enabled the CDC to monitor for changing trends over time.

HOW DID INFLUENZA ANTIVIRAL SUSCEPTIBILITY PATTERNS CHANGE DURING THE PREVIOUS INFLUENZA SEASON?

Antiviral susceptibility patterns changed very little in 2021–2022 compared with the previous season (2020–2021). During the 2021–2022 and 2020–2021 seasons, only a very small of viruses were found to be resistant to oseltamivir. Almost all of the flu viruses tested during 2021–2022 continued to be susceptible to the antiviral drugs recommended for the treatment of flu by the CDC. Resistance to the adamantane class of antiviral drugs among flu A (H3N2) and A (H1N1) pdm09 viruses remained widespread (flu B viruses are not susceptible to adamantane drugs.)

The CDC conducts ongoing surveillance and testing of flu viruses for antiviral-reduced susceptibility and resistance among seasonal and novel flu A viruses (of animal origin that have infected people), and guidance is updated as needed.

Because there were no dramatic changes in antiviral susceptibility patterns during the 2021–2022 flu season, the guidance on the use of flu antiviral drugs for the 2022–2023 flu season remains unchanged. The latest guidance for clinicians on the use of antiviral drugs for flu is available on the CDC website at www.cdc.gov/flu/professionals/antivirals/index.htm.

WHAT CAN PEOPLE DO TO PROTECT THEMSELVES AGAINST FLU VIRUSES WITH REDUCED SUSCEPTIBILITY AND ANTIVIRAL RESISTANCE?

Getting a yearly seasonal flu vaccination is the best way to reduce the risk of flu and its potentially serious complications. Flu vaccines protect against influenza A viruses of two subtypes, A(H1N1) pdm09 and A(H3N2), and type B viruses from two lineages. The CDC recommends that everyone aged six months and older get vaccinated each year. If you are in a group at higher risk of serious flu-related complications and become ill with flu symptoms, call your doctor right away because you might benefit from early treatment with a flu antiviral drug. If you are not at higher risk of flu complications, if possible, stay home from work, school, and errands when you are sick. This will help prevent you from spreading your illness to others.

WHAT IMPLICATIONS DO REDUCED SUSCEPTIBILITY AND ANTIVIRAL RESISTANCE HAVE FOR THE U.S. ANTIVIRAL STOCKPILE THAT WAS CREATED AS PART OF THE U.S. PANDEMIC PLAN?

Monitoring for antiviral drug susceptibility and resistance will be essential to determine the role of antivirals and specific antivirals during the next influenza pandemic. Available FDA-approved and authorized flu antiviral drugs can be used in the event that a novel flu A virus, such as avian flu A(H7N9) virus, gains the ability to spread easily among people in a sustained manner and is susceptible to these antiviral drugs. During the 2009 H1N1 pandemic, neuraminidase inhibitor antiviral drugs were released from the strategic national stockpile (SNS) and used to treat infection with the pandemic virus, now referred to as flu A(H1N1) pdm09 virus.

In addition, an investigational antiviral drug was made available by FDA emergency use authorization for the treatment of hospitalized pandemic influenza patients in the United States through clinician requests to the CDC. Antivirals in the SNS are for use during public health emergencies in the United States, such as a flu pandemic, but not for seasonal flu epidemics. The CDC no longer oversees the SNS.[5]

Section 65.5 | Ineffectiveness of Antibiotics for Colds or Flu

The Centers for Disease Control and Prevention (CDC) has news for parents this cold and flu season: Antibiotics do not work for a cold or the flu. Antibiotics kill bacteria, not viruses. And colds, flu, and most sore throats are caused by viruses. Antibiotics do not touch viruses—never have, never will. And it is not really news. It is a long-documented medical fact.

But tell that to parents seeking relief for a child's runny nose. Research shows that most Americans have either missed the message about appropriate antibiotic use or they simply do not believe it. It is a case of mistaken popular belief winning out over fact. According to public opinion research, there is a perception that "antibiotics cure everything."

Americans believe in the power of antibiotics so much that many patients go to the doctor expecting to get a prescription. And they do. Why? Physicians are often too pressured for time to engage in lengthy explanations of why antibiotics will not work. And, when the diagnosis is uncertain—as many symptoms for viral and bacterial infections are similar—doctors are more likely to yield to patient demands for antibiotics.

[5] "Influenza Antiviral Drug Resistance," Centers for Disease Control and Prevention (CDC), October 25, 2022. Available online. URL: www.cdc.gov/flu/treatment/antiviralresistance.htm. Accessed June 13, 2023.

RISK OF ANTIBIOTIC-RESISTANCE

The problem is taking antibiotics when they are not needed can do more harm than good. Widespread inappropriate use of antibiotics is fueling an increase in drug-resistant bacteria. Sick individuals are not the only people who can suffer the consequences. Families and entire communities feel the impact when disease-causing germs become resistant to antibiotics.

The most obvious consequence of inappropriate antibiotic use is its effect on the sick patient. When antibiotics are incorrectly used to treat children or adults with viral infections, such as colds and flu, they are not getting the best care for their condition. A course of antibiotics will not fight the virus, make the patient feel better, yield a quicker recovery, or keep others from getting sick.

A less obvious consequence of antibiotic overuse is the boost it gives to drug-resistant disease-causing bacteria. Almost every type of bacteria has become stronger and less responsive to antibiotic treatment when it is really needed. These antibiotic-resistant bacteria can quickly spread to family members, school-mates, and coworkers—threatening the community with a new strain of infectious disease that is more difficult to cure and more expensive to treat.

According to the CDC, antibiotic resistance is one of the world's most pressing public health problems. Americans of all ages can lower this risk by talking to their doctors and using antibiotics appropriately during this cold and flu season.

WHAT TO DO FOR COLDS AND FLU

- Children and adults with viral infections recover when the illness has run its course. Colds caused by viruses may last for two weeks or longer.
- Measures that can help a person with a cold or flu feel better are as follows:
  - Increase fluid intake.
  - Use a cool mist vaporizer or saline nasal spray to relieve congestion.

    - Soothe throat with ice chips, sore throat spray, or lozenges (for older children and adults).
- Viral infections may sometimes lead to bacterial infections. Patients should keep their doctor informed if their illness gets worse or lasts a long time.[6]

[6] "Sniffle or Sneeze? No Antibiotics Please," Centers for Disease Control and Prevention (CDC), November 2, 2003. Available online. URL: www.cdc.gov/antibiotic-use/community/downloads/sniffle-sneeze-matte.pdf. Accessed July 4, 2023.

Chapter 66 | Avoiding Drug Interactions

There are more opportunities today than ever before to learn about your health and to take better care of yourself. It is also more important than ever to know about the medicines you take. If you take several different medicines, see more than one doctor, or have certain health conditions, you and your doctors need to be aware of all the medicines you take. Doing so will help you to avoid potential problems such as drug interactions.

Drug interactions may make your drug less effective, cause unexpected side effects, or increase the action of a particular drug. Some drug interactions can even be harmful to you. Reading the label every time you use a nonprescription or prescription drug and taking the time to learn about drug interactions may be critical to your health. You can reduce the risk of potentially harmful drug interactions and side effects with a little bit of knowledge and common sense. Drug interactions fall into the following three broad categories:

- **Drug–drug interactions**. These interactions occur when two or more drugs react with each other. This drug–drug interaction may cause you to experience an unexpected side effect. For example, mixing a drug you take to help you sleep (a sedative) and a drug you take for allergies (an antihistamine) can slow your reactions and make driving a car or operating machinery dangerous.
- **Drug–food/beverage interactions**. These interactions result from drugs reacting with foods or beverages. For example, mixing alcohol with some drugs may cause you to feel tired or slow your reactions.

- **Drug–condition interactions**. These interactions may occur when an existing medical condition makes certain drugs potentially harmful. For example, if you have high blood pressure, you could experience an unwanted reaction if you take a nasal decongestant.

DRUG INTERACTIONS AND OVER-THE-COUNTER MEDICINES

Over-the-counter (OTC) drug labels contain information about ingredients, uses, warnings, and directions that is important to read and understand. The label also includes important information about possible drug interactions. Furthermore, drug labels may change as new information becomes known. That is why it is especially important to read the label every time you use a drug.

- The "Active Ingredients" and "Purpose" sections list:
  - the name and amount of each active ingredient
  - the purpose of each active ingredient
- The "Uses" section of the label:
  - tells you what the drug is used for
  - helps you find the best drug for your specific symptoms
- The "Warnings" section of the label provides important drug interaction and precaution information such as:
  - when to talk to a doctor or pharmacist before use
  - the medical conditions that may make the drug less effective or not safe
  - under what circumstances the drug should not be used
  - when to stop taking the drug
- The "Directions" section of the label tells you:
  - the length of time and the amount of the product that you may safely use
  - any special instructions on how to use the product
- The "Other Information" section of the label tells you:
  - required information about certain ingredients, such as sodium content, for people with dietary restrictions or allergies
- The "Inactive Ingredients" section of the label tells you:
  - the name of each inactive ingredient (such as colorings, binders, etc.)

- The "Questions?" or "Questions or Comments?" section of the label (if included):
  - provides telephone numbers of a source to answer questions about the product

LEARNING MORE ABOUT DRUG INTERACTIONS

Talk to your doctor or pharmacist about the drugs you take. When your doctor prescribes a new drug, discuss all OTC and prescription drugs, dietary supplements, vitamins, botanicals, minerals, and herbals you take, as well as the foods you eat. Ask your pharmacist for the package insert for each prescription drug you take. The package insert provides more information about potential drug interactions.

Before taking a drug, ask your doctor or pharmacist the following questions:

- Can I take it with other drugs?
- Should I avoid certain foods, beverages, or other products?
- What are possible drug interaction signs I should know about?
- How will the drug work in my body?
- Is there more information available about the drug or my condition (on the Internet or in health and medical literature)?

Know how to take drugs safely and responsibly. Remember, the drug label will tell you:

- what the drug is used for
- how to take the drug
- how to reduce the risk of drug interactions and unwanted side effects

If you still have questions after reading the drug product label, ask your doctor or pharmacist for more information.[1]

---

[1] "Drug Interactions: What You Should Know," U.S. Food and Drug Administration (FDA), September 25, 2013. Available online. URL: www.fda.gov/drugs/resources-you-drugs/drug-interactions-what-you-should-know. Accessed July 4, 2023.

Chapter 67 | Complementary and Alternative Medicine for Contagious Diseases

Chapter Contents

Section 67.1 | Complementary and Alternative Medicine for Flu and Colds

Many Americans use medical treatments that are not part of mainstream medicine. When you are using these types of care, it may be called "complementary," "integrative," or "alternative medicine."

Complementary medicine is used together with mainstream medical care. An example is using acupuncture to help with the side effects of cancer treatment. When health-care providers and facilities offer both types of care, it is called "integrative medicine." Alternative medicine is used instead of mainstream medical care.

The claims that nonmainstream practitioners make can sound promising. However, researchers do not know how safe many of these treatments are or how well they work. Studies are underway to determine the safety and usefulness of many of these practices.[1]

SOME BASICS ABOUT FLU AND COLDS

Each year, Americans get more than 1 billion colds, and between 5 and 20 percent of Americans get the flu. The two diseases have some symptoms in common, and both are caused by viruses. However, they are different conditions, and the flu is more severe. Unlike the flu, colds generally do not cause serious complications, such as pneumonia, or lead to hospitalization.

No vaccine can protect you against the common cold, but vaccines can protect you against the flu. Everyone over the age of six months should be vaccinated against the flu each year. Vaccination is the best protection against getting the flu.

Prescription antiviral drugs may be used to treat the flu in people who are very ill or who are at high risk of flu complications. They are not a substitute for getting vaccinated. Vaccination is the first line of defense against the flu; antivirals are the second. If you think you have caught the flu, you may want to check with your

[1] MedlinePlus, "Complementary and Integrative Medicine," National Institutes of Health (NIH), May 21, 2020. Available online. URL: https://medlineplus.gov/complementaryandintegrativemedicine.html. Accessed September 11, 2023.

health-care provider to see whether antiviral medicine is appropriate for you. Call promptly. The drugs work best if they are used early in the illness.

WHAT DO WE KNOW ABOUT THE EFFECTIVENESS OF COMPLEMENTARY APPROACHES FOR FLU AND COLDS?

- No complementary health approach has been shown to be helpful for the flu.
- For colds:
    - Complementary approaches that have shown some promise include oral zinc products, rinsing the nose and sinuses (with a neti pot or other device), honey (as a nighttime cough remedy for children), vitamin C (for people under severe physical stress), probiotics, and meditation.
    - Approaches for which the evidence is conflicting, inadequate, or mostly negative include vitamin C (for most people), echinacea, garlic, and American ginseng.

WHAT DO PEOPLE KNOW ABOUT THE SAFETY OF COMPLEMENTARY APPROACHES FOR COLDS AND FLU?

- People can get severe infections if they use neti pots or other nasal rinsing devices improperly. Tap water is not safe for use as a nasal rinse unless it has been filtered, treated, or processed in specific ways.
- Zinc products used in the nose (such as nasal gels and swabs) have been linked to a long-lasting or even permanent loss of the sense of smell.
- Using a dietary supplement to prevent colds often involves taking it for long periods of time. However, little is known about the long-term safety of some dietary supplements studied for the prevention of colds, such as American ginseng and probiotics.
- Complementary approaches that are safe for some people may not be safe for others. Your age, health, special circumstances (such as pregnancy), and medicines

or supplements that you take may affect the safety of complementary approaches.

WHAT SCIENCE SAYS ABOUT COMPLEMENTARY HEALTH APPROACHES FOR THE FLU

No complementary approach has been shown to prevent the flu or relieve flu symptoms. Complementary approaches that have been studied for the flu include the following. In all instances, there is not enough evidence to show whether the approach is helpful.

- American ginseng
- Chinese herbal medicines
- echinacea
- elderberry
- green tea
- oscillococcinum
- vitamin C
- vitamin D

WHAT SCIENCE SAYS ABOUT COMPLEMENTARY HEALTH APPROACHES FOR COLDS

The following complementary health approaches have been studied for colds.

American Ginseng

- Several studies have evaluated the use of American ginseng to prevent colds. A 2011 evaluation of these studies concluded that the herb has not been shown to reduce the number of colds that people catch although it may shorten the length of colds. The researchers who conducted the evaluation concluded that there was insufficient evidence to support the use of American ginseng for preventing colds.
- Taking American ginseng in an effort to prevent colds means taking it for prolonged periods of time. However, little is known about the herb's long-term safety. American ginseng may interact with the anticoagulant (blood-thinning) drug warfarin.

Echinacea

- At least 24 studies have tested echinacea to see whether it can prevent colds or relieve cold symptoms. A comprehensive 2014 assessment of this research concluded that echinacea has not been convincingly shown to be beneficial. However, at least some echinacea products might have a weak effect.
- One reason why it is hard to reach definite conclusions about this herb is that echinacea products vary greatly. They may contain different species (types) of the plant and be made from different plant parts (the aboveground parts, the root, or both). They may also be manufactured in different ways, and some products contain other ingredients in addition to echinacea. Research findings on one echinacea product may not apply to other products.
- Few side effects have been reported in studies of echinacea. However, some people are allergic to this herb, and in one study in children, taking echinacea was linked to an increase in rashes.

Garlic

- A 2014 evaluation of the research on garlic concluded that there is not enough evidence to show whether this herb can help prevent colds or relieve their symptoms.
- Garlic can cause bad breath, body odor, and other side effects. Because garlic may interact with anticoagulant drugs (blood thinners), people who take these drugs should consult their health-care providers before taking garlic.

Honey

- Honey's traditional reputation as a cough remedy has some science to back it up. A small amount of research suggests that honey may help decrease nighttime coughing in children.

- Honey should never be given to infants under the age of one year because it may contain spores of the bacterium that cause infant botulism. Honey is considered safe for older children.

Meditation

- Reducing stress and improving general health may protect against colds and other respiratory infections. In a study funded by the National Center for Complementary and Integrative Health (NCCIH), adults aged 50 and older were randomly assigned to training in mindfulness meditation, which can reduce stress; an exercise training program, which may improve physical health; or a control group that did not receive any intervention. The study participants kept track of their illnesses during the cold and flu season. People in the meditation group had shorter and less severe acute respiratory infections (most of which were colds) and lost fewer days of work because of these illnesses than those in the control group. Exercise also had some benefits, but not as much as meditation.
- This study is the first to suggest that meditation may reduce the impact of colds. Because it is the only study of its kind, its results should not be regarded as conclusive.
- Meditation is generally considered to be safe for healthy people. However, there have been reports that it might worsen symptoms in people with certain chronic physical or mental health problems. If you have an ongoing health issue, talk with your health-care provider before starting meditation.

Probiotics

- A 2015 evaluation of 13 studies found some evidence suggesting that probiotics might reduce the number of colds or other upper respiratory tract infections that people catch and the length of the illnesses, but the quality of the evidence was low or very low.

- In people who are generally healthy, probiotics have a good safety record. Side effects, if they occur at all, usually consist only of mild digestive symptoms, such as gas. However, information on the long-term safety of probiotics is limited, and safety may differ from one type of probiotic to another. Probiotics have been linked to severe side effects, such as dangerous infections, in people with serious underlying medical problems.

Saline Nasal Irrigation

- Saline nasal irrigation means rinsing your nose and sinuses with salt water. People may do this with a neti pot (a device that comes from the Ayurvedic tradition) or with other devices, such as bottles, sprays, pumps, or nebulizers. Saline nasal irrigation may be used for sinus congestion, allergies, or colds.
- There is limited evidence that saline nasal irrigation can help relieve cold symptoms. Studies of this technique have been too small to allow researchers to reach definite conclusions.
- Saline nasal irrigation used to be considered safe, with only minor side effects such as nasal discomfort or irritation. However, in 2011, a severe disease caused by an amoeba (a type of microorganism) was linked to nasal irrigation with tap water. The U.S. Food and Drug Administration (FDA) has warned that tap water that is not filtered, treated, or processed in specific ways is not safe for use in nasal rinsing devices and has explained how to use and clean these devices safely.

Vitamin C

- An evaluation of the large amount of research done on vitamin C and colds (29 studies involving more than 11,000 people) concluded that taking vitamin C does not prevent colds in the general population and shortens colds only slightly. Taking vitamin C only after you start to feel cold symptoms does not affect the length or severity of the cold.

- Unlike the situation in the general population, vitamin C does seem to reduce the number of colds in people exposed to short periods of extreme physical stress (such as marathon runners and skiers). In studies of these groups, taking vitamin C cut the number of colds in half.
- Taking too much vitamin C can cause diarrhea, nausea, and stomach cramps. People with the iron storage disease, hemochromatosis, should avoid high doses of vitamin C. People who are being treated for cancer or taking cholesterol-lowering medications should talk with their health-care providers before taking vitamin C supplements.

Zinc

- Zinc has been used for colds in forms that are taken orally (by mouth), such as lozenges, tablets, or syrup, or used intranasally (in the nose), such as swabs or gels.
    - oral zinc:
        - A 2012 evaluation of 17 studies of various types of zinc lozenges, tablets, or syrup found that zinc can reduce the duration of colds in adults. Two evaluations of three studies of high-dose zinc acetate lozenges in adults, conducted in 2015 and 2016, found that they shortened colds.
        - Some participants in studies that tested zinc for colds reported that the zinc caused a bad taste or nausea.
        - Long-term use of high doses of zinc can cause low copper levels, reduced immunity, and low levels of high-density lipoprotein (HDL) cholesterol (the "good" cholesterol). Zinc may interact with drugs, including antibiotics and penicillamine (a drug used to treat rheumatoid arthritis).
    - intranasal zinc:
        - The use of zinc products inside the nose, such as gels or swabs, may cause loss of the sense of smell, which may be long-lasting or permanent. In 2009, the FDA

warned consumers to stop using several intranasal zinc products marketed as cold remedies because of this risk.

- Prior to the warnings about effects on the sense of smell, a few studies of intranasal zinc had suggested a possible benefit against cold symptoms. However, the risk of a serious and lasting side effect outweighs any possible benefit in the treatment of a minor illness.

OTHER COMPLEMENTARY APPROACHES

In addition to the complementary approaches described above, several other approaches have been studied for colds. In all instances, there is insufficient evidence to show whether these approaches help to prevent colds or relieve cold symptoms.

- andrographis (andrographis paniculata)
- Chinese herbal medicines
- green tea
- guided imagery
- hydrotherapy
- vitamin D
- vitamin E[2]

Section 67.2 | Understanding Probiotics

WHAT ARE PROBIOTICS?

Probiotics are live microorganisms that are intended to have health benefits when consumed or applied to the body. They can be found in yogurt and other fermented foods, dietary supplements, and beauty products.

Although people often think of bacteria and other microorganisms as harmful "germs," many are actually helpful. Some

[2] "Flu and Colds: In Depth," National Center for Complementary and Integrative Health (NCCIH), November 2016. Available online. URL: www.nccih.nih.gov/health/flu-and-colds-in-depth. Accessed June 29, 2023.

bacteria help digest food, destroy disease-causing cells, or produce vitamins. Many of the microorganisms in probiotic products are the same as or similar to microorganisms that naturally live in our bodies.

WHAT TYPES OF BACTERIA ARE IN PROBIOTICS?

Probiotics may contain a variety of microorganisms. The most common are bacteria that belong to groups called "*Lactobacillus*" and "*Bifidobacterium*." Other bacteria may also be used as probiotics, and so may yeasts such as *Saccharomyces boulardii*.

Different types of probiotics may have different effects. For example, if a specific kind of *Lactobacillus* helps prevent an illness, that does not necessarily mean that another kind of *Lactobacillus* or any of the *Bifidobacterium* probiotics would do the same thing.

ARE PREBIOTICS THE SAME AS PROBIOTICS?

No, prebiotics are not the same as probiotics. Prebiotics are nondigestible food components that selectively stimulate the growth or activity of desirable microorganisms.

WHAT ARE SYNBIOTICS?

Synbiotics are products that combine probiotics and prebiotics.

HOW POPULAR ARE PROBIOTICS?

The 2012 National Health Interview Survey (NHIS) showed that about 4 million (1.6%) U.S. adults had used probiotics or prebiotics in the past 30 days. Among adults, probiotics or prebiotics were the third most commonly used dietary supplement other than vitamins and minerals. The use of probiotics by adults quadrupled between 2007 and 2012. The 2012 NHIS also showed that 300,000 children aged 4–17 (0.5%) had used probiotics or prebiotics in the 30 days before the survey.

HOW MIGHT PROBIOTICS WORK?

Probiotics may have a variety of effects on the body, and different probiotics may act in different ways. Probiotics might:

- help your body maintain a healthy community of microorganisms or help your body's community of microorganisms return to a healthy condition after being disturbed
- produce substances that have desirable effects
- influence your body's immune response

HOW ARE PROBIOTICS REGULATED IN THE UNITED STATES?

Government regulation of probiotics in the United States is complex. Depending on a probiotic product's intended use, the U.S. Food and Drug Administration (FDA) might regulate it as a dietary supplement, a food ingredient, or a drug.

Many probiotics are sold as dietary supplements, which do not require FDA approval before they are marketed. Dietary supplement labels may make claims about how the product affects the structure or function of the body without FDA approval, but they are not allowed to make health claims, such as saying the supplement lowers your risk of getting a disease, without the FDA's consent.

If a probiotic is going to be marketed as a drug for the treatment of a disease or disorder, it has to meet stricter requirements. It must be proven safe and effective for its intended use through clinical trials and be approved by the FDA before it can be sold.

WHAT HAS SCIENCE SHOWN ABOUT THE EFFECTIVENESS OF PROBIOTICS FOR HEALTH CONDITIONS?

A great deal of research has been done on probiotics, but much remains to be learned about whether they are helpful and safe for various health conditions.

Probiotics have shown promise for a variety of health purposes, including prevention of antibiotic-associated diarrhea (including diarrhea caused by *Clostridium difficile*), prevention of necrotizing enterocolitis and sepsis in premature infants, treatment of infant colic, treatment of periodontal disease, and induction or maintenance of remission in ulcerative colitis.

However, in most instances, we still do not know which probiotics are helpful and which are not. We also do not know how much of the probiotic people would have to take or who would be most likely to benefit. Even for the conditions that have been studied the most, researchers are still working toward finding the answers to these questions.

The following summarizes the research on probiotics for some of the conditions for which they have been studied.

Gastrointestinal Conditions

ANTIBIOTIC-ASSOCIATED DIARRHEA

- Probiotics have been studied for antibiotic-associated diarrhea in general, as well as for antibiotic-associated diarrhea caused by one specific bacterium, *C. difficile.*
- A 2017 review of 17 studies (3,631 total participants) in people who were not hospitalized indicated that giving probiotics to patients along with antibiotics was associated with a decrease of about half in the likelihood of antibiotic-associated diarrhea. However, this conclusion was considered tentative because the quality of the studies was only moderate. Patients who were given probiotics had no more side effects than patients who did not receive them.
- Probiotics may be helpful for antibiotic-associated diarrhea in young and middle-aged people, but a benefit has not been demonstrated in elderly people, according to a 2016 review of 30 studies (7,260 participants), five of which focused on people aged 65 or older. It is uncertain whether probiotics actually do not work in elderly people or whether no effect was seen because there were only a few studies of people in this age group.
- A review of 23 studies (with 3,938 participants) of probiotics to prevent antibiotic-associated diarrhea in children provided moderate-quality evidence that probiotics had a protective effect. No serious side effects were observed in children who were otherwise healthy, except for the infection for which they were being treated.

CLOSTRIDIUM DIFFICILE INFECTION

- The bacterium *C. difficile* can infect the colon (large intestine) of patients who have received antibiotics, causing diarrhea that can range from mild to severe. *C. difficile* infection is difficult to treat and sometimes comes back after treatment. It is more common in people who take antibiotics long-term and in elderly people, and it can spread in hospitals and nursing homes. *C. difficile* infection affects about half a million people a year in the United States and causes about 15,000 deaths.
- A 2017 analysis of 31 studies (8,672 total patients) concluded that it is moderately certain that probiotics can reduce the risk of *C. difficile* diarrhea in adults and children who are receiving antibiotics. Most of these studies involved hospital patients. The analysis also concluded that the use of probiotics along with antibiotics appears to be safe, except for patients who are very weak or have poorly functioning immune systems.
- The types of probiotics that would be most useful in reducing the risk of *C. difficile* diarrhea, the length of time for which they should be taken, and the most appropriate doses are uncertain.

CONSTIPATION

- A 2014 review of 14 studies (1,182 participants) of probiotics for constipation in adults showed some evidence of benefit, especially for *Bifidobacterium lactis*.
- A 2017 evaluation of nine studies (778 participants) of probiotics for constipation in elderly people indicated that probiotics produced a small but meaningful benefit. The type of bacteria most often tested was *Bifidobacterium longum*. The researchers who performed the evaluation suggested that probiotics might be helpful for chronic constipation in older people as an addition to the usual forms of treatment.
- A 2017 review looked at seven studies of probiotics for constipation in children (515 participants). The studies

were hard to compare because of differences in the groups of children studied, the types of probiotics used, and other factors. The reviewers did not find evidence that any of the probiotics tested in the children were helpful. A second 2017 review, which included four of the same studies and two others (498 total participants in the six studies examined), took a more optimistic view of the evidence, noting that overall, probiotics did increase stool frequency and that the effect was more noticeable in Asian than European children.

DIARRHEA CAUSED BY CANCER TREATMENT

- Diarrhea is a common side effect of chemotherapy or radiotherapy for cancer. It has been suggested that probiotics might help prevent or treat this type of diarrhea. However, a 2018 review of 12 studies (1,554 participants) found that the evidence for a beneficial effect of probiotics was inconclusive.

DIVERTICULAR DISEASE

- In diverticulosis, small pouches develop at weak spots in the wall of the colon (large intestine). In most cases, this does not cause any symptoms. If symptoms (such as bloating, constipation, diarrhea, or cramping) do occur, the condition is called "diverticular disease." If any of the pouches become inflamed, the condition is called "diverticulitis." Patients with diverticulitis can have severe abdominal pain and may develop serious complications.
- A 2016 review of 11 studies (764 participants) of probiotics for diverticular disease was unable to reach conclusions on whether the probiotics were helpful because of the poor quality of the studies.

INFLAMMATORY BOWEL DISEASE

- Inflammatory bowel disease is a term for a group of conditions that cause a portion of the digestive system to become inflamed; the most common types are ulcerative colitis and Crohn's disease. Symptoms may include abdominal pain, diarrhea (which may be bloody), loss of appetite, weight loss, and fever. The symptoms can range from mild to severe, and they may come and go. Treatment includes medicines and, in some cases, surgery.

- A 2014 review of 21 studies in patients with ulcerative colitis (1,700 participants) indicated that adding probiotics, prebiotics, or synbiotics to conventional treatment could be helpful in inducing or maintaining remission of the disease. The same review also looked at 14 studies (746 participants) of probiotics, prebiotics, or synbiotics for Crohn's disease and did not find evidence that they were beneficial.

IRRITABLE BOWEL SYNDROME

- A 2018 review of 53 studies (5,545 total participants) of probiotics for irritable bowel syndrome (IBS) concluded that probiotics may have beneficial effects on global IBS symptoms and abdominal pain, but it was not possible to draw definite conclusions about their effectiveness or to identify which species, strains, or combinations of probiotics are most likely to be helpful.

TRAVELER'S DIARRHEA

- A 2018 review evaluated 11 studies (5,143 participants) of probiotics or prebiotics for the prevention of traveler's diarrhea and found evidence that they may be helpful. However, the review did not assess the quality of the studies and did not include data on side effects.
- A 2017 clinical practice guideline by the International Society of Travel Medicine stated that there is insufficient evidence to recommend probiotics or prebiotics to prevent or treat traveler's diarrhea. The guidelines acknowledged that there is evidence suggesting a small benefit but pointed out that studies vary greatly in terms

of factors such as the probiotic strains used, the causes of the diarrhea, and geographic locations. Also, some studies had weaknesses in their design.

Conditions in Infants

INFANT COLIC

- Colic is excessive, unexplained crying in young infants. Babies with colic may cry for three hours a day or more, but they eat well and grow normally. The cause of colic is not well understood, but studies have shown differences in the microbial community in the digestive tract between infants who have colic and those who do not, which suggests that microorganisms may be involved.
- A 2018 review of seven studies (471 participants) of probiotics for colic, five of which involved the probiotic *Lactobacillus reuteri* DSM 17938, found that this probiotic was associated with successful treatment (defined as a reduction of more than half in daily crying time). However, the effect was mainly seen in exclusively breastfed infants.
- No harmful effects were seen in a review of four studies (345 participants) of *L. reuteri* DSM 17938 for colic or in a small study funded by the National Centre for Complementary and Integrative Health (NCCIH) that included repeated physical examinations and blood tests in infants with colic who were given this probiotic, as well as parents' reports of symptoms.

NECROTIZING ENTEROCOLITIS

- Necrotizing enterocolitis is a serious, sometimes fatal disease that occurs in premature infants. It involves injury or damage to the intestinal tract, causing the death of intestinal tissue. Its exact cause is unknown, but an abnormal reaction to food components and the microorganisms that live in a premature baby's digestive tract may play a role.

- A 2017 review of 23 studies (7,325 infants) showed that probiotics helped prevent necrotizing enterocolitis in very-low-birth-weight infants. However, the results of individual studies varied; not all showed a benefit. Probiotics that included both *Lactobacillus* and *Bifidobacterium* seemed to produce the best results, but it was not possible to identify the most beneficial strains within these large groups of bacteria.
- None of the infants in the studies described above developed harmful short-term side effects from the probiotics. However, the long-term effects of receiving probiotics at such a young age are uncertain. Outside of these studies, there have been instances when probiotics did have harmful effects in newborns. In several instances, babies developed bloodstream infections from microorganisms intentionally included in a probiotic product, and in one case, a premature baby died after being infected with a mold that had contaminated a probiotic dietary supplement.

SEPSIS IN INFANTS

- Sepsis is a serious illness in which the body has a harmful, overwhelming response to an infection. It can cause major organs and body systems to stop working properly and can be life-threatening. The risk of sepsis is highest in infants, children, the elderly, and people with serious medical problems. One group particularly at risk for sepsis is premature infants.
- A review of 37 studies (9,416 participants) found that probiotics were helpful in reducing the risk of sepsis in premature infants.

Dental Disorders

DENTAL CARIES (TOOTH DECAY)

- A small amount of research, all in infants and young children, has examined the possibility that probiotics might be helpful in preventing dental caries (also called "cavities" or "tooth decay"). A review of seven studies (1,715 total participants) found that the use of probiotics was associated with fewer cavities in four of the seven studies, but the quality of the evidence was low, and no definite conclusions about the effectiveness of probiotics could be reached.

PERIODONTAL DISEASES (GUM DISEASE)

- Periodontal diseases result from infections and inflammation of the gums and bones that surround and support the teeth. If the disease is severe, the gums can pull away from the teeth; bone can be lost; and teeth may loosen or fall out.
- A 2016 review of 12 studies (452 participants) that evaluated probiotics for periodontal disease found evidence that they could be a helpful addition to treatment by reducing disease-causing bacteria and improving clinical signs of the disease. However, effects may differ for different probiotics.

Conditions Related to Allergy

ALLERGIC RHINITIS (HAY FEVER)

- A review of 23 studies (1,919 participants) in which probiotics were tested for treating allergic rhinitis found some evidence that they may be helpful in improving symptoms and quality of life. However, because the studies tested different probiotics and measured different effects, no recommendations about the use of probiotics could be made. Few side effects of probiotics were reported in these studies.

ASTHMA

- A review of 11 studies (910 participants) of probiotics for asthma in children had inconclusive results.

ATOPIC DERMATITIS

- Atopic dermatitis is an itchy chronic skin disorder that is associated with allergies but not caused by them. It is most common in infants and may start as early as age two to six months. Many people outgrow it by early adulthood. Atopic dermatitis is one of several types of eczema.
- A 2017 review of 13 studies (1,271 participants) of probiotics for the treatment of atopic dermatitis in infants and children did not find consistent evidence of a beneficial effect. A review of 9 studies (269 participants) in adults provided preliminary evidence that some strains of probiotics might be beneficial for symptoms of atopic dermatitis.

Prevention of Allergies

- It is been suggested that changes in people's lifestyles and environment may have led to reduced contact with microorganisms early in life and that this decrease may have contributed to an increase in allergies. This is sometimes called the "hygiene hypothesis" although factors unrelated to hygiene, such as smaller family size and the use of antibiotics, may also play a role. Studies have been done in which probiotics were given to pregnant women and/or young infants in the hope of preventing the development of allergies.
- A 2015 review of 17 studies (4,755 participants) that evaluated the use of probiotics during pregnancy or early infancy found that infants exposed to probiotics had a lower risk of developing atopic dermatitis, especially if they were exposed to a mixture of probiotics. However, probiotics did not have an effect on the risks of asthma, wheezing, or hay fever (allergic rhinitis).

Other Conditions

ACNE

- Research has identified mechanisms by which probiotics, either taken orally or used topically (applied to the skin), might influence acne. However, there has been very little research in people on probiotics for acne, and the 2016 guidelines for managing acne of the American Academy of Dermatology (AAD) state that the existing evidence is not strong enough to justify any recommendations about the use of probiotics.

HEPATIC ENCEPHALOPATHY

- When the liver is damaged and unable to remove toxic substances from the blood, the toxins can build up in the bloodstream and affect the nervous system. This may lead to impairments of brain function called "hepatic encephalopathy."
- A 2017 review looked at 21 studies (1,420 participants) of probiotics for hepatic encephalopathy and concluded that they were generally of low quality. There was evidence that compared with a placebo (an inactive substance) or no treatment, probiotics probably had beneficial effects on hepatic encephalopathy, but it was uncertain whether probiotics were better than lactulose, a conventional treatment for liver disease.

UPPER RESPIRATORY INFECTIONS

- Probiotics have been tested for their effects against upper respiratory infections (a group that includes the common cold, middle ear infections, sinusitis, and various throat infections). A 2015 evaluation of 12 studies with 3,720 total participants indicated that people taking probiotics may have fewer and shorter upper respiratory infections.
- However, the quality of the evidence was low because some of the studies were poorly conducted.

URINARY TRACT INFECTIONS

A 2015 review of nine studies (735 participants) of probiotics for the prevention of urinary tract infections did not find evidence of a beneficial effect.

CAN PROBIOTICS BE HARMFUL?

- Probiotics have an extensive history of apparently safe use, particularly in healthy people. However, few studies have looked at the safety of probiotics in detail, so there is a lack of solid information on the frequency and severity of side effects.
- The risk of harmful effects from probiotics is greater in people with severe illnesses or compromised immune systems. When probiotics are being considered for high-risk individuals, such as premature infants or seriously ill hospital patients, the potential risks of probiotics should be carefully weighed against their benefits.
- Possible harmful effects of probiotics include infections, the production of harmful substances by the probiotic microorganisms, and the transfer of antibiotic-resistance genes from probiotic microorganisms to other microorganisms in the digestive tract.
- Some probiotic products have been reported to contain microorganisms other than those listed on the label. In some instances, these contaminants may pose serious health risks.[3]

Section 67.3 | Dietary Supplements

WHAT IS A DIETARY SUPPLEMENT?

Dietary supplements are substances you might use to add nutrients to your diet or to lower your risk of health problems such as osteoporosis or arthritis. Dietary supplements come in the form of pills, capsules, powders, gel capsules and tablets, extracts, or liquids. They might contain vitamins, minerals, fiber, amino acids, herbs or other plants, or enzymes. Sometimes, the ingredients in dietary

[3] "Probiotics: What You Need to Know," National Center for Complementary and Integrative Health (NCCIH), August 1, 2019. Available online. URL: www.nccih.nih.gov/health/probiotics-what-you-need-to-know. Accessed June 29, 2023.

supplements are added to foods and drinks. A doctor's prescription is not needed to buy dietary supplements.[4]

FEDERAL REGULATION OF DIETARY SUPPLEMENTS

- Federal regulations state that companies are responsible for having evidence that their dietary supplements are safe and for ensuring that product labels are truthful and not misleading. Manufacturers are required to produce dietary supplements in a quality manner, ensure that they do not contain contaminants or impurities, and label them accurately.
- However, rules for manufacturing and distributing dietary supplements are less strict than those for prescription or over-the-counter (OTC) drugs.
    - The U.S. Food and Drug Administration (FDA), which regulates dietary supplements, requires that companies submit safety data about any new ingredient not sold in the United States in a dietary supplement before 1994. In all other cases, the FDA is not authorized to review dietary supplements for safety and effectiveness before they are marketed.
    - The FDA can take action against adulterated or misbranded dietary supplements only after the product is on the market. In contrast, companies must show the FDA evidence that their prescription and OTC drugs are safe and effective before the drugs are marketed.
- Once a dietary supplement is on the market, the FDA tracks side effects reported by consumers, supplement companies, and others. You can report any safety concerns you may have about a dietary supplement through the U.S. Department of Health and Human Services (HHS) Safety Reporting Portal (SRP)(www.safetyreporting.hhs.gov/SRP2/en/Home.aspx?sid=9fec20aa-cf60-4ff0-b227-ca0c9048edae).

[4] National Institute on Aging (NIA), "Dietary Supplements for Older Adults," National Institutes of Health (NIH), April 23, 2021. Available online. URL: www.nia.nih.gov/health/dietary-supplements-older-adults. Accessed June 29, 2023.

- If the FDA finds a product to be unsafe, it can take legal action against the manufacturer or distributor and may issue a warning or require that the product be removed from the marketplace. However, the FDA says it cannot test all products marketed as dietary supplements that may have potentially harmful hidden ingredients. In 2023, the FDA launched the Dietary Supplement Ingredient Directory (www.fda.gov/food/dietary-supplements/dietary-supplement-ingredient-directory), a web page where the public can look up ingredients used in products marketed as dietary supplements and find what the FDA has said about that ingredient, as well as whether the agency has taken any action with regard to the ingredient.

Health and Structure/Function Claims

- The labels on dietary supplements cannot claim that the product can diagnose, treat, cure, mitigate, or prevent any disease; claims like these are only permitted for drugs. However, some types of claims related to health or the way that the product affects the structure or function of the body may appear on dietary supplement labels.
  - **Health claims**. It describes a relationship between a substance in the supplement and reduced risk of a disease or condition. They must be based on scientific evidence. For example, if a supplement label says "Calcium may reduce the risk of the bone disease osteoporosis," that is a health claim.
  - **Structure/function claims**. It describes the effect of a substance on maintaining the body's normal structure or function. For example, if a supplement label says "Calcium builds strong bones," that is a structure/function claim. Structure/function claims on dietary supplement labels must be accompanied by this disclaimer: "This statement has not been evaluated by the FDA. This product is not intended

to diagnose, treat, cure, mitigate, or prevent any disease."

- **Advertising.** The U.S. Federal Trade Commission (FTC), which regulates advertising, requires that advertising be truthful and not misleading.

WHAT SCIENCE SAYS ABOUT THE EFFECTIVENESS OF DIETARY SUPPLEMENTS

- Some dietary supplements can be good for your health, while others have not been proven to work. For information on the effectiveness of different supplements, see the National Center for Complementary and Integrative Health (NCCIH; www.nccih.nih.gov/health/dietary-and-herbal-supplements) web page about dietary supplements.
- Studies of some supplements have not supported claims made about them. For example, in several studies, echinacea did not help cure colds, and Ginkgo biloba was not useful for dementia. Many times the research on a dietary supplement is conflicting, such as whether the supplements glucosamine and chondroitin improve symptoms of osteoarthritis.
- Strong evidence to back up claims made for dietary supplements is often lacking. For example, a 2022 review identified 27 ingredients frequently included in supplements with claims related to immune function, such as "supports healthy immune system" or "natural immune booster." The reviewers searched the scientific literature for rigorous studies in people on the effectiveness of each ingredient, and they found evidence of this type for only eight of them. Some of the studies suggested possible benefits, but the evidence was not strong enough to allow definite conclusions to be reached. Additional research is needed, so consumers will know whether a dietary supplement promoted for immune health can help protect them from getting sick.

WHAT SCIENCE SAYS ABOUT THE SAFETY AND SIDE EFFECTS OF DIETARY SUPPLEMENTS

- What is on the label may not be what is in the product. For example, the FDA has found prescription drugs, including anticoagulants (e.g., warfarin), anticonvulsants (e.g., phenytoin), and others, in products being sold as dietary supplements. You can see a list of some of those products on the FDA's Health Fraud Product Database (www.fda.gov/consumers/health-fraud-scams/health-fraud-product-database) web page.
- A government study of 127 dietary supplements marketed for weight loss or to support the immune system found that 20 percent made illegal claims.
- Some dietary supplements may harm you if you have a particular medical condition or risk factor or are taking certain prescription or OTC medications. For example, the herbal supplement St. John's wort makes many medications less effective.
- Dietary supplements result in an estimated 23,000 emergency room visits every year in the United States, according to a 2015 study. Many of the patients are young adults having heart problems from weight-loss or energy products and older adults having swallowing problems from taking large vitamin pills.
- Although it is still rare, more cases are being reported of acute (sudden) liver damage in people taking dietary supplements in the United States and elsewhere. The liver injury can be severe, can require an emergency liver transplant, and is sometimes fatal.
- Many dietary supplements (and some prescription drugs) come from natural sources, but "natural" does not always mean "safe." For example, the kava plant is a member of the pepper family, but taking kava supplements can cause liver disease.
- A manufacturer's use of the term "standardized" (or "verified" or "certified") does not necessarily guarantee product quality or consistency.

SAFETY CONSIDERATIONS

- If you are going to have surgery, be aware that certain dietary supplements may increase the risk of bleeding or affect your response to anesthesia. Talk to your health-care providers as far in advance of the operation as possible and tell them about all dietary supplements that you are taking.
- If you are pregnant, nursing a baby, trying to get pregnant, or considering giving a child a dietary supplement, consider that many dietary supplements have not been tested on pregnant women, nursing mothers, or children.
- If you are taking a dietary supplement, follow the instructions on the label. If you have side effects, stop taking the supplement and contact your health-care provider. You may also want to contact the supplement manufacturer.[5]

Section 67.4 | CAM for Hepatitis C

WHAT IS HEPATITIS C?

Hepatitis C is a contagious liver disease. It is caused by the hepatitis C virus. People can get hepatitis C through contact with blood from a person who is already infected or, less commonly, through having sex with an infected person. The infection usually becomes chronic. Chronic hepatitis C is often treated with drugs that can eliminate the virus. This may slow or stop liver damage, but the drugs may cause side effects, and for some people, treatment is ineffective. An estimated 3.2 million Americans have chronic hepatitis C.

---

[5] "Using Dietary Supplements Wisely," National Center for Complementary and Integrative Health (NCCIH), January 2019. Available online. URL: www.nccih.nih.gov/health/using-dietary-supplements-wisely. Accessed June 29, 2023.

USE OF HERBAL SUPPLEMENTS AND OTHER COMPLEMENTARY APPROACHES FOR HEPATITIS C

Several herbal supplements have been studied for hepatitis C, and a substantial number of people with hepatitis C have tried herbal supplements. For example, a survey of 1,145 participants in the Hepatitis C Long-Term Treatment Against Cirrhosis (HALT-C) trial, a study supported by the National Institutes of Health (NIH), found that 23 percent of the participants were using herbal products. Although participants reported using many different herbal products, silymarin (milk thistle) was by far the most common. Another study, which surveyed 120 adults with hepatitis C, found that many used a variety of complementary health approaches, including multivitamins, herbal remedies, massage, deep breathing exercises, meditation, progressive relaxation, and yoga*.

**A mind and body practice with origins in ancient Indian philosophy. The various styles of yoga typically combine physical postures, breathing techniques, and meditation or relaxation.*

WHAT SCIENCE SAYS

No dietary supplement has been shown to be effective for hepatitis C. This section summarizes what is known about the safety and effectiveness of milk thistle and some of the other dietary supplements studied for hepatitis C.

- Milk thistle (scientific name: *Silybum marianum*) is a plant from the aster family. Silymarin is an active component of milk thistle that is believed to be responsible for the herb's health-related properties. Milk thistle has been used in Europe for treating liver disease and jaundice since the 16th century. In the United States, silymarin is the most popular dietary supplement taken by people with liver disease. However, two rigorously designed studies of silymarin in people with hepatitis C did not show any benefit.
- A 2012 controlled clinical trial, cofounded by the National Center for Complementary and Integrative

Health (NCCIH) and the National Institute of Diabetes and Digestive and Kidney Diseases (NIDDK), showed that two higher-than-usual doses of silymarin were no better than placebo in reducing the high blood levels of an enzyme that indicates liver damage. In the study, 154 people who had not responded to standard antiviral treatment for chronic hepatitis C were randomly assigned to receive 420 mg of silymarin, 700 mg of silymarin, or placebo three times per day for 24 weeks. At the end of the treatment period, blood levels of the enzyme were similar in all three groups.

- Results of the HALT-C study mentioned above suggested that silymarin used by hepatitis C patients was associated with fewer and milder symptoms of liver disease and a somewhat better quality of life, but there was no change in virus activity or liver inflammation. The researchers emphasized that this was a retrospective study (one that examined the medical and lifestyle histories of the participants). The finding of improved quality of life in patients taking silymarin was not confirmed in the more rigorous 2012 study described previously.

WHAT DO WE KNOW ABOUT SAFETY?

- **Safety**. Available evidence from clinical trials in people with liver disease suggests that milk thistle is generally well-tolerated. Side effects can include a laxative effect, nausea, diarrhea, abdominal bloating and pain, and occasional allergic reactions. In NIH-funded studies of silymarin in people with hepatitis C that were completed in 2010 and 2012, the frequency of side effects was similar in people taking silymarin and those taking placebos. However, these studies were not large enough to show with certainty that silymarin is safe for people with chronic hepatitis C.

Other supplements have been studied for hepatitis C, but overall, no benefits have been clearly demonstrated. These supplements include the following:

- **Probiotics**. These are live microorganisms that are intended to have a health benefit when consumed. Research has not produced any clear evidence that probiotics are helpful in people with hepatitis C. Most people can use probiotics without experiencing any side effects—or with only mild gastrointestinal side effects, such as intestinal gas—but there have been some case reports of serious adverse effects in people with underlying serious health conditions.
- **Zinc**. Preliminary studies, most of which were conducted outside the United States, have examined the use of zinc for hepatitis C. Zinc supplements might help correct zinc deficiencies associated with hepatitis C or reduce some symptoms, but the evidence for these possible benefits is limited. Zinc is generally considered to be safe when used appropriately, but it can be toxic if taken in excessive amounts.
- **Combination of certain supplements with conventional drug therapy**. A few preliminary studies have looked at the effects of combining supplements such as lactoferrin, S-Adenosyl-L-methionine (SAMe), or zinc with conventional drug therapy for hepatitis C. The evidence is not sufficient to draw clear conclusions about benefits or safety.
- **Glycyrrhizin**. This—a compound found in licorice root—has been tested in a few clinical trials in hepatitis C patients, but there is not enough evidence to determine if it is helpful. In large amounts, glycyrrhizin or licorice can be dangerous in people with a history of hypertension (high blood pressure), kidney failure, or cardiovascular diseases.
- **TJ-108, Schisandra, oxymatrine, and thymus extract**. Preliminary studies have examined the potential of the following products for treating chronic hepatitis

C: TJ-108 (a mixture of herbs used in Japanese Kampo medicine), Schisandra, oxymatrine (an extract from the sophora root), and thymus extract. The limited research on these products has not produced convincing evidence that they are helpful for hepatitis C.

- **Colloidal silver**. This has been suggested as a treatment for hepatitis C, but there is no research to support its use for this purpose. Colloidal silver is known to cause serious side effects, including permanent bluish discoloration of the skin, called "argyria."[6]

[6] "Hepatitis C: A Focus on Dietary Supplements," National Center for Complementary and Integrative Health (NCCIH), November 2014. Available online. URL: https://files.nccih.nih.gov/s3fs-public/Hepatitis_C_11-12-2015.pdf. Accessed June 29, 2023.

Part 6 | Prevention and Control Measures for Contagious Diseases

Chapter 68 | Personal Hygiene Practices

Many diseases and conditions can be prevented or controlled through appropriate personal hygiene and by regularly washing parts of the body and hair with soap and water. Good body washing practices can prevent the spread of hygiene-related diseases.

KEEPING HANDS CLEAN

Handwashing is one of the best ways to protect yourself and your family from getting sick.

How Germs Spread

Washing hands can keep you healthy and prevent the spread of respiratory and diarrheal infections. Germs can spread from person to person or from surface to people when you:

- touch your eyes, nose, and mouth with unwashed hands
- prepare or eat food and drinks with unwashed hands
- touch surfaces or objects that have germs on them
- blow your nose, cough, or sneeze into your hands and then touch other people's hands or common objects

Key Times to Wash Hands

You can help yourself and your loved ones stay healthy by washing your hands often, especially during these key times when you are likely to get and spread germs:

- before, during, and after preparing food
- before and after eating food

- before and after caring for someone at home who is sick with vomiting or diarrhea
- before and after treating a cut or wound
- after using the toilet
- after changing diapers or cleaning up a child who has used the toilet
- after blowing your nose, coughing, or sneezing
- after touching an animal, animal feed, or animal waste
- after handling pet food or pet treats
- after touching garbage

If soap and water are not readily available, use a hand sanitizer with at least 60 percent alcohol to clean your hands.

Follow Five Steps to Wash Your Hands the Right Way

Washing your hands is easy, and it is one of the most effective ways to prevent the spread of germs. Clean hands can help stop germs from spreading from one person to another and in our communities—including your home, workplace, schools, and childcare facilities.

Follow these five steps every time:

- Wet your hands with clean, running water (warm or cold), turn off the tap, and apply soap.
- Lather your hands by rubbing them together with the soap. Lather the backs of your hands, between your fingers, and under your nails.
- Scrub your hands for at least 20 seconds. Need a timer? Hum the "Happy Birthday" song from beginning to end twice.
- Rinse your hands well under clean, running water.
- Dry your hands using a clean towel or an air dryer.

Use Hand Sanitizer When You Cannot Use Soap and Water

Washing hands with soap and water is the best way to get rid of germs in most situations. If soap and water are not readily available, you can use an alcohol-based hand sanitizer that contains at least

60 percent alcohol. You can tell if the sanitizer contains at least 60 percent alcohol by looking at the product label.

Sanitizers can quickly reduce the number of germs on hands in many situations, but:

- sanitizers do not get rid of all types of germs
- hand sanitizers may not be as effective when hands are visibly dirty or greasy
- hand sanitizers might not remove harmful chemicals, such as pesticides, from hands and heavy metals

Caution: Swallowing alcohol-based hand sanitizer can cause alcohol poisoning if more than a couple of mouthfuls are swallowed. Keep it out of reach of young children and supervise their use.

How to Use Hand Sanitizer

- Apply the gel product to the palm of one hand (read the label to learn the correct amount).
- Cover all surfaces of hands.
- Rub your hands and fingers together until they are dry. This should take around 20 seconds.

NAIL HYGIENE

Appropriate hand hygiene includes diligently cleaning and trimming fingernails, which may harbor dirt and germs and can contribute to the spread of some infections, such as pinworms. Fingernails should be kept short, and the undersides should be cleaned frequently with soap and water. Because of their length, longer fingernails can harbor more dirt and bacteria than short nails, thus potentially contributing to the spread of infection.

Before clipping or grooming nails, all equipment (e.g., nail clippers and files) should be properly cleaned. Sterilizing equipment before use is especially important when nail tools are shared among a number of people, as is common in commercial nail salons.

Infections of the fingernails or toenails are often characterized by swelling of the surrounding skin, pain in the surrounding area, or thickening of the nail. In some cases, these infections may be serious and need to be treated by a physician.

To help prevent the spread of germs and nail infections, do the following:

- Keep nails short and trim them often.
- Scrub the underside of nails with soap and water (or a nail brush) every time you wash your hands.
- Clean any nail grooming tools before use.
- In commercial settings such as nail salons, sterilize nail grooming tools before use.
- Avoid biting or chewing nails.
- Avoid cutting cuticles, as they act as barriers to prevent infection.
- Never rip or bite a hangnail. Instead, clip it with a clean, sanitized nail trimmer.

FACIAL CLEANLINESS

Facial cleanliness is important to your health. Use soap and clean, running water to remove dirt, oil, and unwanted debris from your face.

Many diseases and conditions can be prevented or controlled through appropriate personal hygiene and by frequently washing parts of the face. Appropriate facial hygiene practices include not only washing the face but also properly caring for teeth, mouth, eyes, contact lenses, and ears.

Think before Touching Your Face

Your hands can make your face dirty. Thinking before touching your face can help stop the spread of germs. On average, people touch their faces 23 times per hour. Unwashed hands can easily spread germs to your face after touching contaminated surfaces or objects. Protect yourself by:

- washing your hands at key times (such as before touching your face or putting in contact lenses)
- using a tissue for your nose

- using a tissue to scratch or rub your eyes or to adjust your glasses
- preventing itchiness by using facial moisturizer for dry skin and eye drops for dry eyes

Keep Your Face Mask Clean

Wearing a mask that covers your mouth and nose can be an important way to prevent the spread of respiratory illness. Keeping your mask clean will help keep your skin healthy. Wash reusable masks before wearing them and as soon as they become dirty. If you use a disposable face mask, throw it away after wearing it once.

Face Washing Is Key in Preventing the Spread of Some Diseases

Respiratory illnesses can be caused by many different bacteria and viruses. Typically, respiratory infections, such as the common cold, flu, and COVID-19, can spread through droplets in the air when an infected person coughs or sneezes. They can also be spread by direct contact with bacteria, viruses, and other disease-causing germs. When you touch your face, the germs on your hands can enter your mucous membranes through your nose, eyes, and mouth, causing infection. Protect yourself by washing your hands before touching your face.

Pink eye (conjunctivitis) spreads easily from person to person. Good hygiene practices, such as handwashing, face washing, and not touching or rubbing eyes, are important for limiting the spread of pink eye.

Trachoma is rare in the United States, but it is the world's leading cause of preventable blindness. It spreads through close personal contact. It often infects entire families and communities. Poor facial hygiene can lead to the spread of this disease through eye-seeking flies and contaminated fingers. The promotion of good hygiene practices, such as handwashing and face washing at least once a day with water, is a key step in breaking the cycle of trachoma transmission.

COUGHING AND SNEEZING

Covering coughs and sneezes and keeping hands clean can help prevent the spread of serious respiratory illnesses such as influenza, respiratory syncytial virus (RSV), whooping cough, and COVID 19. Germs can be easily spread by:

- coughing, sneezing, or talking
- touching your face with unwashed hands after touching contaminated surfaces or objects
- touching surfaces or objects that may be frequently touched by other people

To help stop the spread of germs, do the following:

- Cover your mouth and nose with a tissue when you cough or sneeze.
- Throw used tissues in the trash.
- If you do not have a tissue, cough or sneeze into your elbow, not your hands.

Remember to immediately wash your hands after blowing your nose, coughing, or sneezing.

Washing your hands is one of the most effective ways to prevent yourself and your loved ones from getting sick, especially at key times when you are likely to get and spread germs.

- Wash your hands with soap and water for at least 20 seconds.
- If soap and water are not readily available, use an alcohol-based hand sanitizer that contains at least 60 percent alcohol to clean hands.

To help prevent the spread of respiratory disease, you can also avoid close contact with people who are sick. If you are ill, you should try to distance yourself from others, so you do not spread your germs. Distancing includes staying home from work or school when possible.

FOOT HYGIENE

Many diseases and foot problems can be prevented through healthy personal hygiene and taking care of your feet. Healthy foot hygiene practices include not only washing your feet but also clipping your toenails and wearing well-fitting, protective footwear.

Basic Care for Healthy Feet

HOW TO PROTECT YOUR FEET

- Wash your feet every day and dry them completely.
- Clip your toenails short and keep them clean.
- Change your socks at least once a day.
- Check your feet regularly for cuts, sores, swelling, dryness, and infected toenails and apply treatment as needed.
- When visiting a salon for foot care, choose a salon that is clean and licensed by your state's cosmetology board. Make sure the salon sterilizes instruments after each use (such as nail clippers, scissors, and other tools).

Foot Hygiene Is Key in Promoting Good Health

Several foot-related conditions are directly related to hygiene:

- **Athlete's foot, or tinea pedis.** This is an infection of the skin and feet that can be caused by a variety of fungi that thrive in warm, dark, and moist environments. Although tinea pedis can affect any part of the foot, the infection most often affects the space between the toes. Good hygiene practices, such as keeping your feet and toes clean and dry and changing your shoes and socks regularly, help prevent or control tinea pedis.
- **Diabetes.** This disease can damage the nerves and affect blood flow in the feet and legs. Poor foot hygiene can put you at an increased risk for infection.
- **Fungal nail infections.** These infections are common infections of the fingernails or toenails that can cause the nail to become discolored and thick and more likely to crack and break. Small cracks in your nail or the surrounding skin can allow these germs to enter your nail and cause an infection.
- **Hookworm infection.** Hookworm is a parasitic worm (also called a "helminth"). Globally, it is one of the most

common roundworms found in humans. Hookworm infection is most common in resource-limited settings with poor access to water, sanitation, and hygiene. The best way to avoid hookworm infection is not to walk barefoot in areas where hookworm is common and where the soil may be contaminated by human poop (feces).

Fish Pedicures and Fish Spas

During a fish pedicure, also known as a "fish spa treatment," customers place their feet in a tub of water filled with small fish called "Garra rufa." Garra rufa are sometimes referred to as "doctor fish" because they eat away dead skin found on people's feet, leaving newer skin exposed.

Garra rufa are native to the Middle East, where they have been used as a medical treatment for people with skin diseases, such as psoriasis.

WHY HAVE SOME STATES BANNED THE USE OF FISH PEDICURES?

Each state has the authority to ban fish pedicures, and some states have done that.

Reasons for the bans include the following:

- The fish pedicure tubs cannot be sufficiently cleaned between customers when the fish are present.
- The fish themselves cannot be disinfected or sanitized between customers, and there is no effective way to disinfect the tubs. Because of the cost of the fish, salon owners are likely to use the same fish multiple times with different customers, which increases the risk of spreading infections.
- Chinese Chinchin, another species of fish that is often mislabeled as Garra rufa and used in fish pedicures, grows teeth and can draw blood, increasing the risk of infection.
- Fish pedicures do not meet the legal definition of a pedicure.
- Some state regulations specify that fish at a salon must be contained in an aquarium.

- The fish must be starved to get them to eat skin, which might be considered animal cruelty.
- According to the U.S. Fish and Wildlife Service, Garra rufa could pose a threat to native plant and animal life if released into the wild because the fish is not native to the United States.

HAIR AND SCALP HYGIENE

Maintaining a healthy scalp and hair through good hygiene and proper hair care can help prevent and control many diseases and conditions. Use soap and clean, running water to remove dirt, oil, and unwanted residue from your head.

Break up the Buildup

Like the rest of your skin, the scalp produces a natural oil called "sebum" that moisturizes and protects your skin from infection. Some people produce more sebum than others. When the body produces too much sebum, it can build up on your scalp. If you shower less frequently, dead skin, dirt, product residue, and sweat may also build up on your scalp. This can result in greasy hair, increased risk for infection, and unpleasant odor. Practice the following habits to improve your scalp and hair care routine:

- Use an exfoliator on the scalp to break up the buildup.
- Select a shampoo and conditioner that work for your hair type.
- Wash your hair regularly.
- Brush regularly to prevent tangled hair and to help break apart buildup.

Washing Your Scalp Helps Control Scalp Conditions and Infections

Ringworm on the scalp spreads through direct contact with an infected animal or person or from the environment. Good hygiene practices, such as not sharing combs, towels, or other personal items and washing your hands regularly, can help protect you.

Head lice spread most commonly by direct head-to-head (hair-to-hair) contact. However, much less frequently, they can spread through shared clothing or other belongings. This can happen if lice crawl onto those items or eggs attached to shed hairs fall on the items. Good hygiene practices are important for preventing and controlling the spread of head lice. For example, do not share combs, brushes, or towels. Machine wash clothes and linens used by people with head lice.

MENSTRUAL HYGIENE

Menstruation (also called a "period") is a normal biological process experienced by millions around the world each month. A period happens when the uterus sheds blood and tissue from the uterine lining and leaves your body through the vagina.

Practice Healthy Habits during Your Period

Good menstrual health and hygiene practices can prevent infections, reduce odors, and help you stay comfortable during your period.

You can choose many types of menstrual products to absorb or collect blood during your period, including sanitary pads, tampons, menstrual cups, menstrual discs, and period underwear. Follow these tips when you are using menstrual products, in addition to the instructions that come with the product:

- Wash your hands before and after using the restroom and before using a menstrual product.
- Discard used disposable menstrual products properly. Wrap them with toilet paper, a tissue, or other material and then toss them into a trash bin. Do not flush menstrual products down the toilet.
- Change sanitary pads every few hours, no matter how light the flow. Change them more frequently if your period is heavy.
- Change tampons every 4–8 hours. Do not wear a single tampon for more than 8 hours at a time.
    - Use the lowest-absorbency tampon needed. If you can wear one tampon for up to 8 hours without changing, the absorbency may be too high.

- Clean menstrual cups every day after use. Sanitize menstrual cups after your period is over by rinsing them thoroughly and then placing them in boiling water for one to two minutes.
- Most reusable period underwear is machine washable. Follow product directions on the best way to clean.

Menstrual Hygiene Is Key in Promoting Good Health

These hygiene practices can help you stay healthy and comfortable during your period:

- **Wear lightweight, breathable clothing (such as cotton underwear).** Tight fabrics can trap moisture and heat, allowing germs to thrive.
- **Change your menstrual products regularly.** Trapped moisture provides a breeding ground for bacteria and fungi. Wearing a pad or period underwear for too long can lead to a rash or an infection.
- **Keep your genital area clean.** Wash the outside of your vagina (vulva) and bottom every day. When you go to the bathroom, wipe from the front of your body toward the back, not the other way. Use only water to rinse your vulva. The vagina is a self-cleaning organ. Changing the natural pH balance of your vagina by washing or using chemicals to cleanse out the vagina can be harmful and may result in a yeast infection or bacterial vaginosis (BV).
- **Use unscented toilet paper, tampons, or pads.** Scented hygiene products can irritate the skin and impact your natural pH balance.
- **Drink enough liquids.** This can help wash out your urinary tract and help prevent infections, such as vaginal candidiasis.
- **Track and monitor your period.** Your menstrual cycle is a valuable marker of your overall health. Irregular periods can be a sign of conditions such as diabetes, thyroid dysfunction, and celiac disease. You can track your period on a calendar or with an app on your phone designed for this purpose.

- **Visit a health-care provider for your annual checkup.** An annual well-woman exam is a full checkup that includes a Papanicolaou (Pap) smear, a pelvic exam, and a breast exam. These exams are essential for good reproductive health as they can catch early signs of cancer or other health issues.

Talk to a doctor if you experience a change in odor, have extreme or unusual pain, or have more severe period symptoms than usual (such as a heavier flow or longer period).

Menstrual Hygiene Day: May 28

Each year on May 28, Menstrual Hygiene Day (https://menstrualhygieneday.org/) is observed to highlight good menstrual hygiene practices during your period and to raise awareness about the importance of access to menstrual products, period education, and sanitation facilities.

What You Can Do

Everyone can participate in Menstrual Hygiene Day by:

- spreading awareness in your community about the importance of good menstrual hygiene habits
- visiting the WASH United's Menstrual Hygiene Day site (https://menstrualhygieneday.org/) for more information and resources
- joining a worldwide conversation on social media using #MHDay2023
- learning more about other hygiene practices to keep you healthy[1]

[1] "Personal Hygiene" Centers for Disease Control and Prevention (CDC), December 1, 2022. Available online. URL: www.cdc.gov/hygiene/personal-hygiene/index.html. Accessed September 14, 2023.

Chapter 69 | **Influence of Social and Cultural Environment on Public Health**

WHAT ARE SOCIAL DETERMINANTS OF HEALTH?

Social determinants of health (SDOH) are the nonmedical factors that influence health outcomes. They are the conditions in which people are born, grow, work, live, and age, and the wider set of forces and systems shaping the conditions of daily life. These forces and systems include economic policies and systems, development agendas, social norms, social policies, racism, climate change, and political systems.[1]

SDOH can be grouped into five domains.

Economic Stability

In the United States, 1 in 10 people live in poverty, and many people cannot afford things, such as healthy foods, health care, and housing.

People with steady employment are less likely to live in poverty and more likely to be healthy, but many people have trouble finding and keeping a job. People with disabilities, injuries, or conditions, such as arthritis, may be especially limited in their ability to work.

[1] "Social Determinants of Health at CDC," Centers for Disease Control and Prevention (CDC), December 8, 2022. Available online. URL: www.cdc.gov/about/sdoh/index.html. Accessed July 26, 2023.

In addition, many people with steady work still do not earn enough to afford the things they need to stay healthy.

Employment programs, career counseling, and high-quality childcare opportunities can help more people find and keep jobs. In addition, policies to help people pay for food, housing, health care, and education can reduce poverty and improve health and well-being.

Education Access and Quality

People with higher levels of education are more likely to be healthier and live longer.

Children from low-income families, children with disabilities, and children who routinely experience forms of social discrimination—such as bullying—are more likely to struggle with math and reading. They are also less likely to graduate from high school or go to college. This means they are less likely to get safe, high-paying jobs and more likely to have health problems.

In addition, some children live in places with poorly performing schools, and many families cannot afford to send their children to college. The stress of living in poverty can also affect children's brain development, making it harder for them to do well in school. Interventions to help children and adolescents do well in school and help families pay for college can have long-term health benefits.

Health Care Access and Quality

Many people in the United States do not get the health-care services they need.

About 1 in 10 people in the United States do not have health insurance. People without insurance are less likely to have a primary care provider, and they may not be able to afford the health-care services and medications they need. Strategies to increase insurance coverage rates are critical for making sure more people get important health-care services, such as preventive care and treatment for chronic illnesses.

Sometimes, people do not get recommended health-care services, such as cancer screenings, because they do not have a primary care provider. Other times, it is because they live too far away from health-care providers who offer them. Interventions to increase access to health-care professionals and improve communication—in person or remotely—can help more people get the care they need.

Neighborhood and Built Environment

The neighborhoods people live in have a major impact on their health and well-being.

Many people in the United States live in neighborhoods with high rates of violence, unsafe air or water, and other health and safety risks. Racial/ethnic minorities and people with low incomes are more likely to live in places with these risks. In addition, some people are exposed to things at work that can harm their health, such as secondhand smoke or loud noises.

Interventions and policy changes at the local, state, and federal levels can help reduce these health and safety risks and promote health. For example, providing opportunities for people to walk and bike in their communities—such as adding sidewalks and bike lanes—can increase safety and help improve health and quality of life.

Social and Community Context

People's relationships and interactions with family, friends, coworkers, and community members can have a major impact on their health and well-being.

Many people face challenges and dangers they cannot control—unsafe neighborhoods, discrimination, or trouble affording the things they need. This can have a negative impact on health and safety throughout life.

Positive relationships at home, at work, and in the community can help reduce these negative impacts. But some people—such as children whose parents are in jail and adolescents who are bullied—often do not get support from loved ones or others. Interventions to help people get the social and community support they need are critical for improving health and well-being.

SDOH have a major impact on people's health, well-being, and quality of life. Examples of SDOH include the following:

- safe housing, transportation, and neighborhoods
- racism, discrimination, and violence
- education, job opportunities, and income
- access to nutritious foods and physical activity opportunities
- polluted air and water
- language and literacy skills

SDOH also contribute to wide health disparities and inequities. For example, people who do not have access to grocery stores with healthy foods are less likely to have good nutrition. That raises their risk of health conditions, such as heart disease, diabetes, and obesity—and even lowers life expectancy relative to people who do have access to healthy foods.

Just promoting healthy choices will not eliminate these and other health disparities. Instead, public health organizations and their partners in sectors, such as education, transportation, and housing, need to take action to improve the conditions in people's environments.[2]

WHAT IS THE CDC DOING TO ADDRESS SOCIAL DETERMINANTS OF HEALTH?

Because health equity is a priority for the Centers for Disease Control and Prevention (CDC), the agency has taken multiple steps to ensure that efforts to address SDOH are built into the agency's work and not confined to a single program, the CDC center, or public health topic.

In the fall of 2021, the CDC leadership started an agencywide process to build and expand crosscutting efforts to address SDOH. This effort was led by the National Center for Chronic Disease

[2] Office of Disease Prevention and Health Promotion (ODPHP), "Social Determinants of Health," U.S. Department of Health and Human Services (HHS), August 19, 2020. Available online. URL: https://health.gov/healthypeople/priority-areas/social-determinants-health. Accessed August 11, 2023.

Prevention and Health Promotion (NCCDPHP) and resulted in a framework of six pillars:

- **Data and surveillance.** Embed a consistent SDOH approach to standardization, collection, analysis, and dissemination of data across the agency.
- **Evaluation and evidence building.** Advance evaluation and build evidence for strategies that address SDOH to reduce disparities and promote health equity.
- **Partnerships and collaboration.** Establish criteria, actionable steps, and strategies for partnerships, collaborations, and relationships that result in improved health outcomes over the long term.
- **Community engagement.** Foster meaningful, sustained community engagement across all phases of CDC intervention planning and implementation.
- **Infrastructure and capacity.** Strengthen and sustain infrastructure, such as workforce, training, and access to financial resources, required to address SDOH and reduce health disparities.
- **Policy and law.** Identify evidence, tools, and resources to enhance communication about policies that affect SDOH with policymakers and other stakeholders.

The CDC is using this framework to help agency leadership make decisions about where to invest SDOH resources.

WHY IS ADDRESSING SOCIAL DETERMINANTS OF HEALTH IMPORTANT FOR THE CDC AND PUBLIC HEALTH?

Addressing differences in SDOH makes progress toward health equity, a state in which every person has the opportunity to attain their highest level of health. SDOH have been shown to have a greater influence on health than either genetic factors or access to health-care services. For example, poverty is highly correlated with poorer health outcomes and higher risk of premature death. SDOH, including the effects of centuries of racism, are key drivers of health inequities within communities of color. The impact is pervasive and deeply embedded in our society, creating inequities in access to a range of social and economic benefits—such as housing, education, wealth, and employment. These inequities put people at higher risk of poor health.

The CDC is coordinating efforts to focus its resources on the areas where federal public health investments can accelerate progress and make the most difference. SDOH are multifaceted public health problems, which provide an opportunity for collaboration with many sectors (e.g., transportation, education, housing, and health care) and types of organizations (e.g., public agencies, private industries, and community-based organizations).

The CDC's Racial and Ethnic Approaches to Community Health (REACH) (www.cdc.gov/nccdphp/dnpao/state-local-programs/reach/index.htm) focuses on reducing high rates of chronic diseases for specific racial and ethnic groups in urban, rural, and tribal communities. Since 1999, the program has worked across sectors in racial and ethnic minority communities to reduce tobacco use, improve access to healthy foods, change the built environment to promote physical activity, and connect people to clinical care.

PUBLIC HEALTH ACTIONS THAT AFFECT SOCIAL DETERMINANTS OF HEALTH

Convene

Bring together community members and organizations to identify local concerns. The CDC has a long history of convening partners through national conferences, webinars, collaborative publications, and guideline development. The CDC also encourages other public health organizations to act as conveners by including coalition-building or community engagement activities as a requirement in some funded projects.

Integrate

Collect and use multiple sources of data, including public health data, to help develop strategies for set direction. For example, public health departments can provide geographic information system (GIS) maps of community needs and assets based on CDC PLACES data and environmental justice data.

Influence

Lead approaches to develop policies and solutions or leverage funding through various mechanisms to implement and expand priority actions. For example, when CDC Director Dr. Rochelle Walensky, an American physician-scientist, announced that racism is a public health threat, it reinforced actions that communities were already taking and supported many others as they took subsequent actions.

THE CDC'S ROLE IN ADDRESSING SOCIAL DETERMINANTS OF HEALTH

The CDC is committed to addressing health inequities and their root causes, including SDOH. In April 2021, Dr. Walensky declared racism a public health threat, and the agency is currently engaged in an all-encompassing health equity initiative. As the federal government's leading public health agency, the CDC has a unique role in contributing to work on SDOH.[3]

[3] See footnote [1].

Chapter 70 | Vaccine Types and Ingredients

WHAT ARE VACCINES?

Vaccines are injections (shots), liquids, pills, or nasal sprays that you take to teach your body's immune system to recognize and defend against harmful germs. For example, there are vaccines to protect against diseases caused by:

- viruses, such as the ones that cause the flu and COVID-19
- bacteria, including tetanus, diphtheria, and pertussis[1]

Scientific research has led to the development of numerous types of vaccines that safely elicit immune responses that protect against infection, and researchers continue to investigate novel vaccine strategies for the prevention of existing and emerging infectious diseases. Recent decades have brought major advances in understanding the complex interactions between the microbes that cause disease and their human hosts. These insights, as well as advances in laboratory techniques and technologies, have aided the development of new types of vaccines.

WHOLE-PATHOGEN VACCINES

Traditional vaccines consist of entire pathogens that have been killed or weakened so that they cannot cause disease. Such whole-pathogen vaccines can elicit strong protective immune responses.

---

[1] MedlinePlus, "Vaccines," National Institutes of Health (NIH), February 22, 2022. Available online. URL: https://medlineplus.gov/vaccines.html. Accessed September 13, 2023.

Many of the vaccines in clinical use today fall into this category. However, not every disease-causing microbe can be effectively targeted with a whole-pathogen vaccine.

Scientists first described the ability of inactivated, or killed, microbes to induce immunity in the nineteenth century. This led to the development of inactivated vaccines, which are produced by killing the pathogen with chemicals, heat, or radiation. One contemporary example is Havrix, an inactivated vaccine against the hepatitis A virus that was developed by the National Institute of Allergy and Infectious Diseases (NIAID) and partners and licensed in the United States in 1995.

Advances in tissue culture techniques in the 1950s enabled the development of live-attenuated vaccines, which contain a version of the living microbe that has been weakened in the laboratory. The measles, mumps, and rubella (MMR) vaccine is one example. These vaccines elicit strong immune responses that can confer life-long immunity after only one or two doses. Live-attenuated vaccines are relatively easy to create for certain viruses but difficult to produce for more complex pathogens such as bacteria and parasites.

Modern genetic engineering techniques have enabled the creation of chimeric viruses, which contain genetic information from and display the biological properties of different parent viruses. A NIAID-developed live-attenuated chimeric vaccine consisting of a dengue virus backbone with Zika virus surface proteins is undergoing early-stage testing in humans.

SUBUNIT VACCINES

Instead of the entire pathogen, subunit vaccines include only the components, or antigens, that best stimulate the immune system. Although this design can make vaccines safer and easier to produce, it often requires the incorporation of adjuvants to elicit a strong protective immune response because the antigens alone are not sufficient to induce adequate long-term immunity.

Including only the essential antigens in a vaccine can minimize side effects, as illustrated by the development of a new generation of pertussis (whooping cough) vaccines. The first pertussis vaccines, introduced in the 1940s, comprised inactivated *Bordetella pertussis* bacteria. Although effective, whole-cell pertussis vaccines frequently caused minor adverse reactions such as fever and swelling at the injection site. This caused many people to avoid the vaccine, and by the 1970s, decreasing vaccination rates had brought about an increase in new infections. Basic research at the NIAID and elsewhere, as well as NIAID-supported clinical work, led to the development of acellular (not containing cells) pertussis vaccines that are based on individual, purified *B. pertussis* components. These vaccines are similarly effective as whole-cell vaccines but much less likely to cause adverse reactions.

Some vaccines to prevent bacterial infections are based on the polysaccharides, or sugars, that form the outer coating of many bacteria. The first licensed vaccine against *Haemophilus influenzae* type b (Hib), invented at the National Institute of Child Health and Human Development of the National Institutes of Health (NIH) and further developed by NIAID-supported researchers, was a polysaccharide vaccine. However, its usefulness was limited, as it did not elicit strong immune responses in infants—the age group with the highest incidence of Hib disease. The NIH researchers next developed a so-called conjugate vaccine in which the Hib polysaccharide is attached, or "conjugated," to a protein antigen to offer improved protection. This formulation greatly increased the ability of the immune systems of young children to recognize the polysaccharide and develop immunity. Today conjugate vaccines are available to protect against Hib, pneumococcal, and meningococcal infections.

Other vaccines against bacterial illnesses, such as diphtheria and tetanus vaccines, aim to elicit immune responses against disease-causing proteins, or toxins, secreted by the bacteria. The antigens in these so-called toxoid vaccines are chemically inactivated toxins, known as "toxoids."

In the 1970s, advances in laboratory techniques ushered in the era of genetic engineering. A decade later, recombinant deoxyribonucleic acid (DNA) technology—which enables DNA from two or more sources to be combined—was harnessed to develop the first recombinant protein vaccine, the hepatitis B vaccine. The vaccine antigen is a hepatitis B virus protein produced by yeast cells into which the genetic code for the viral protein has been inserted.

Vaccines to prevent human papillomavirus (HPV) infection are also based on recombinant protein antigens. In the early 1990s, scientists at the NIH's National Cancer Institute discovered that proteins from the outer shell of HPV can form particles that closely resemble the virus. These virus-like particles (VLPs) prompt an immune response similar to that elicited by the natural virus, but VLPs are noninfectious because they do not contain the genetic material the virus needs to replicate inside cells. The NIAID scientists have designed an experimental VLP vaccine to prevent chikungunya that elicited robust immune responses in an early-stage clinical trial.

Scientists at the NIAID and other institutions are also developing new strategies to present protein subunit antigens to the immune system. As part of efforts to develop a universal flu vaccine, NIAID scientists designed an experimental vaccine featuring the protein ferritin, which can self-assemble into microscopic pieces called "nanoparticles" that display a protein antigen. An experimental nanoparticle-based influenza vaccine is being evaluated in an early-stage trial in humans. The nanoparticle-based technology is also being assessed as a platform for the development of vaccines against Middle East respiratory syndrome (MERS) coronavirus, respiratory syncytial virus (RSV), and Epstein-Barr virus (EBV).

Other relatively recent advances in laboratory techniques, such as the ability to solve atomic structures of proteins, also have contributed to advances in subunit vaccine development. For example, by solving the three-dimensional structure of a protein on the RSV surface bound to an antibody, NIAID scientists identified a key area of the protein that is highly sensitive to neutralizing antibodies. They were then able to modify the RSV protein to stabilize the structural form in which it displays the neutralization-sensitive site.

While most subunit vaccines focus on a particular pathogen, scientists are also developing vaccines that could offer broad protection against various diseases. The NIAID investigators in 2017 launched an early-phase clinical trial of a vaccine to prevent mosquito-borne diseases such as malaria, Zika, chikungunya, and dengue fever. The experimental vaccine, designed to trigger an immune response to mosquito saliva rather than a specific virus or parasite, contains four recombinant proteins from mosquito salivary glands.

NUCLEIC ACID VACCINES

Another investigational approach to vaccination involves introducing genetic material encoding the antigen or antigens against which an immune response is sought. The body's own cells then use this genetic material to produce the antigens. Potential advantages of this approach include the stimulation of broad long-term immune responses, excellent vaccine stability, and relative ease of large-scale vaccine manufacture. Many such vaccines are in the research pipeline although none are currently licensed for human use.

The DNA plasmid vaccines comprise a small circular piece of DNA called a "plasmid" that carries genes encoding proteins from the pathogen of interest. The manufacturing process for DNA plasmid vaccines is well-established, allowing experimental vaccines to be quickly developed to address emerging or reemerging infectious diseases. The NIAID's Vaccine Research Center has developed candidate DNA vaccines to address several viral disease threats during outbreaks, including severe acute respiratory syndrome (SARS) coronavirus (SARS-CoV) in 2003, H5N1 avian influenza in 2005, H1N1 pandemic influenza in 2009, and Zika virus in 2016. The time from selection of the viral genes to be included in the vaccine to initiation of clinical studies in humans was shortened from 20 months with SARS-CoV to slightly longer than three months with Zika virus.

Vaccines based on the messenger ribonucleic acid (mRNA), an intermediary between DNA and protein, are also being developed. Recent technological advances have largely overcome issues with the instability of mRNA and the difficulty of delivering it into cells, and some mRNA vaccines have demonstrated encouraging early results. For example, NIAID-supported researchers developed an experimental mRNA vaccine that protected mice and monkeys against Zika virus infection after a single dose.

Rather than delivering DNA or mRNA directly to cells, some vaccines use a harmless virus or bacterium as a vector, or carrier, to introduce genetic material into cells. Several such recombinant vector vaccines are approved to protect animals from infectious diseases, including rabies and distemper. Many of these veterinary vaccines are based on a technology developed by NIAID researchers in the 1980s that uses weakened versions of a poxvirus to deliver the pathogen's genetic material. Today, NIAID-supported scientists are developing and evaluating recombinant vectored vaccines to protect humans from viruses such as human immunodeficiency virus (HIV), Zika virus, and Ebola virus.[2]

[2] "Vaccine Types," National Institute of Allergy and Infectious Diseases (NIAID), July 1, 2019. Available online. URL: www.niaid.nih.gov/research/vaccine-types. Accessed July 5, 2023.

Chapter 71 | Vaccines: What They Are and How They Work

Chapter Contents

VACCINES PROTECT AGAINST DISEASES

Different vaccines work in different ways, but every vaccine helps the body's immune system learn how to fight germs. It typically takes a few weeks for protection to develop after vaccination, but that protection can last a lifetime. A few vaccines, such as those for tetanus or seasonal flu, require occasional booster doses to maintain the body's defenses.

STRENGTHENING YOUR BABY'S IMMUNE SYSTEM

Immunity is the body's way of preventing disease. Because a baby's immune system is not fully developed at birth, babies face a greater risk of becoming infected and getting seriously ill. Vaccines help teach the immune system how to defend against germs. Vaccination protects your baby by helping build up their natural defenses.

- Children are exposed to thousands of germs every day. This happens through the food they eat, the air they breathe, and the things they put in their mouth.
- Babies are born with immune systems that can fight most germs, but some germs cause serious or even deadly diseases a baby cannot handle. For those, babies need the help of vaccines.
- Vaccines use very small amounts of antigens to help your child's immune system recognize and learn to fight serious diseases. Antigens are the parts of a germ that cause the body's immune system to go to work.

VACCINE INGREDIENTS

Today's vaccines use only the ingredients they need to be as safe and effective as possible. A vaccine could include any of these kinds of ingredients:

- Adjuvants such as aluminum salts help boost the body's response to a vaccine (also found in antacids, antiperspirants, etc.).

- Stabilizers such as sugars or gelatin help keep a vaccine effective after it is manufactured (naturally present in the body and found in foods such as Jell-O®).
- Formaldehyde helps prevent bacterial contamination during manufacturing. Formaldehyde is naturally present in the body at levels higher than vaccines (also found in the environment, preservatives, and household products).
- Thimerosal is a preservative used in the vaccine manufacturing process. It is no longer used to make any vaccine except multidose vials of the flu vaccine. Single-dose vials of the flu vaccine are available as an alternative.

VACCINES ARE SAFE

Before a new vaccine is ever given to people, extensive lab testing is done. Once testing in people begins, it can still take years before clinical studies are complete and the vaccine is licensed.

After a vaccine is licensed, the U.S. Food and Drug Administration (FDA), the Centers for Disease Control and Prevention (CDC), the National Institutes of Health (NIH), and other federal agencies continue routine monitoring and investigate any potential safety concerns.

MILD SIDE EFFECTS ARE EXPECTED

Vaccines, such as medicine, can have some side effects. But most people who get vaccinated have only mild side effects or none at all. The most common side effects include fever, tiredness, body aches, redness, swelling, and tenderness where the shot was given. Mild reactions usually go away on their own within a few days. Serious, long-lasting side effects are extremely rare. We know they are rare because the CDC tracks and investigates reports of serious side effects.

WHY YOUR CHILD SHOULD GET VACCINATED

Vaccines can prevent common diseases that used to seriously harm or even kill infants, children, and adults. Without vaccines, your child is at risk of becoming seriously ill or even dying from childhood diseases, such as measles and whooping cough.

It is always better to prevent a disease than to treat one after it occurs.

- Vaccination is a safe, highly effective, and easy way to help keep your family healthy.
- The recommended vaccination schedule balances when a child is likely to be exposed to a disease and when a vaccine will be most effective.
- Vaccines are tested to ensure they can be given safely and effectively at the recommended ages.

The CDC vaccine information statements (VISs; www.cdc.gov/vaccines/hcp/vis/current-vis.html) explain both the benefits and risks of a vaccine. Your health-care provider can give you the VIS for any vaccine.[1]

Section 71.2 | Understanding Vaccine Mechanisms

Diseases that vaccines prevent can be dangerous or even deadly. Vaccines greatly reduce the risk of infection by working with the body's natural defenses to safely develop immunity to disease.

THE IMMUNE SYSTEM: THE BODY'S DEFENSE AGAINST INFECTION

To understand how vaccines work, it is helpful to first look at how the body fights illnesses. When germs, such as bacteria or viruses, invade the body, they attack and multiply. This invasion is called an "infection," and the infection is what causes illnesses. The immune system uses several tools to fight infection. Blood contains red blood cells, for carrying oxygen to tissues and organs, and white

[1] "Making the Vaccine Decision: Addressing Common Concerns," Centers for Disease Control and Prevention (CDC), July 19, 2023. Available online. URL: www.cdc.gov/vaccines/parents/why-vaccinate/vaccine-decision.html. Accessed August 7, 2023.

or immune cells, for fighting infection. These white cells consist primarily of macrophages, B lymphocytes, and T lymphocytes:

- **Macrophages.** These are white blood cells that swallow up and digest germs, plus dead or dying cells. The macrophages leave behind parts of the invading germs called "antigens." The body identifies antigens as dangerous and stimulates the body to attack them.
- **B lymphocytes.** Antibodies attack the antigens left behind by the macrophages. Antibodies are produced by defensive white blood cells called "B lymphocytes."
- **T lymphocytes.** These are another type of defensive white blood cells. They attack cells in the body that have already been infected.

The first time the body encounters a germ, it can take several days to make and use all the germ-fighting tools needed to get over the infection. After the infection, the immune system remembers what it learned about how to protect the body against that disease.

The body keeps a few T lymphocytes, called "memory cells" that go into action quickly if the body encounters the same germ again. When the familiar antigens are detected, B lymphocytes produce antibodies to attack them.

HOW VACCINES WORK

Vaccines help develop immunity by imitating an infection. This type of infection, however, does not cause illness, but it does cause the immune system to produce T lymphocytes and antibodies. Sometimes, after getting a vaccine, the imitation infection can cause minor symptoms, such as fever. Such minor symptoms are normal and should be expected as the body builds immunity.

Once the imitation infection goes away, the body is left with a supply of "memory" T lymphocytes, as well as B lymphocytes that will remember how to fight that disease in the future. However, it typically takes a few weeks for the body to produce T lymphocytes and B lymphocytes after vaccination. Therefore, it is possible that a person who was infected with a disease just before or just after vaccination could develop symptoms and get a disease because the vaccine has not had enough time to provide protection.

TYPES OF VACCINES

Scientists take many approaches to designing vaccines. These approaches are based on information about the germs (viruses or bacteria) the vaccine will prevent, such as how it infects cells and how the immune system responds to it. Practical considerations, such as regions of the world where the vaccine would be used, are also important because the strain of a virus and environmental conditions, such as temperature and risk of exposure, may be different in various parts of the world. The vaccine delivery options available may also differ geographically. Today, there are five main types of vaccines that infants and young children commonly receive:

- **Live, attenuated vaccines.** These vaccines fight viruses. These vaccines contain a version of the living virus that has been weakened so that it does not cause serious disease in people with healthy immune systems. Because live, attenuated vaccines are the closest thing to a natural infection, they are good teachers for the immune system. Examples of live, attenuated vaccines include measles, mumps, and rubella (MMR) vaccine and varicella (chickenpox) vaccine. Even though these vaccines are very effective, not everyone can receive them. Children with weakened immune systems—for example, those who are undergoing chemotherapy—cannot get live vaccines.
- **Inactivated vaccines.** These vaccines also fight viruses. These vaccines are made by inactivating, or killing, the virus during the process of making the vaccine. The inactivated polio vaccine is an example of this type of vaccine. Inactivated vaccines produce immune responses in different ways than live, attenuated vaccines. Often, multiple doses are necessary to build up and/or maintain immunity.
- **Toxoid vaccines.** These vaccines prevent diseases caused by bacteria that produce toxins (poisons) in

the body. In the process of making these vaccines, the toxins are weakened, so they cannot cause illness. Weakened toxins are called "toxoids." When the immune system receives a vaccine containing a toxoid, it learns how to fight off the natural toxin. The diphtheria, tetanus, and acellular pertussis (DTaP) vaccine contains diphtheria and tetanus toxoids.

- **Subunit vaccines**. These vaccines include only parts of the virus or bacteria, or subunits, instead of the entire germ. Because these vaccines contain only the essential antigens and not all the other molecules that make up the germ, side effects are less common. The pertussis (whooping cough) component of the DTaP vaccine is an example of a subunit vaccine.
- **Conjugate vaccines**. These vaccines fight different types of bacteria. These bacteria have antigens with an outer coating of sugar-like substances called "polysaccharides." This type of coating disguises the antigen, making it hard for a young child's immature immune system to recognize it and respond to it. Conjugate vaccines are effective for these types of bacteria because they connect (or conjugate) the polysaccharides to antigens that the immune system responds to very well. This linkage helps the immature immune system react to the coating and develop an immune response. An example of this type of vaccine is the *Haemophilus influenzae* type b (Hib) vaccine.

VACCINES REQUIRE MORE THAN ONE DOSE

There are four reasons that babies—and even teens or adults for that matter—who receive a vaccine for the first time may need more than one dose:

- For some vaccines (primarily inactivated vaccines), the first dose does not provide as much immunity as possible. So more than one dose is needed to build more complete immunity. The vaccine that protects against the bacteria Hib, which causes meningitis, is a good example.

- In other cases, such as the DTaP vaccine, which protects against diphtheria, tetanus, and pertussis, the initial series of four shots that children receive as part of their infant immunizations helps them build immunity. After a while, however, that immunity begins to wear off. At that point, a "booster" dose is needed to bring immunity levels back up. This booster dose is needed at four through six years old for DTaP. Another booster against these diseases is needed at 11 or 12 years of age. This booster for older children—and teens and adults, too—is called "Tdap."
- For some vaccines (primarily live vaccines), studies have shown that more than one dose is needed for everyone to develop the best immune response. For example, after one dose of the MMR vaccine, some people may not develop enough antibodies to fight off infection. The second dose helps make sure that almost everyone is protected.
- Finally, in the case of the flu vaccine, adults and children (older than six months) need to get a dose every year. Children aged six months through eight years who have never gotten the flu vaccine in the past or have only gotten one dose in past years need two doses the first year they are vaccinated against the flu for best protection. Then annual flu shots are needed because the disease-causing viruses may be different from year to year. Every year, the flu vaccine is designed to prevent the specific viruses that experts predict will be circulating.

THE BOTTOM LINE

Some people believe that naturally acquired immunity—immunity from having the disease itself—is better than the immunity provided by vaccines. However, natural infections can cause severe complications and be deadly. This is true even for diseases that most people consider mild, such as chickenpox. It is impossible to predict who will get serious infections that may lead to hospitalization.

Vaccines, like any medication, can cause side effects. The most common side effects are mild. However, many vaccine-preventable disease symptoms can be serious or even deadly. Although many of these diseases are rare in this country, they do circulate around the world and can be brought into the United States, putting unvaccinated children at risk. Even with advances in health care, the diseases that vaccines prevent can still be very serious, and vaccination is the best way to prevent them.[2]

[2] "Understanding How Vaccines Work," Centers for Disease Control and Prevention (CDC), February 2013. Available online. URL: www.cdc.gov/vaccines/hcp/patient-ed/conversations/downloads/vacsafe-understand-bw-office.pdf. Accessed July 5, 2023.

Chapter 72 | Questions and Answers about Immunizations

Most parents choose to vaccinate their children according to the recommended schedule, but many parents may still have questions about the vaccines recommended for their child.

VACCINE SAFETY

Are Vaccines Safe?

Yes. Vaccines are very safe. The United States' long-standing vaccine safety system ensures that vaccines are as safe as possible. Currently, the United States has the safest vaccine supply in its history. Millions of children safely receive vaccines each year. The most common side effects are very mild, such as pain or swelling at the injection site.

What Are the Risks and Benefits of Vaccines?

Vaccines can prevent infectious diseases that once killed or harmed many infants, children, and adults. Without vaccines, your child is at risk of getting seriously ill and suffering pain, disability, and even death from diseases such as measles and whooping cough. The main risks associated with getting vaccines are side effects, which are almost always mild (redness and swelling at the injection site) and go away within a few days. Serious side effects after vaccination, such as a severe allergic reaction, are very rare, and doctors and clinic staff are trained to deal with them. The disease-prevention benefits of getting vaccines are much greater than the possible side effects for almost all children. The only exceptions to this are cases in which a child has a serious chronic medical condition, such as cancer or a disease that weakens the immune system, or has had a severe allergic reaction to a previous vaccine dose.

Is There a Link between Vaccines and Autism?

No. Scientific studies and reviews continue to show no relationship between vaccines and autism.

SIDE EFFECTS

What are the common Side Effects of Vaccines?

Vaccines, such as any medication, may cause some side effects. Most of these side effects are very minor, such as soreness where the shot was given, fussiness, or a low-grade fever. These side effects typically only last a couple of days and are treatable. For example, you can apply a cool, wet washcloth on the sore area to ease discomfort.

Can Vaccines Overload Your Baby's Immune System?

Vaccines do not overload the immune system. Every day, a healthy baby's immune system successfully fights off thousands of germs. Antigens are parts of germs that cause the body's immune system to go to work to build antibodies, which fight off diseases.

The antigens in vaccines come from the germs themselves, but the germs are weakened or killed, so they cannot cause serious illness. Even if babies receive several vaccinations in one day, vaccines contain only a tiny fraction of the antigens they encounter every day in their environment. Vaccines give your child the antibodies they need to fight off serious vaccine-preventable diseases.

SCHEDULE FOR VACCINES

Why Do Vaccines Start So Early?

The recommended schedule protects infants and children by providing protection early in life before they come into contact with life-threatening diseases. Children receive vaccinations early because they are susceptible to diseases at a young age.

Should Your Child Get Shots If He/She Is Sick?

Talk with your child's doctor, but children can usually get vaccinated even if they have a mild illness such as a cold, earache, mild fever, or diarrhea. If the doctor says it is okay, your child can still get vaccinated.

Should You Delay Some Vaccines or Follow a Nonstandard Schedule?

Children do not receive any known benefits from following schedules that delay vaccines. Infants and young children who follow immunization schedules that spread out or leave out shots are at risk of developing diseases during the time you delay their shots.

Why Should You Not Delay Some Vaccines If You Are Planning for Your Baby to Get Them All Eventually?

Young children have the highest risk of having a serious case of disease that could cause hospitalization or death. Delaying or spreading out vaccine doses leaves your child unprotected during the time when they need vaccine protection the most. For example, diseases such as *Haemophilus influenzae* type b (Hib) or pneumococcus almost always occur in the first two years of a baby's life. And some diseases, such as hepatitis B and whooping cough (pertussis), are more serious when babies get them.

The Centers for Disease Control and Prevention (CDC) recommends all children receive vaccines according to the recommended immunization schedule to provide them with maximum protection.

If You Are Breastfeeding, Do You Vaccinate Your Baby on Schedule?

Yes, even breastfed babies need to be protected with vaccines at the recommended ages. The immune system is not fully developed at birth, which puts newborns at greater risk for infections.

Breast milk provides important protection from some infections as your baby's immune system is developing. For example, babies who are breastfed have a lower risk of ear infections, respiratory tract infections, and diarrhea. However, breast milk does not protect children against all diseases. Even in breastfed infants, vaccines are the most effective way to prevent many diseases. Your baby needs the long-term protection that can only come from following the CDC's recommended schedule (www.cdc.gov/vaccines/schedules/easy-to-read/child-easyread.html).

Can You Wait to Vaccinate Your Baby Since He/She Is Not in Childcare?

No, even young children who are cared for at home can be exposed to vaccine-preventable diseases, so it is important for them to get all their vaccines at the recommended ages. Children can catch these illnesses from any number of people or places, including from parents, brothers or sisters, or visitors to their home; on playgrounds; or even at the grocery store. Regardless of whether your baby is cared for outside the home, your baby comes in contact with people throughout the day, some of whom may have a vaccine-preventable disease.

Many of these diseases can be especially dangerous to young children, so it is safest to vaccinate your child at the recommended ages.

Can You Wait until Your Child Goes to School to Catch Up on Immunizations?

No. Before entering school, young children can be exposed to vaccine-preventable diseases. Children under age five are especially susceptible to diseases because their immune systems have not built up the necessary defenses to fight infection.

Why Do Adolescents Need Vaccines?

Vaccines are recommended throughout our lives to protect against serious diseases. As protection from childhood vaccines wears off, adolescents need vaccines that will extend protection. Adolescents need protection from additional infections as well before the risk of exposure increases.

Why Are Multiple Doses Needed for Each Vaccine?

Getting every recommended dose of each vaccine provides your child with the best protection possible. Depending on the vaccine, your child will need more than one dose to build high enough immunity to help prevent disease or to boost immunity that fades over time. Your child may also receive more than one dose to make sure they are protected if they did not get immunity from a first dose or to protect them against germs that change over time, such as flu. Every dose is important because each protects against an infectious disease that can be especially serious for infants and very young children.

PROTECTION FROM DISEASES

Do Infants Have Natural Immunity?

Babies may get some temporary protection from mom during the last few weeks of pregnancy but only for diseases to which mom is immune. Breastfeeding may also protect your baby temporarily from minor infections, such as colds. These antibodies do not last long, leaving your baby vulnerable to disease.

Have We Not Gotten Rid of Most of These Diseases in This Country?

Some vaccine-preventable diseases, such as pertussis (whooping cough) and chickenpox, remain common in the United States. On the other hand, other diseases vaccines prevent are no longer common in this country because of vaccines. If we stopped vaccinating, the few cases we have in the United States could very quickly become tens or hundreds of thousands of cases. Even though many serious vaccine-preventable diseases are uncommon in the United States, some are common in other parts of the world. Even if your family does not travel internationally, you could come into contact with international travelers anywhere in your community. Children who do not receive all vaccinations and are exposed to a disease can become seriously sick and spread it through a community.[1]

[1] "Common Questions about Vaccines," Centers for Disease Control and Prevention (CDC), August 7, 2023. Available online. URL: www.cdc.gov/vaccines/parents/FAQs.html. Accessed September 15, 2023.

Chapter 73 | Childhood Immunizations: Ten Vaccines for Fourteen Diseases

CHICKENPOX

Two doses of the chickenpox shot are recommended for children by doctors as the best way to protect against chickenpox (varicella).

When Should Your Child Get the Chickenpox Shot?

Your child should get one dose at each of the following ages:

- first dose: 12–15 months
- second dose: 4–6 years

Older children or adolescents should also get two doses of the chickenpox vaccine if they have never had chickenpox or were never vaccinated. They should also get a second shot if they have had only one chickenpox shot.

Why Should Your Child Get the Chickenpox Shot?

Chickenpox is usually mild, but it can be serious in infants under 12 months of age, adolescents, adults, pregnant people, and people with a weakened immune system. Some people get so sick that they need to be hospitalized. It does not happen often, but people can die from chickenpox. Most people who are vaccinated with two doses of varicella vaccine will be protected for life.

What Are the Side Effects?

Most children do not have any side effects from the shot. The side effects that do occur are usually mild and may include the following:

- soreness, redness, or swelling where the shot was given
- fever
- mild rash

The Chickenpox Shot Is Safe

The chickenpox shot is safe, and it is effective at protecting against chickenpox. Vaccines, like any medicine, can have side effects. These are usually mild and go away on their own.

DIPHTHERIA

Five doses of a diphtheria, tetanus, and acellular pertussis (DTaP) shot for children and one tetanus, diphtheria, and pertussis (Tdap) shot for preteens are recommended by doctors as the best way to protect against diphtheria.

When Should Your Child Get a Diphtheria Shot?

Your child should get one dose of DTaP at each of the following ages:

- first dose: 2 months
- second dose: 4 months
- third dose: 6 months
- fourth dose: 15–18 months
- fifth dose: 4–6 years

Your child should get one dose of Tdap at the following age:

- first dose: 11 or 12 years

Why Should Your Child Get a Diphtheria Shot?

Your child should get a diphtheria shot because it:

- protects against diphtheria, which can be very serious and even deadly, as well as tetanus and whooping cough (pertussis)

- prevents your child from developing a thick coating in the back of the nose or throat from diphtheria that can make it hard to breathe or swallow
- keeps your child from missing school or childcare and you from missing work

Which Vaccines Protect against Diphtheria?

Two shots help protect children against diphtheria: DTaP and Tdap. Both also help protect against tetanus and whooping cough. These shots do not offer lifetime protection. People need booster shots to keep up protection.

Diphtheria Shots Are Safe

Diphtheria shots are safe and effective at preventing diphtheria. Vaccines, like any medicine, can have side effects. These are usually mild and go away on their own.

What Are the Side Effects?

Most children do not have any side effects from DTaP or Tdap. The side effects that do occur from DTaP are usually mild and may include the following:

- soreness or swelling where the shot was given
- fever
- fussiness
- feeling tired
- loss of appetite
- vomiting

More serious side effects are very rare, but DTaP can include the following:

- a fever over 105 °F (55 °C)
- nonstop crying for three hours or more
- seizures (jerking, twitching of the muscles, or staring)

The side effects from Tdap are usually mild and may include the following:

- pain, redness, or swelling where the shot was given

- mild fever
- headache
- feeling tired
- nausea, vomiting, diarrhea, and stomachache

Some preteens and teens might faint after getting Tdap or any other shot.

To prevent fainting and injuries related to fainting, people should be seated or lying down during vaccination and remain in that position for 15 minutes after the vaccine is given.

FLU (INFLUENZA)

A yearly flu vaccine is the best way to protect your child from flu and its potentially serious complications.

Why Should Your Child Get a Flu Vaccine?

Your child should get a flu vaccine because it:

- reduces the risk of flu illness and hospitalization among children
- saves your child's life
- makes the illness less severe among people who get vaccinated but still get sick with the flu
- reduces the risk of illness, which can keep your child from missing school or childcare and you from having to miss work
- reduces the high risk of developing serious flu complications, especially if your child is younger than five years or of any age with certain chronic conditions
- helps prevent the spreading of the flu to family and friends, including babies younger than six months who are too young to get a flu vaccine

When Should Your Child Get a Flu Vaccine?

Doctors recommend that your child get a flu vaccine every year in the fall, starting when he or she is six months old. Some children aged six months through eight years may need two doses for best protection.

- The Centers for Disease Control and Prevention (CDC) recommends a flu vaccine by the end of October before the flu begins spreading in your community. Getting vaccinated later, however, can still be beneficial, and vaccination should continue to be offered throughout the flu season, even into January or later.
- Children aged six months through eight years getting a flu vaccine for the first time and those who have only previously gotten one dose of flu vaccine should get two doses of vaccine. The first dose should be given as soon as the vaccine becomes available.
- If your child previously got two doses of flu vaccine (at any time), he only needs one dose of flu vaccine this season.

The CDC recommends a yearly flu vaccine for everyone aged six months and older. Pregnant women should get a flu vaccine during each pregnancy. Flu vaccines given during pregnancy help protect both the mother and her baby from the flu.

What Vaccines Protect against Flu?

For the 2020–2021 flu season, the CDC recommends a yearly flu vaccination for everyone six months and older.

- Flu shots can be given to your child aged six months and older.
- The nasal spray vaccine can be given to people aged 2–49. However, certain people with underlying medical conditions should not get the nasal spray vaccine.

Your child's doctor will know which vaccines are right for your child.

Should You Get Vaccinated If You Are Pregnant?

Yes. Changes in your immune, heart, and lung functions during pregnancy make you more likely to get seriously ill from the flu.

The CDC recommends pregnant women get a yearly seasonal flu shot by the end of October, if possible, to ensure the best protection against the flu. You can be vaccinated during any trimester of your pregnancy. Getting vaccinated can also help protect your baby after birth from the flu. (Mom passes antibodies onto the developing baby during her pregnancy.)

Flu Vaccines Are Very Safe

Flu vaccines have a good safety record. Hundreds of millions of Americans have safely received flu vaccines for more than 50 years, and there has been extensive research supporting the safety of flu vaccines.

Vaccines, like any medicine, can have side effects. When they occur, flu vaccine side effects are generally mild and go away on their own within a few days.

What Are the Side Effects?

Common side effects from the flu shot may include the following:

- soreness, redness, and/or swelling where the shot was given
- headache
- fever
- nausea
- muscle aches

Side effects from the nasal spray flu vaccine may include the following:

- runny nose
- wheezing
- headache
- vomiting
- muscle aches

If these problems occur, they usually begin soon after vaccination and are mild and short-lived.

To prevent fainting and injuries related to fainting, adolescents should be seated or lying down during vaccination and remain in that position for 15 minutes after the vaccine is given.

Why Does Your Child Need a Flu Vaccine Every Year?

Flu viruses are constantly changing, so new vaccines are made each year to protect against the flu viruses that are likely to cause the most illness. Also, the protection provided by flu vaccination wears off over time. Your child's flu vaccine will protect against the flu all season, but they will need a vaccine again next flu season for the best protection against the flu.

HEPATITIS A

Two doses of the hepatitis A vaccine are recommended for children by doctors as the best way to protect against hepatitis A.

Why Should Your Child Get the Hepatitis A Shot?

Your child should get the hepatitis A shot because it:

- protects your child from hepatitis A, a potentially serious disease
- protects other people from the disease because children under six years old with hepatitis A usually do not have symptoms, but they often pass the disease to others without anyone knowing they were infected
- keeps your child from missing school or childcare and you from missing work

When Should Your Child Get the Hepatitis A Shot?

Your child will need two doses of the hepatitis A shot for best protection. He or she should get one dose at each of the following ages:

- first dose: 12 through 23 months
- second dose: 6 months after the last dose

The Hepatitis A Shot Is Safe

The hepatitis A vaccine is very safe, and it is effective at preventing the hepatitis A disease. Vaccines, like any medicine, can have side effects. These are usually mild and go away on their own.

What Are the Side Effects?

The most common side effects are usually mild and last one or two days. They include the following:

- sore arm from the shot
- headache
- tiredness
- fever
- loss of appetite (not wanting to eat)

HEPATITIS B

Three doses of the hepatitis B shot are recommended for children by doctors as the best way to protect against hepatitis B.

When Should Your Child Get the Shot?

Your child should get one dose at each of the following ages:

- first dose: shortly after birth
- second dose: 1–2 months
- third dose: 6–18 months

Why Should Your Child Get the Hepatitis B Shot?

Your child should get the hepatitis A shot because it:

- protects your child from hepatitis B, a potentially serious disease
- protects other people from the disease because children with hepatitis B usually do not have symptoms, but they may pass the disease to others without anyone knowing they were infected
- prevents your child from developing liver disease and cancer from hepatitis B
- keeps your child from missing school or childcare and you from missing work

The Hepatitis B Shot Is Safe

The hepatitis B shot is very safe and is effective at preventing hepatitis B. Vaccines, like any medicine, can have side effects. These are usually mild and go away on their own.

What Are the Side Effects?

The most common side effects of the hepatitis B vaccine are mild and include the following:

- low fever (less than 101 °F (38.3 °C))
- sore arm from the shot

HAEMOPHILUS INFLUENZAE TYPE B

Three doses or four doses, depending on the brand, of a *Haemophilus influenzae* type b (Hib) vaccine are recommended for children by doctors as the best way to protect against Hib disease.

When Should Your Child Get a Hib Shot?

Your child should get one dose at each of the following ages:

- first dose: 2 months
- second dose: 4 months
- third dose: 6 months for some brands
- fourth dose: 12–15 months

Why Should Your Child Get a Hib Shot?

Your child should get the Hib shot because it:

- protects your child from Hib disease, which can cause lifelong disability and be deadly
- protects your child from the most common type of Hib disease, meningitis (an infection of the lining of the brain and spinal cord)
- keeps your child from missing school or childcare and you from missing work

Hib Shots Are Safe

Hib shots are safe and effective at preventing Hib disease. Vaccines, like any medicine, can have side effects. These are usually mild and go away on their own.

What Are the Side Effects?

Most children do not have any side effects from the shot. The side effects that do occur are usually mild and may include the following:

- redness, swelling, warmth, or pain where the shot was given
- fever

HUMAN PAPILLOMAVIRUS

The human papillomavirus (HPV) vaccination is recommended for children aged 11–12 years to protect against cancers caused by HPV infection.

When Should Your Child Get the Shot?

11–12 YEARS

- Two doses of the HPV shot are needed, 6–12 months apart.
- If the shots are given less than 5 months apart, a third dose is needed.

IF STARTED AFTER 15TH BIRTHDAY

- Three doses of the HPV shot should be given over six months.
- If your teen has not gotten the vaccine yet, talk to his/her doctor about getting it as soon as possible.

Your child can get the first dose of the HPV vaccine at the same visit they get vaccines to protect against meningitis and whooping cough.

Why Does Your Child Need the Human Papillomavirus Shot?

Your child should get the HPV shot because it:

- protects against infections that can lead to certain cancers
- protects against abnormal cells that can lead to cancer (precancers) and the lasting effects of testing and treatment for these precancers
- protects your child long before they are ever exposed to cancer-causing infections

The Human Papillomavirus Shot Is Safe

The HPV shot is very safe, and it is effective at protecting against HPV infection. Vaccines, like any medicine, can have side effects. These are usually mild and go away on their own.

With over 135 million doses distributed in the United States, the HPV vaccine has a reassuring safety record that is backed by over 15 years of monitoring and research.

What Are the Side Effects?

The most common side effects of the HPV vaccine are mild and include the following:

- pain, redness, or swelling in the arm where the shot was given
- fever
- dizziness or fainting*
- nausea
- headache or feeling tired
- muscle or joint pain

It is important to tell the doctor or nurse if your child has any severe allergies, including an allergy to latex or yeast.

**Fainting after any vaccine, including the HPV vaccine, is more common among adolescents. To prevent fainting and injuries related to fainting, adolescents should be seated or lying down during vaccination and for 15 minutes after the shot.*

MEASLES

Two doses of the measles, mumps, and rubella (MMR) vaccine are recommended for children by health-care providers as the best way to protect against measles, mumps, and rubella.

When Should Your Child Get the Measles, Mumps, and Rubella Shot?

Your child should get one dose at each of the following ages:

- first dose: 12–15 months
- second dose: 4–6 years

Before traveling to another country, infants 6–11 months should get one dose of the MMR shot.

Why Should Your Child Get the Measles, Mumps, and Rubella Shot?

Your child should get the MMR shot because it:

- protects your child from measles, a potentially serious disease, as well as mumps and rubella
- protects your child from getting an uncomfortable rash and high fever from measles
- keeps your child from missing school or childcare and you from missing work

The Measles Shot Is Safe

The measles shot is very safe and is effective at preventing measles. Vaccines, like any medicine, can have side effects. These are usually mild and go away on their own.

There Is No Link between the Measles, Mumps, and Rubella Shot and Autism

Scientists in the United States and other countries have carefully studied the MMR shot. None has found a link between autism and the MMR shot.

What Are the Side Effects of the Shot?

Most children do not have any side effects from the shot. The side effects that do occur are usually mild and may include the following:

- soreness, redness, or swelling where the shot was given
- fever
- mild rash
- temporary pain and stiffness in the joints

More serious side effects are rare. These may include a high fever that could cause a seizure.

MENINGOCOCCAL DISEASE

Two doses of the meningococcal shot called "MenACWY" are recommended for preteens and teens by doctors as the best way to protect against meningococcal disease.

When Should Your Child Get the MenACWY Shot?

Your child should get one dose at each of the following ages:

- first dose: 11–12 years
- second dose: 16 years

Teens may also get a meningococcal B (MenB) shot, preferably at ages 16–18. Multiple doses are needed for the best protection, and the same vaccine must be used for all doses. If you are interested, talk to your child's doctor.

Why Should Your Child Get Meningococcal Shots?

Your child should get the MMR shot because it:

- protects against the bacteria that cause meningococcal disease
- protects your child from infections of the lining of the brain and spinal cord as well as bloodstream infections
- protect your child from long-term disabilities that often come with surviving meningococcal disease

What Vaccines Protect against Meningococcal Disease?

- Meningococcal conjugate (MenACWY) vaccine protects against four types (serogroups A, C, W, and Y) of *Neisseria meningitidis* bacteria.
- Serogroup B meningococcal (MenB) vaccine protects against one type (serogroup B) of *Neisseria meningitidis* bacteria.

Meningococcal Shots Are Safe

Meningococcal shots are safe and effective at preventing meningococcal disease. Vaccines, like any medicine, can have side effects. These are usually mild and go away on their own.

What Are the Side Effects?

About half of people who get a MenACWY vaccine have mild side effects following vaccination:

- redness or soreness where the shot is given
- muscle pain
- headache
- tiredness

These reactions usually get better on their own within one to two days, but serious reactions are possible.

Following a MenB shot, more than half of people who get the vaccine will have mild problems, including:

- soreness, redness, or swelling where the shot is given
- fatigue (feeling tired)
- headache
- muscle or joint pain
- fever or chills
- nausea or diarrhea

These reactions usually get better on their own within three to five days, but serious reactions are possible. Note that teens can get both meningococcal vaccines during the same visit but in different arms.

Some preteens and teens might faint after getting a meningococcal vaccine or any other shot. To prevent fainting and injuries related to fainting, people should be seated or lying down during vaccination and remain in that position for 15 minutes after the vaccine is given.

MUMPS

Two doses of the MMR shot are recommended for children by doctors as the best way to protect against measles, mumps, and rubella.

When Should Your Child Get the MMR Shot?

Your child should get one dose at each of the following ages:

- first dose: 12–15 months
- second dose: 4–6 years

Before traveling to another country, infants 6–11 months should get one dose of the MMR shot.

Why Should Your Child Get the Measles, Mumps, and Rubella Shot?

Your child should get the MMR shot because it:

- protects your child from mumps, a potentially serious disease, as well as measles and rubella
- protects your child from getting a fever and swollen glands under the ears or jaw from mumps
- keeps your child from missing school or childcare and you from missing work

Almost everyone who has not had the MMR shot will get mumps if they are exposed to the mumps virus.

The Measles, Mumps, and Rubella Shot Is Safe

The MMR shot is very safe and is effective at preventing mumps. Vaccines, like any medicine, can have side effects. These are usually mild and go away on their own.

There Is No Link between the Measles, Mumps, and Rubella Shot and Autism

Scientists in the United States and other countries have carefully studied the MMR shot. None has found a link between autism and the MMR shot.

What Are the Side Effects of the Shot?

Most children do not have any side effects from the shot. The side effects that do occur are usually mild and may include the following:

- soreness, redness, or swelling where the shot was given
- fever
- mild rash
- temporary pain and stiffness in the joints

More serious side effects are rare. These may include a high fever that could cause a seizure.

PNEUMOCOCCAL DISEASE

Four doses of a pneumococcal shot (pneumococcal conjugate vaccine PCV13 or PCV15) are recommended for children by doctors as the best way to protect against pneumococcal disease.

When Should Your Child Get a Pneumococcal Shot?

Your child should get one dose at each of the following ages:

- first dose: 2 months
- second dose: 4 months
- third dose: 6 months
- fourth dose: 12–15 months

Why Should Your Child Get the Pneumococcal Shot?

Your child should get the pneumococcal shot because it:

- protects your child from potentially serious and even deadly infections caused by pneumococcal

disease, such as pneumococcal meningitis (infection of the tissue covering the brain and spinal cord) and pneumonia (lung infection)
- keeps your child from missing school or childcare and you from missing work

Pneumococcal Shots Are Safe

Pneumococcal shots are safe and effective at preventing pneumococcal disease. Vaccines, like any medicine, can have side effects. These are usually mild and go away on their own.

What Types of Pneumococcal Vaccines Are There?

All babies and young children should receive a pneumococcal conjugate vaccine (PCV13 or PCV15). Some children with medical conditions that increase their risk of pneumococcal disease should also receive the pneumococcal polysaccharide vaccine (PPSV23). The number of doses depends on the medical condition. Talk to your child's doctor about which vaccines they recommend.

What Are the Side Effects?

Most children do not have any side effects from the shot. The side effects that do occur are usually mild and may include the following:

- fussiness
- feeling tired
- loss of appetite (not wanting to eat)
- redness, swelling, or soreness where the shot was given
- fever or chills
- headache
- muscle aches or joint pain

POLIO

Four doses of the polio shot for children are recommended by doctors as the best way to protect against polio.

When Should Your Child Get the Polio Shot?

Your child will need one dose at each of the following ages:

- first dose: 2 months
- second dose: 4 months
- third dose: 6–18 months
- fourth dose: 4–6 years

Why Should Your Child Get the Polio Shot?

Your child should get the polio shot because it:

- protects your child from polio, a potentially serious disease
- protects your child from developing lifelong paralysis from polio

The Polio Shot Is Safe

The polio shot is very safe and is effective at preventing polio. Vaccines, like any medicine, can have side effects. These are usually mild and go away on their own.

What Are the Side Effects?

- redness, swelling, or pain where the shot was given

ROTAVIRUS

Two or more doses of a rotavirus vaccine are recommended for children by doctors as the best way to protect against rotavirus.

When Should Your Baby Get the Drops?

Your baby should get either of the following two rotavirus vaccines:

- RotaTeq® (RV5) is given in three doses at ages two months, four months, and six months.
- Rotarix® (RV1) is given in two doses at ages two months and four months.

There are two brands of rotavirus vaccine: RotaTeq® and Rotarix®. Both brands of the rotavirus vaccines are given by mouth (drops), not by a shot.

Why Should Your Baby Get the Rotavirus Drops?

Your child should get the rotavirus drops because it:

- protects your baby from rotavirus, a potentially serious disease
- protects your baby from developing diarrhea, vomiting, and stomach pain caused by rotavirus
- keeps your child from missing school or childcare and you from missing work

The Rotavirus Vaccine Is Safe

The rotavirus vaccine is very safe and effective at preventing rotavirus. Vaccines, like any medicine, can have side effects. These are usually mild and go away on their own.

What Are the Side Effects?

Side effects are rare and usually mild and may include fussiness, diarrhea, and vomiting.

Some studies have shown a small rise in cases of intussusception within a week after the first or second dose of the rotavirus vaccine. Intussusception is a type of bowel blockage that is treated in a hospital. Some babies might need surgery. Studies estimate a risk ranging from about one intussusception case in every 20,000 infants to one intussusception case in every 100,000 infants after vaccination.

RUBELLA

Two doses of the MMR shot are recommended for children by doctors as the best way to protect against rubella.

When Should Your Child Get the Measles, Mumps, and Rubella Shot?

Your child should get one dose at each of the following ages:

- first dose: 12–15 months
- second dose: 4–6 years

Before traveling to another country, infants 6–11 months should get one dose of the MMR shot.

Why Should Your Child Get the Rubella Shot?

Your child should get the rubella shot because it:

- protects your child from rubella, a potentially serious disease, as well as measles and mumps
- prevents your child from spreading rubella to a pregnant woman whose unborn baby could develop serious birth defects or die if the mother gets rubella
- prevents your child from getting a rash and fever from rubella
- keeps your child from missing school or childcare and you from missing work to care for your sick child

The Measles, Mumps, and Rubella Shot Is Safe

The MMR shot is very safe and is effective at preventing rubella. Vaccines, like any medicine, can have side effects. These are usually mild and go away on their own.

There Is No Link between the MMR Shot and Autism

Scientists in the United States and other countries have carefully studied the MMR shot. None has found a link between autism and the MMR shot.

What Are the Side Effects of the Shot?

Most children do not have any side effects from the shot. The side effects that do occur are usually very mild and may include the following:

- fever
- soreness, redness, or swelling where the shot was given

- temporary pain and stiffness in the joints (mostly in teens and adults)
- mild rash

More serious side effects are rare. These may include a high fever that could cause a seizure.

TETANUS

Five doses of a DTaP shot for children and one Tdap shot for preteens are recommended by doctors as the best way to protect against tetanus.

When Should Your Child Get a Tetanus Shot?

Your child should get one dose of DTaP at each of the following ages:

- first dose: 2 months
- second dose: 4 months
- third dose: 6 months
- fourth dose: 15–18 months
- fifth dose: 4–6 years

Your child should also get one dose of Tdap at the following age:

- sixth dose: 11–12 years

Why Should Your Child Get a Tetanus Shot?

Your child should get the tetanus shot because it:

- protects your child from tetanus, which can be a serious and even deadly disease, as well as diphtheria and whooping cough (pertussis)
- protects your child from painful muscle stiffness from tetanus
- keeps your child from missing school or childcare and you from missing work

What Vaccines Protect against Tetanus?

There are two vaccines that help protect children against tetanus: DTaP and Tdap. Both also protect against diphtheria and whooping cough. These shots do not offer lifetime protection. People need booster shots to keep up protection.

Tetanus Shots Are Safe

Tetanus shots are safe and effective at preventing tetanus. Vaccines, like any medicine, can have side effects. These are usually mild and go away on their own.

What Are the Side Effects?

Most children do not have any side effects from DTaP or Tdap. The side effects that do occur from DTaP are usually mild and may include the following:

- soreness or swelling where the shot was given
- fever
- fussiness
- feeling tired
- loss of appetite
- vomiting

More serious side effects are very rare, but the DTaP vaccine can cause the following:

- a fever over 105 °F (40.56 °C)
- nonstop crying for three hours or more
- seizures (jerking, twitching of the muscles, or staring)

The side effects from Tdap are usually mild and may include the following:

- pain, redness, or swelling where the shot was given
- mild fever
- headache
- feeling tired
- nausea, vomiting, diarrhea, and stomachache

Some preteens and teens might faint after getting Tdap or any other shot.

To prevent fainting and injuries related to fainting, people should be seated or lying down during vaccination and remain in that position for 15 minutes after the vaccine is given.

WHOOPING COUGH (PERTUSSIS)

Five doses of the DTaP shot for children and one Tdap shot for preteens are recommended by doctors as the best way to protect against whooping cough (pertussis).

When Should Your Child Get a Whooping Cough Shot?

Your child should get one dose of DTaP at each of the following ages:

- first dose: 2 months
- second dose: 4 months
- third dose: 6 months
- fourth dose: 15–18 months
- fifth dose: 4–6 years

Your child should get one dose of Tdap at the following age:

- first dose: 11–12 years

Why Should Your Child Get a Whooping Cough Shot?

Your child should get the whooping cough shot because it:

- helps protect your child from whooping cough, a potentially serious and even deadly disease as well as diphtheria and tetanus
- helps prevent your child from having violent coughing fits from whooping cough
- helps protect your newborn when they are most vulnerable to serious disease and complications
- keeps your child from missing school or childcare and you from missing work

What Vaccines Protect against Whooping Cough?

There are two vaccines that help protect children against whooping cough: DTaP and Tdap. Both also protect against diphtheria and tetanus. These shots do not offer lifetime protection.

Whooping Cough Shots Are Safe

Whooping cough shots are safe and effective at preventing whooping cough. Vaccines, like any medicine, can have side effects. These are usually mild and go away on their own.

What Are the Side Effects?

Most children do not have any side effects from DTaP or Tdap. The side effects that do occur with DTaP are usually mild and may include the following:

- soreness or swelling where the shot was given
- fever
- fussiness
- feeling tired
- loss of appetite
- vomiting

More serious side effects are very rare, but the DTaP vaccine can cause the following:

- a fever over 105 °F (40.56 °C)
- nonstop crying for three hours or more
- seizures (jerking, twitching of the muscles, or staring)

The side effects from Tdap are usually mild and may include the following:

- pain, redness, or swelling where the shot was given
- mild fever
- headache
- feeling tired
- nausea, vomiting, diarrhea, and stomachache

Some preteens and teens might faint after getting Tdap or any other shot. To prevent fainting and injuries related to fainting, people should be seated or lying down during vaccination and remain in that position for 15 minutes after the vaccine is given.[1]

[1] "Vaccines for Your Children," Centers for Disease Control and Prevention (CDC), August 5, 2019. Available online. URL: www.cdc.gov/vaccines/parents/diseases/index.html. Accessed July 6, 2023.

Chapter 74 | Adolescent Immunization Facts

It is important that young people see health-care providers regularly. Regular checkups ensure that adolescents receive the recommended clinical preventive services, which are immunizations, screening tests, and health counseling recommended for people their age. Routine health-care visits help prevent unhealthy behaviors, promote healthy decision-making, and reduce the likelihood of developing major health issues now and in the future. Preventive health visits also provide an opportunity to help teens learn how to use the health-care system when they are adults.

Clinical preventive services for adolescents that are recommended by the U.S. Preventive Services Task Force (USPSTF), the Advisory Committee on Immunization Practices (ACIP), and the American Academy of Pediatrics (AAP) Bright Future are covered without co-payments or deductibles in health insurance plans. Yet many teens do not receive all the recommended preventive services they need. Families take babies and young children in for immunizations and checkups, but regular checkups are important for adolescents too. Most medical groups agree that routine visits to see a health-care provider, whether the young person is healthy or sick, are important for adolescents' health. Although annual wellness checkups are ideal, any visit to the health-care provider's office or other health-care location can be an opportunity to receive preventive care.

WHERE DO ADOLESCENTS RECEIVE PREVENTIVE HEALTH CARE?

Preventive services for adolescents are provided in different places, including:

- health-care providers' offices (e.g., pediatricians, internal and family medicine physicians)
- community health centers
- university clinics
- school-based health centers
- local health departments

Adolescents often see multiple providers to address different health-care needs. For instance, they may get vision or height and weight screenings from their school nurse or during a sports physical. Some preventive services, such as an annual flu shot, can be obtained in other locations, such as local drug and grocery stores. If adolescents receive preventive services in multiple settings, it can be difficult to keep track of which services have been received and which are still needed. An easy way to keep up to date on the full range of preventive services is to schedule an annual visit with a health-care provider.[1]

COVID-19 VACCINES

The following COVID-19 vaccines, categorized into three vaccine types, are currently authorized by the U.S. Food and Drug Administration (FDA) and available for use in the United States:

- messenger ribonucleic acid (mRNA) vaccines
    - Moderna COVID-19 Vaccine, Bivalent
    - Pfizer-BioNTech COVID-19 Vaccine, Bivalent
- protein subunit vaccine
    - Novavax COVID-19 Vaccine, Adjuvanted

The monovalent formulations of the two mRNA COVID-19 vaccines (COMIRNATY/Moderna COVID-19 Vaccine and

[1] Office of Population Affairs (OPA), "Clinical Preventive Services," U.S. Department of Health and Human Services (HHS), March 14, 2017. Available online. URL: https://opa.hhs.gov/adolescent-health/physical-health-developing-adolescents/clinical-preventive-services. Accessed August 23, 2023.

SPIKEVAX/Pfizer-BioNTech COVID-19 Vaccine) should no longer be used for COVID-19 vaccination.

All currently available mRNA COVID-19 vaccines in the United States are formulated as a bivalent vaccine based on the original (ancestral) strain of severe acute respiratory syndrome coronavirus 2 (SARS-CoV-2) and the Omicron BA.4 and BA.5 (BA.4/BA.5) variants of SARS-CoV-2.

Novavax COVID-19 Vaccine is formulated as a monovalent vaccine based on the original (ancestral strain) of SARS-CoV-2. Janssen COVID-19 Vaccine is no longer available in the United States.

None of the currently FDA-authorized COVID-19 vaccines are live virus vaccines.[2]

Table 74.1 lists the recommended immunizations for children aged 7–18; for information about missed childhood vaccinations, see Table 74.2.

ADDITIONAL INFORMATION

- If your child misses a shot recommended for their age, talk to your child's doctor as soon as possible to see when the missed shot can be given.
- If your child has any medical conditions that put them at risk for infection or is traveling outside the United States, talk to your child's doctor about additional vaccines that they may need.

Talk with your child's doctor if you have questions about any shot recommended for your child.[3]

[2] "Interim Clinical Considerations for Use of COVID-19 Vaccines in the United States," Centers for Disease Control and Prevention (CDC), June 14, 2023. Available online. URL: www.cdc.gov/vaccines/covid-19/clinical-considerations/interim-considerations-us.html. Accessed August 23, 2023.

[3] "Recommended Vaccinations for Children 7 to 18 Years Old, Parent-Friendly Version," Centers for Disease Control and Prevention (CDC), February 10, 2023. Available online. URL: www.cdc.gov/vaccines/schedules/easy-to-read/adolescent-easyread.html. Accessed August 24, 2023.

Table 74.1. Recommended Vaccines for Children Aged 7–18

<table>
<tr><th>Vaccine</th><th>7 Years</th><th>8 Years</th><th>9 Years</th><th>10 Years</th><th>11 Years</th><th>12 Years</th><th>13 Years</th><th>14 Years</th><th>15 Years</th><th>16 Years</th><th>17 Years</th><th>18 Years</th></tr>
<tr><td>COVID-19*</td><td colspan="12">COVID-19*: The vaccine is recommended for all children unless your doctor tells you that your child cannot safely receive the vaccine.</td></tr>
<tr><td>Flu**
(one or two doses yearly; influenza)</td><td>The vaccine is recommended for all children unless your doctor tells you that your child cannot safely receive the vaccine.</td><td colspan="11">The vaccine is recommended for all children unless your doctor tells you that your child cannot safely receive the vaccine.</td></tr>
<tr><td>Tetanus, diphtheria, and pertussis (Tdap)</td><td colspan="4">The vaccine should be given if a child is catching up on missed vaccines. A vaccine series does not need to be restarted, regardless of the time that has elapsed between doses.</td><td colspan="2">The vaccine is recommended for all children unless your doctor tells you that your child cannot safely receive the vaccine.</td><td colspan="6">The vaccine should be given if a child is catching up on missed vaccines. A vaccine series does not need to be restarted, regardless of the time that has elapsed between doses.</td></tr>
</table>

Table 74.1. Continued

Vaccine	7 Years	8 Years	9 Years	10 Years	11 Years	12 Years	13 Years	14 Years	15 Years	16 Years	17 Years	18 Years
Human papillomavirus (HPV[†])			The vaccine series can begin at this age.		The vaccine is recommended for all children unless your doctor tells you that your child cannot safely receive the vaccine.		The vaccine should be given if a child is catching up on missed vaccines. A vaccine series does not need to be restarted, regardless of the time that has elapsed between doses.					
Meningococcal disease (MenACWY)					The vaccine should be given if a child is catching up on missed vaccines. A vaccine series does not need to be restarted, regardless of the time that has elapsed between doses.		The vaccine should be given if a child is catching up on missed vaccines. A vaccine series does not need to be restarted, regardless of the time that has elapsed between doses.			The vaccine should be given if a child is catching up on missed vaccines. A vaccine series does not need to be restarted, regardless of the time that has elapsed between doses.	The vaccine should be given if a child is catching up on missed vaccines. A vaccine series does not need to be restarted, regardless of the time that has elapsed between doses.	

Table 74.1. Continued

Vaccine	7 Years	8 Years	9 Years	10 Years	11 Years	12 Years	13 Years	14 Years	15 Years	16 Years	17 Years	18 Years
Meningococcal disease (MenB)											Children not at increased risk may get the vaccine if they wish after speaking to a provider.	

*COVID-19: * The number of doses recommended depends on your child's age and the type of COVID-19 vaccine used.*
*Flu: ** Two doses given at least four weeks apart are recommended for children aged six months through eight years who are getting influenza (flu) vaccine for the first time and for some other children in this age group.*
HPV: † Those aged 11–12 years should get a two-shot series separated by 6–12 months. The series can begin at nine years of age. A three-shot series is recommended for those with weakened immune systems and those who start the series after their 15th birthday.

Table 74.2. Catching Up on Missed Childhood Vaccination for Children Aged 7–18

Vaccine	7 Years	8 Years	9 Years	10 Years	11 Years	12 Years	13 Years	14 Years	15 Years	16 Years	17 Years	18 Years
Measles, mumps, and rubella (MMR)	The vaccine should be given if a child is catching up on missed vaccines. A vaccine series does not need to be restarted, regardless of the time that has elapsed between doses.											
Varicella (Chickenpox)	The vaccine should be given if a child is catching up on missed vaccines. A vaccine series does not need to be restarted, regardless of the time that has elapsed between doses.											
Hepatitis A (HepA)	The vaccine should be given if a child is catching up on missed vaccines. A vaccine series does not need to be restarted, regardless of the time that has elapsed between doses.											
Hepatitis B (HepB)	The vaccine should be given if a child is catching up on missed vaccines. A vaccine series does not need to be restarted, regardless of the time that has elapsed between doses.											
Inactivated polio vaccine (IPV; Polio)	The vaccine should be given if a child is catching up on missed vaccines. A vaccine series does not need to be restarted, regardless of the time that has elapsed between doses.											

Chapter 75 | Adult Immunization Recommendations

ADULTS NEED VACCINES, TOO

Getting vaccinated is one of the safest ways for you to protect your health. Vaccines help prevent getting and spreading serious diseases that could result in poor health, missed work, medical bills, and not being able to care for the family. Everyone should make sure they are up-to-date on these routine vaccines:

- COVID-19 vaccine
- flu vaccine (influenza)
- tetanus, diphtheria, and whooping cough (Tdap) vaccine or tetanus and diphtheria (Td) vaccine

VACCINES YOU NEED BETWEEN THE AGES OF 19 AND 26

All adults aged 19–26 should make sure they are up-to-date on the following vaccines:

- chickenpox vaccine (varicella)
- COVID-19 vaccine
- flu vaccine (influenza)
- hepatitis B vaccine
- human papillomavirus (HPV) vaccine
- measles, mumps, and rubella (MMR) vaccine
- Tdap vaccine or Td vaccine

You may need other vaccines based on other factors, too. Talk with your doctor to learn which vaccines are recommended for you, which may include meningococcal group B (MenB) vaccine (meningococcal disease)—for adults up to 23 years of age. Under the Affordable Care Act (ACA), insurance plans that cover children allow parents to add or keep children on the health insurance policy until they turn 26 years old.

VACCINES YOU NEED BETWEEN THE AGES OF 27 AND 49

All adults aged 27–49 should make sure they are up-to-date on the following vaccines:

- COVID-19 vaccine
- flu vaccine (influenza)
- hepatitis B vaccine
- MMR vaccine
- Tdap vaccine or Td vaccine

You may need other vaccines based on your age or other factors, too. Talk with your doctor to learn which vaccines are recommended for you. These may include:

- chickenpox vaccine (varicella)—if born in 1980 or later
- HPV vaccine

VACCINES YOU NEED BETWEEN THE AGES OF 50 AND 64

All adults aged 50–64 should make sure they are up-to-date on the following vaccines:

- COVID-19 vaccine
- flu vaccine (influenza)
- shingles vaccine (zoster)
- Tdap or Td vaccine

You may need other vaccines, too, based on your age or other factors. Talk with your doctor to learn which vaccines are recommended for you. These may include:

- hepatitis B vaccine—recommended for all adults up to 59 years of age
- MMR vaccine—if born in 1957 or later

VACCINES YOU NEED AT THE AGES OF 65 AND OLDER

As we get older, our immune systems tend to weaken over time, putting us at higher risk for certain diseases. All adults aged 65 and older should make sure they are up-to-date on the following vaccines:

- COVID-19 vaccine
- flu vaccine (influenza)
- pneumococcal vaccine
- shingles vaccine (zoster)
- Tdap or Td vaccine

LIFE EVENTS, JOB, AND TRAVEL

Pregnancy

Get the whooping cough vaccine during each pregnancy.

- Tdap vaccine—between 27 and 36 weeks of pregnancy to help protect your baby against whooping cough.

Make sure you are up-to-date on other vaccines, too:

- COVID-19 vaccine
- flu vaccine (influenza), especially if you are pregnant during flu season, which is October through May
- hepatitis B vaccine

Talk with your ob-gyn or midwife to find out which vaccines are recommended to help protect you and your baby.

International Travelers

Get vaccinated before you travel. The vaccines recommended or required for an international traveler depend on several factors, including age, health, and itinerary.

Take the following steps to make sure you are prepared for your trip:

- Make sure you are up-to-date with all recommended vaccines. Talk with your health-care provider and get any vaccines that you may have missed. Take a short quiz and get a list of vaccines you may need based on your lifestyle, travel habits, and other factors.

- Learn the recommended and required vaccines for your destination. Visit Travelers' Health: Destinations (wwwnc.cdc.gov/travel/destinations/list) for more information about recommendations and requirements for the locations you will be visiting during your travel.
- Get vaccinated at least four to six weeks before your trip. Planning ahead will give you enough time to build up immunity and get the best protection.

Find a travel clinic. Many state and local health departments provide travel vaccinations. Get more travel vaccination information as well as information on where to find travel vaccinations at the Travelers' Health Clinic page of the Centers for Disease Control and Prevention (CDC; wwwnc.cdc.gov/travel/page/find-clinic).

Immigrants, Refugees, and International Adoptions

IMMIGRANTS

Whether you are applying for an immigrant visa overseas or for legal permanent residence within the United States, you need to meet the Vaccination criteria for U.S. immigration.

REFUGEES

Refugees are not required to have vaccinations before arrival in the United States, but you can start getting certain vaccinations through the Vaccination program for U.S.-bound refugees.

INTERNATIONAL ADOPTIONS

- **Adoptees aged 10 years and under**. Immigration law allows for adoptive parents to sign an affidavit stating they will be vaccinated after arrival to the United States.
- **Adoptees over 10 years of age**. Immigration law requires proof of vaccination during the overseas medical examination.
- **Parents or close contacts traveling internationally to adopt a child**. Make sure you are fully vaccinated according to the CDC's Advisory Committee on

Immunization Practices (ACIP) recommendations. Some vaccine-preventable diseases, such as hepatitis A, are more common in other countries than in the United States.

OTHER HEALTH CONDITIONS

Diabetes Type I and Type II

People with diabetes (both type 1 and type 2) are at higher risk for serious problems, including hospitalization or death, from certain vaccine-preventable diseases. Vaccines are one of the safest ways for you to protect your health, even if you are taking prescription medications. In addition to vaccines recommended for all adults (COVID-19, flu (influenza), and Tdap or Td), make sure you are up-to-date on the following vaccine:

- pneumococcal vaccine

You may need other vaccines based on your age or other factors, too. Talk with your doctor to find out which vaccines are recommended for you. These may include:

- chickenpox vaccine (varicella)—recommended for all adults born in 1980 or later
- hepatitis B vaccine—recommended for all adults up to 59 years of age and for some adults aged 60 and older with known risk factors
- HPV vaccine—recommended for all adults up to 26 years of age and for some adults aged 27–45
- MMR vaccine—recommended for all adults born in 1957 or later
- shingles vaccine (zoster)—recommended for all adults aged 50 and older

Heart Disease, Stroke, or Other Cardiovascular Diseases

People with heart disease and those who have suffered a stroke are at higher risk for serious problems or complications from certain vaccine-preventable diseases. Other vaccine-preventable diseases, such as the flu, can even increase the risk of another heart attack. In addition to vaccines recommended for all adults (COVID-19, flu (influenza), and Tdap or Td), make sure you are up-to-date on the following vaccine:

- pneumococcal vaccine

You may need other vaccines based on your age or other factors, too. Talk with your cardiologist or primary care doctor to find out which vaccines are recommended for you. These may include:

- chickenpox vaccine (varicella)—recommended for all adults born in 1980 or later
- hepatitis B vaccine—recommended for all adults up to 59 years of age and for some adults aged 60 and older with known risk factors
- HPV vaccine—recommended for all adults up to 26 years of age and for some adults aged 27–45
- MMR vaccine—recommended for all adults born in 1957 or later
- shingles vaccine (zoster)—recommended for all adults aged 50 and older

Human Immunodeficiency Virus Infections

Vaccines are especially critical for people with chronic health conditions, such as human immunodeficiency virus (HIV) infection. Vaccine recommendations may differ based on CD4 count. In addition to vaccines recommended for all adults (COVID-19, flu (influenza), and Tdap or Td), make sure you are up-to-date on the following vaccines:

- hepatitis A vaccine
- hepatitis B vaccine
- meningococcal conjugate vaccine (MenACWY)
- pneumococcal vaccine
- shingles vaccine (zoster)

If your CD4 count is 200 or greater (If CD4 percentages are available, CD4 percentage should be 15% or greater), in addition to the vaccines listed above, you may need the following vaccines:

- chickenpox vaccine (varicella)—recommended for all adults born in 1980 or later

- MMR vaccine—recommended for all adults born in 1957 or later

You may need other vaccines based on your age or other factors, too. Talk with your doctor to find out which vaccines are recommended for you. This may include:

- HPV vaccine—recommended for all adults up to 26 years of age and for some adults aged 27–45

Liver Disease

Vaccines are especially critical for people with health conditions such as liver disease. Getting vaccinated is one of the safest ways for you to protect your health, even if you are taking prescription medications for liver disease. In addition to vaccines recommended for all adults (COVID-19, flu (influenza), and Tdap or Td), make sure you are up-to-date on the following vaccines:

- hepatitis A vaccine
- hepatitis B vaccine
- pneumococcal vaccine

You may need other vaccines based on your age or other factors, too. Talk with your doctor to find out which vaccines are recommended for you. These may include:

- chickenpox vaccine (varicella)—recommended for all adults born in 1980 or later
- HPV vaccine—recommended for all adults up to 26 years of age and for some adults aged 27–45
- MMR vaccine—recommended for all adults born in 1957 or later
- shingles vaccine (zoster)—recommended for all adults aged 50 and older

Lung Disease

People with lung disease (including asthma or chronic obstructive pulmonary disease (COPD)) are at higher risk for serious problems, including hospitalization or death, from certain vaccine-preventable diseases. Getting vaccinated is one of the safest ways for you to protect your health, even if you are taking prescription medications for your condition. In addition to vaccines recommended for all adults (COVID-19, flu (influenza), and Tdap or Td), make sure you are up-to-date on the following vaccine:

- pneumococcal vaccine

You may need other vaccines based on your age or other factors, too. Talk with your doctor to find out which vaccines are recommended for you. These may include:

- chickenpox vaccine (varicella)—recommended for all adults born in 1980 or later
- hepatitis B vaccine—recommended for all adults up to 59 years of age and for some adults aged 60 and older with known risk factors
- HPV vaccine—recommended for all adults up to 26 years of age and for some adults aged 27–45
- MMR vaccine—recommended for all adults born in 1957 or later
- shingles vaccine (zoster)—recommended for all adults aged 50 and older

End-Stage Kidney Disease

Getting vaccinated is one of the safest ways for you to protect your health, even if you are taking prescription medications for end-stage renal (kidney) disease or on hemodialysis. In addition to vaccines recommended for all adults (COVID-19, flu (influenza), and Tdap or Td), make sure you are up-to-date on the following vaccines:

- hepatitis B vaccine
- pneumococcal vaccine

You may need other vaccines based on your age or other factors, too. Talk with your doctor to find out which vaccines are recommended for you. These may include:

- chickenpox vaccine (varicella)—recommended for all adults born in 1980 or later
- HPV vaccine—recommended for all adults up to 26 years of age and for some adults aged 27–45

- MMR vaccine—recommended for all adults born in 1957 or later
- shingles vaccine (zoster)—recommended for all adults aged 50 and older

Weakened Immune System

Vaccines are especially critical for people with a weakened immune system from diseases such as cancer or patients taking immunosuppressive drugs. Having a weakened immune system means that it is more difficult to fight off infections or diseases in the body. In addition to vaccines recommended for all adults (COVID-19, flu (influenza), and Tdap or Td), adults with weakened immune systems caused by immunocompromising conditions such as cancer should make sure they are up-to-date on the following vaccines:

- *Haemophilus influenzae* type b (Hib) vaccine—recommended for adults with complement deficiency, which is a specific type of immune deficiency and for adults who have received a hematopoietic stem cell transplant (HSCT, or a bone marrow transplant)
- pneumococcal vaccines (PCV15 or PCV20 and PPSV23)
- meningococcal vaccines (MenACWY and MenB)—recommended for adults with complement deficiency, which is a specific type of immune deficiency
- shingles vaccine (zoster)

You may need other vaccines based on your age or other factors, too. Talk with your doctor to find out which vaccines are recommended for you. These may include:

- hepatitis B vaccine—recommended for all adults up to 59 years of age and for some adults aged 60 and older with known risk factors
- HPV vaccine—recommended for all adults up to 26 years of age and for some adults aged 27–45[1]

---

[1] "What Vaccines Are Recommended for You," Centers for Disease Control and Prevention (CDC), September 8, 2023. Available online. URL: www.cdc.gov/vaccines/adults/rec-vac/index.html. Accessed August 23, 2023.

Chapter 76 | Possible Side Effects from Vaccines

Any vaccine can cause side effects. For the most part, these are minor (e.g., a sore arm or low-grade fever) and go away within a few days. Listed below are vaccines licensed in the United States and the side effects that have been associated with each of them.

Remember, vaccines are continually monitored for safety, and like any medication, vaccines can cause side effects. However, a decision not to immunize a child also involves risk and could put the child and others who come into contact with him or her at risk of contracting a potentially deadly disease.

DIPHTHERIA, TETANUS, AND ACELLULAR PERTUSSIS VACCINE

What Are the Risks from the Diphtheria, Tetanus, and Acellular Pertussis Vaccine?

- Soreness or swelling where the shot was given, fever, fussiness, feeling tired, loss of appetite, and vomiting sometimes happen after diphtheria, tetanus, and acellular pertussis (DTaP) vaccination.
- More serious reactions, such as seizures, nonstop crying for three hours or more, or high fever (over 105 °F (40.556 °C)), after DTaP vaccination happen much less often. Rarely, vaccination is followed by swelling of the entire arm or leg, especially in older children when they receive their fourth or fifth dose.

As with any medicine, there is a very remote chance of a vaccine causing a severe allergic reaction, other serious injury, or death.

HEPATITIS A VACCINE

What Are the Risks from the Hepatitis A Vaccine?

- Soreness or redness where the shot is given, fever, headache, tiredness, or loss of appetite can happen after hepatitis A vaccination.

HEPATITIS B VACCINE

What Are the Risks from the Hepatitis B Vaccine?

- Soreness where the shot is given or fever can happen after hepatitis B vaccination.

HAEMOPHILUS INFLUENZAE TYPE B VACCINE

What Are the Risks from the *Haemophilus influenzae* Type B Vaccine?

- Redness, warmth, and swelling where the shot is given and fever can happen after *Haemophilus influenzae* type B vaccination.

HUMAN PAPILLOMAVIRUS GARDASIL-9 VACCINE

What Are the Risks from the Human Papillomavirus Vaccine?

- Soreness, redness, or swelling where the shot is given can happen after human papillomavirus vaccine (HPV) vaccination.
- Fever or headache can happen after HPV vaccination.

INACTIVATED INFLUENZA VACCINE

What Are the Risks from the Inactivated Influenza Vaccine?

- Soreness, redness, and swelling where the shot is given; fever; muscle aches; and headache can happen after influenza vaccination.
- There may be a very small increased risk of Guillain-Barré syndrome (GBS) after inactivated influenza vaccine (the flu shot).

Young children who get the flu shot along with the pneumococcal vaccine (PCV13) and/or DTaP vaccine at the same time might be slightly more likely to have a seizure caused by fever. Tell your health-care provider if a child who is getting the flu vaccine has ever had a seizure.

LIVE INFLUENZA VACCINE

What Are the Risks from the Live Attenuated Influenza Vaccine?

- Runny nose or nasal congestion, wheezing, and headache can happen after the live attenuated influenza vaccine (LAIV).
- Vomiting, muscle aches, fever, sore throat, and cough are other possible side effects.

If these problems occur, they usually begin soon after vaccination and are mild and short-lived.

MEASLES, MUMPS, AND RUBELLA VACCINE

What Are the Risks from the Measles, Mumps, and Rubella Vaccine?

- A sore arm from the injection or redness where the shot is given, fever, and a mild rash can happen after measles, mumps, and rubella (MMR) vaccination.
- Swelling of the glands in the cheeks or neck or temporary pain and stiffness in the joints (mostly in teenage or adult women) sometimes occur after MMR vaccination.
- More serious reactions happen rarely. These can include seizures (often associated with fever) or temporary low platelet count that can cause unusual bleeding or bruising.
- In people with serious immune system problems, this vaccine may cause an infection that may be life-threatening. People with serious immune system problems should not get the MMR vaccine.

MEASLES, MUMPS, RUBELLA, AND VARICELLA VACCINE

What Are the Risks from the Measles, Mumps, Rubella, and Varicella Vaccine?

- Sore arm from the injection, redness where the shot is given, fever, and a mild rash can happen after measles, mumps, rubella, and varicella (MMRV) vaccination.
- Swelling of the glands in the cheeks or neck or temporary pain and stiffness in the joints sometimes occur after MMRV vaccination.
- Seizures, often associated with fever, can happen after the MMRV vaccine. The risk of seizures is higher after MMRV than after separate MMR and varicella vaccines when given as the first dose of the two-dose series in younger children. Your health-care provider can advise you about the appropriate vaccines for your child.
- More serious reactions happen rarely, including temporary low platelet count, which can cause unusual bleeding or bruising.
- In people with serious immune system problems, this vaccine may cause an infection that may be life-threatening. People with serious immune system problems should not get the MMRV vaccine.

If a person develops a rash after MMRV vaccination, it could be related to either the measles or the varicella component of the vaccine. The varicella vaccine virus could be spread to an unprotected person. Anyone who gets a rash should stay away from infants and people with a weakened immune system until the rash goes away. Talk with your health-care provider to learn more.

Some people who are vaccinated against chickenpox get shingles (herpes zoster) years later. This is much less common after vaccination than after chickenpox disease.

MENINGOCOCCAL ACWY VACCINE

What Are the Risks from Meningococcal Vaccines?

- Redness or soreness where the shot is given can happen after meningococcal ACWY vaccination.

- A small percentage of people who receive the meningococcal ACWY vaccine experience muscle pain, headache, or tiredness.

MENINGOCOCCAL B VACCINE

What Are the Risks from Meningococcal Vaccines?

- Soreness, redness, or swelling where the shot is given; tiredness; fatigue; headache; muscle or joint pain; fever; chills; nausea; or diarrhea can happen after meningococcal B vaccination. Some of these reactions occur in more than half of the people who receive the vaccine.

PNEUMOCOCCAL CONJUGATE VACCINE

What Are the Risks from the Pneumococcal Conjugate Vaccine?

- Redness, swelling, pain, or tenderness where the shot is given; fever; loss of appetite; fussiness (irritability); feeling tired; headache; muscle aches; joint pain; and chills can happen after pneumococcal conjugate vaccination.

Young children may be at increased risk for seizures caused by fever after the pneumococcal conjugate vaccine (PCV13) if it is administered at the same time as the inactivated influenza vaccine. Ask your health-care provider for more information.

PNEUMOCOCCAL POLYSACCHARIDE VACCINE

What Are the Risks from the Pneumococcal Polysaccharide Vaccine?

- Redness or pain where the shot is given, feeling tired, fever, or muscle aches can happen after pneumococcal polysaccharide vaccine (PPSV23).

POLIO VACCINE

- A sore spot with redness, swelling, or pain where the shot is given can happen after polio vaccination.

RABIES VACCINE

What Are the Risks from the Rabies Vaccine?

- Soreness, redness, swelling, or itching at the site of the injection; headache; nausea; abdominal pain; muscle aches; or dizziness can happen after the rabies vaccine.
- Hives, pain in the joints, or fever sometimes happens after booster doses.

ROTAVIRUS VACCINE

What Are the Risks from the Rotavirus Vaccine?

- Irritability or mild, temporary diarrhea or vomiting can happen after rotavirus vaccination.

Intussusception is a type of bowel blockage that is treated in a hospital and could require surgery. It happens naturally in some infants every year in the United States, and usually, there is no known reason for it. There is also a small risk of intussusception from rotavirus vaccination, usually within a week after the first or second vaccine dose. This additional risk is estimated to range from about 1 in 20,000 U.S. infants to 1 in 100,000 U.S. infants who get the rotavirus vaccine. Your health-care provider can give you more information.

ADULT TETANUS AND DIPHTHERIA VACCINE

What Are the Risks from the Adult Tetanus and Diphtheria Vaccine?

- Pain, redness, or swelling where the shot was given; mild fever; headache; feeling tired; nausea; vomiting; diarrhea; or stomachache sometimes happens after adult tetanus and diphtheria (Td) vaccination.

COMBINED TETANUS, DIPHTHERIA, AND PERTUSSIS VACCINE

What Are the Risks from the Combined Tetanus, Diphtheria, and Pertussis Vaccine?

- Pain, redness, or swelling where the shot was given; mild fever; headache; feeling tired; nausea; vomiting; diarrhea;

or stomachache sometimes happens after combined tetanus, diphtheria, and pertussis (Tdap) vaccination.

VARICELLA VACCINE

What Are the Risks from the Varicella Vaccine?

- Sore arm from the injection, redness or rash where the shot is given, or fever can happen after varicella vaccination.
- More serious reactions happen very rarely. These can include pneumonia, infection of the brain and/or spinal cord covering, or seizures that are often associated with fever.
- In people with serious immune system problems, this vaccine may cause an infection that may be life-threatening. People with serious immune system problems should not get the varicella vaccine.

It is possible for a vaccinated person to develop a rash. If this happens, the varicella vaccine virus could be spread to an unprotected person. Anyone who gets a rash should stay away from infants and people with a weakened immune system until the rash goes away. Talk with your health-care provider to learn more.

Some people who are vaccinated against chickenpox get shingles (herpes zoster) years later. This is much less common after vaccination than after chickenpox disease.

YELLOW FEVER VACCINE

What Are the Risks from the Yellow Fever Vaccine?

- Soreness, redness, or swelling where the shot was given is common after yellow fever vaccination.
- Fever sometimes happens.
- Headache and muscle aches can occur.
- More serious reactions happen rarely after yellow fever vaccination. These can include the following:
    - nervous system reactions, such as inflammation of the brain (encephalitis) and/or spinal cord covering (meningitis) or GBS, among others

- life-threatening severe illness with organ dysfunction or failure

People aged 60 and older and people with weakened immune systems might be more likely to experience serious reactions to the yellow fever vaccine.

ZOSTER SHINGLES VACCINE

What Are the Risks from the Shingles Vaccine?

- A sore arm with mild or moderate pain is very common after recombinant shingles vaccine. Redness and swelling can also happen at the site of the injection.
- Tiredness, muscle pain, headache, shivering, fever, stomach pain, and nausea are common after recombinant shingles vaccine.

These side effects may temporarily prevent a vaccinated person from doing regular activities. Symptoms usually go away on their own in two to three days. You should still get the second dose of the recombinant shingles vaccine even if you had one of these reactions after the first dose.

GBS, a serious nervous system disorder, has been reported very rarely after recombinant zoster vaccine.

TRAVEL AND SPECIAL CIRCUMSTANCE VACCINES

Adenovirus Vaccine

WHAT ARE THE RISKS FROM THE ADENOVIRUS VACCINE?

- Headache, upper respiratory tract infection, stuffy nose, sore throat, abdominal pain, cough, nausea, diarrhea, fever, or joint pain can happen after adenovirus vaccination.
- More serious problems including blood in the urine or stool, pneumonia, or inflammation of the stomach or intestines rarely occur after adenovirus vaccination.

Note: Adenovirus vaccine is approved for use only among military personnel.

Anthrax Vaccine

WHAT ARE THE RISKS FROM THE ANTHRAX VACCINE?

- Tenderness, redness, itching, or a lump or bruise where the shot is given
- Muscle aches or short-term trouble moving your arm
- Headaches or fatigue

Cholera Vaccine

WHAT ARE THE RISKS FROM THE CHOLERA VACCINE?

- Tiredness, headache, abdominal pain, nausea, vomiting, lack of appetite, and diarrhea can happen after cholera vaccination.

As with any medicine, there is a very remote chance of a vaccine causing a severe allergic reaction, other serious injury, or death.

Japanese Encephalitis IXIARO Vaccine

WHAT ARE THE RISKS FROM THE JAPANESE ENCEPHALITIS VACCINE?

- Pain, tenderness, redness, or swelling where the shot was given is common after Japanese encephalitis (JE) vaccination.
- Fever sometimes happens (more often in children).
- Headache or muscle aches can occur (mainly in adults).

Studies have shown that severe reactions to JE vaccine are very rare.

Typhoid Vaccine

WHAT ARE THE RISKS FROM THE TYPHOID VACCINE?

- Pain from the shot, redness, or swelling at the site of the injection; fever; headache; and general discomfort can happen after the inactivated typhoid vaccine.
- Fever, headache, abdominal pain, diarrhea, nausea, and vomiting can happen after a live typhoid vaccine.

People sometimes faint after medical procedures, including vaccination. Tell your provider if you feel dizzy or have vision changes or ringing in the ears.

As with any medicine, there is a very remote chance of a vaccine causing a severe allergic reaction, other serious injury, or death. This remains applicable for each of the vaccines mentioned above.[1]

[1] "Vaccines & Immunizations," Centers for Disease Control and Prevention (CDC), April 2, 2020. Available online. URL: www.cdc.gov/vaccines/vac-gen/side-effects.htm. Accessed July 6, 2023.

Chapter 77 | Vaccine Adverse Event Reporting System

The Vaccine Adverse Event Reporting System (VAERS) is the nation's early warning system that monitors the safety of vaccines after they are authorized or licensed for use by the U.S. Food and Drug Administration (FDA). The VAERS is part of the larger vaccine safety system in the United States that helps make sure vaccines are safe. The system is comanaged by the Centers for Disease Control and Prevention (CDC) and the FDA.

The VAERS accepts and analyzes reports of possible health problems—also called "adverse events"—after vaccination. As an early warning system, the VAERS cannot prove that a vaccine caused a problem. Specifically, a report to the VAERS does not mean that a vaccine caused an adverse event. But the VAERS can give the CDC and the FDA important information. If it looks as though a vaccine might be causing a problem, the FDA and the CDC will investigate further and take action if needed.

Anyone can submit a report to the VAERS—health-care professionals, vaccine manufacturers, and the general public. The VAERS welcomes all reports, regardless of seriousness and regardless of how likely the vaccine may have been to have caused the adverse event.

TOP SIX THINGS TO KNOW ABOUT VACCINE ADVERSE EVENT REPORTING SYSTEM

- The VAERS is a national vaccine safety surveillance program that helps detect unusual or unexpected reporting patterns of adverse events for vaccines.
- The VAERS is a passive surveillance system, meaning it relies on people sending in reports of their experiences after vaccination.
- The VAERS accepts reports from anyone, including patients, family members, health-care providers, and vaccine manufacturers.
- Health-care providers and vaccine manufacturers are required by law to report certain events after vaccination.
- The VAERS is not designed to determine if a vaccine caused or contributed to an adverse event. A report to the VAERS does not mean the vaccine caused the event.
- If the VAERS detects a pattern of adverse events following vaccination, other vaccine safety monitoring systems conduct follow-up studies.

HOW THE VACCINE ADVERSE EVENT REPORTING SYSTEM WORKS

The VAERS is part of the larger post-licensure vaccine safety monitoring system in the United States. After vaccines are licensed or authorized for use by the FDA, they are continually monitored for safety by multiple, complementary systems. These systems also conduct safety studies in populations that are larger and more diverse than those typically included in vaccine clinical trials.

As a passive reporting system, the VAERS relies on individuals to send in reports of adverse health events following vaccination. From these reports, VAERS scientists can:

- assess the safety of newly licensed vaccines
- detect new, unusual, or rare adverse events that happen after vaccination
- monitor increases in known side effects, such as arm soreness where a shot was given
- identify potential patient risk factors for particular types of health problems related to vaccines

- identify and address possible reporting clusters
- recognize persistent safe-use problems and administration errors
- watch for unexpected or unusual patterns in adverse event reports
- serve as a monitoring system in public health emergencies

The information collected by the VAERS can quickly provide an early warning of a potential safety problem with a vaccine. Patterns of adverse events, or an unusually high number of adverse events reported after a particular vaccine, are called "signals." If a signal is identified through the VAERS, scientists may conduct further studies to find out if the signal represents an actual risk.

INFORMATION COLLECTED FROM REPORTS

The number of VAERS reports submitted varies each year. In 2019, the VAERS received over 48,000 reports. About 85–90 percent of the reports described mild side effects such as fever, arm soreness, or mild irritability. The remaining reports are classified as serious, which means that the reported adverse event resulted in permanent disability, hospitalization, prolongation of an existing hospitalization, life-threatening illness, congenital deformity/birth defect, or death. While these events can happen after vaccination, they are rarely caused by the vaccine.

Adverse event information collected by the VAERS includes the following:

- the type of vaccine received
- the date of vaccination
- when the adverse event began
- current illnesses and medications
- medical history
- past history of adverse events following vaccination
- demographic information

In some cases, multiple reports are submitted for the same adverse event. For example, the person who experienced the adverse event and their health-care provider could submit a report for the same adverse event. VAERS scientists review the reports, identify any duplicates, and attach them to the original submission. This review process ensures the same adverse event is not counted more than once, even in cases where there are multiple reports of the same adverse event. Only the primary reports are shown in the public data system, not additional or follow-up reports for the same event.

STRENGTHS AND LIMITATIONS OF VACCINE ADVERSE EVENT REPORTING SYSTEM DATA

When evaluating VAERS data, it is important to understand the strengths and limitations.

Strengths of Vaccine Adverse Event Reporting System

- The VAERS accepts reports from anyone. This also allows the VAERS to act as an early warning system to detect rare adverse events.
- The VAERS collects information about the vaccine, the person vaccinated, and the adverse event. Scientists obtain follow-up information on serious reports.
- All data (without identifying patient information) are publicly available.

Limitations of Vaccine Adverse Event Reporting System

- The VAERS is a passive reporting system, meaning that reports about adverse events are not automatically collected. Instead, someone who had or is aware of an adverse event following vaccination must file a report.
- VAERS reports are submitted by anyone and sometimes lack details or contain errors.
- VAERS data alone cannot determine if the vaccine caused the reported adverse event.
- This specific limitation has caused confusion about the publicly available data, specifically regarding the number of reported deaths. In the past, there have been instances

where people misinterpreted reports of death following vaccination as death caused by the vaccines; that is a mistake.

The VAERS accepts all reports of adverse events following vaccination without judging whether the vaccine caused the adverse health event. Some reports to the VAERS might represent true vaccine reactions, and others might be coincidental adverse health events not related to vaccination at all.

Generally, a causal relationship cannot be established using information from VAERS reports alone.

- The number of reports submitted to the VAERS may increase in response to media attention and increased public awareness.
- It is not possible to use VAERS data to calculate how often an adverse event occurs in a population.[1]

[1] "Vaccine Adverse Event Reporting System (VAERS)," Centers for Disease Control and Prevention (CDC), September 8, 2022. Available online. URL: www.cdc.gov/vaccinesafety/ensuringsafety/monitoring/vaers. Accessed July 10, 2023.

Chapter 78 | Vaccination Records

WHY YOU NEED YOUR CHILD'S VACCINE RECORDS

It is important to keep your child's vaccination records (the history of which vaccines they received) up to date and in a safe place. Without documentation, your child might not be allowed to attend school, play sports, or travel abroad. Your child may need their vaccination records later as adults for certain occupations.

School and Childcare

Vaccine requirements for schools or childcare facilities are different in each state. Talk to your school system or childcare facility to learn about the requirements where you live.

Extracurricular Activities and Teams

Some athletic programs, sports teams, summer camps, or other activities require physical examinations and vaccinations. Talk to your child's athletic department or program to learn the requirements.

KEEPING TRACK OF RECORDS

Keep your child's vaccination records in a safe place beginning with their first vaccine. Your child's doctor will keep a record of vaccines given in their clinic. Ask your child's doctor or nurse how they keep vaccination records and how you can get an official copy. You can also ask your child's doctor to enter vaccination information in your state's immunization information system (IIS), a statewide registry for records.

FINDING OFFICIAL VACCINATION RECORDS

If you cannot find a copy or do not have your child's vaccination records, you can try to get an official copy from a few different places.

Your Child's Doctor or Clinic

Doctors and health clinics keep records of the vaccines they give to your child. Keep in mind that they may save records for only a few years. If your child has gotten vaccines at different locations, you may have to contact each of them to get your child's records.

Your State's Immunization Registry

States and some large cities have secure immunization information systems (IIS) that keep vaccination records for the people in the state or city. However, some people's records may not be complete. Contact the IIS in your state or the state where your child received their last vaccine to see if they have your child's records and learn how to request an official copy. Your doctor may also be able to help you get vaccination records from your state's IIS for vaccines that were given at other locations by other providers.

Your Child's School

Most schools keep vaccination records on file. Schools may keep records for a year or two after a student leaves or graduates. Contact your child's school for more information.

IF YOU CANNOT FIND YOUR CHILD'S VACCINE RECORDS

If you cannot find the vaccination records, it is important to stay on the safe side and vaccinate (or revaccinate) your child. It is safe for your child to repeat a vaccine that they received earlier. Sometimes, repeat vaccinations may be required for proof of immunizations. Talk to your child's doctor about how to protect your child.

Alternatively, you can also have your child's blood tested for antibodies to check immunity for some vaccine-preventable diseases. However, these tests are not always completely accurate.

SAVING YOUR CHILD'S VACCINATION RECORDS

It is important to keep your child's vaccination records safe and updated. Schools, summer camps, athletic teams, colleges, international travel, and more may require vaccination records.

Storing Your Child's Records

Keep your child's vaccination records in a safe place where you can easily find them. Some people keep their child's records with other important documents, such as birth certificates and passports.

Updating Your Child's Records

Bring your child's vaccine record to each doctor visit and ask the doctor or nurse to write down the vaccine, date, and dosage. It is also helpful to write down the name of the doctor's office or clinic where your child got the shot, so you know where to get the official records from if you misplace the record.[1]

KEEPING YOUR VACCINE RECORDS UP TO DATE

Your vaccination record (sometimes called your "immunization record") provides a history of all the vaccines you received as a child and adult. This record may be required for certain jobs, travel abroad, or school registration.

HOW TO LOCATE YOUR VACCINATION RECORDS

Unfortunately, there is no national organization that maintains vaccination records. The Centers for Disease Control and Prevention (CDC) does not have this information. The records that exist are

[1] "Vaccines for Your Children," Centers for Disease Control and Prevention (CDC), October 15, 2022. Available online. URL: www.cdc.gov/vaccines/parents/records/keeping-track.html. Accessed July 10, 2023.

the ones you or your parents were given when the vaccines were administered and the ones in the medical record of the doctor or clinic where the vaccines were given.

If you need official copies of vaccination records or if you need to update your personal records, there are several places you can look:

- Ask parents or other caregivers if they have records of your childhood immunizations.
- Try looking through baby books or other saved documents from your childhood.
- Check with your high school and/or college health services for dates of any immunizations. Keep in mind that generally records are kept only for one to two years after students leave the system.
- Check with your previous employers (including the military) that may have required immunizations.
- Check with your doctor or public health clinic. Keep in mind that vaccination records are maintained at the doctor's office for a limited number of years.
- Contact your state's health department. Some states have registries (immunization information systems) that include adult vaccines.

WHAT TO DO IF YOU CANNOT FIND YOUR RECORDS

If you cannot find your personal records or records from the doctor, you may need to get some of the vaccines again. While this is not ideal, it is safe to repeat vaccines. The doctor can also sometimes do blood tests to see if you are immune to certain vaccine-preventable diseases.

TOOLS TO RECORD YOUR VACCINATIONS

Today we move, travel, and change health-care providers more than we did in previous generations. Finding old immunization information can be difficult and time-consuming. Therefore, it is critical that you keep an accurate and up-to-date record of the vaccinations you have received. Keeping an immunization record and storing it with other important documents (or in a safe place) will save you time and unnecessary hassle.

Ask your doctor, pharmacist, or other vaccine provider for an immunization record form or download and use this form (www.immunize.org/catg.d/p2023.pdf). Bring this record with you to health visits and ask your vaccine provider to sign and date the form for each vaccine you receive. That way, you can be sure that the immunization information is current and correct.

If your vaccine provider participates in an immunization registry (www.cdc.gov/vaccines/programs/iis/about.html), ask that your vaccines be documented there as well.[2]

[2] "Vaccine Information for Adults," Centers for Disease Control and Prevention (CDC), May 2, 2016. Available online. URL: www.cdc.gov/vaccines/adults/vaccination-records.html?s_cid=PN-NCIRD-LifeSpan-Pregnancy-MMR-2. Accessed July 10, 2023.

Chapter 79 | Consequences of Vaccine Misinformation

VACCINES

Vaccines are generally made from weakened strains of disease-causing microbes that are not virulent enough to cause an infection. When they are introduced to the body, the immune system learns to produce cells that can defeat the infection, thus making the body capable of resisting the disease in the future.

THE SUCCESS OF VACCINATION

Immunization programs have been very successful at controlling infectious diseases. More than 200 years ago, British physician Edward Jenner pioneered the smallpox vaccine. Smallpox has since been eradicated worldwide, and it is estimated that 5 million lives are saved annually as a result of the smallpox vaccine. This achievement should be compelling evidence that vaccines work and do so astonishingly well.

In total, the United Nations International Children's Emergency Fund (UNICEF) estimates that immunization saves approximately 9 million lives annually the world over. In addition to smallpox, vaccination has brought under control diseases such as diphtheria, tetanus, yellow fever, whooping cough, polio, and measles.

MISINFORMATION ABOUT VACCINES

A report by the Centers for Disease Control and Prevention (CDC) estimated that 77 percent of U.S. children between 19 and 35 months of age were being fully immunized with the recommended vaccinations. Reasons for the remaining 33 percent being either not immunized or under-immunized include limited health-care access, financial barriers, and misconceptions about vaccinations and vaccine safety.

Misinformation about vaccines has existed as long as vaccines themselves. Parents who delay or refuse vaccination because of misinformation can place their own children, as well as other children, at risk of contracting preventable diseases.

The anti-vaccine debate increased in intensity with the publication of a study by Dr. Andrew Wakefield in the scientific journal *Lancet* in 1998, which concluded that autism was linked to the measles, mumps, and rubella (MMR) vaccine. This led to ripples in the medical community and spread panic among some parents, celebrities, and politicians, with a resultant drop in vaccination rates. The study was later declared a fraud, and Wakefield was stripped of his medical license.

WHY WOULD PARENTS WILLINGLY PUT THEIR CHILDREN AT RISK OF VACCINE-PREVENTABLE DISEASES?

- **The absence of societal fear is one factor**. For centuries, people lived in terror of communicable diseases, but immunization resulted in lower incidences of such illnesses, and subsequent generations have not been exposed to diseases such as polio, rubella, and diphtheria. The absence of disease visibility has resulted in a lack of community fear, so in a sense, the immunization program has become a victim of its own success. But, fortunately, the majority of parents have continued to realize that vaccination is essential for the safety of their children and the benefit of community health.
- **The timing of vaccinations makes them scapegoats for various disorders that may occur around the same time as immunization**. Children of vaccination age are often subject to a number of minor illnesses, but just because a disorder is detected at the time of vaccination does not necessarily indicate that vaccination caused the disorder. Additionally, fever is a common side effect of vaccination,

but life-threatening reactions are very rare, and most medical professionals advise that this and other minor side effects should not be a deterrent to the protection offered by immunization.

- **Uninformed people may disseminate misinformation.** Parents rely on multiple resources for information about vaccines, including websites, family members, friends, and celebrities, some of whom could be seriously misinformed.
- **A person often perceives risk based on his or her limited experiences and knowledge.** Someone who has come across the child of a family member or friend who had an adverse reaction to vaccination might perceive it as overly risky. People also tend to tolerate natural risks (infectious diseases) more easily than man-made risks (vaccination side effects). Risks that have clear benefits associated with them are generally tolerated better than risks with benefits that are not immediate or not understood well.

VACCINATION IN THE UNITED STATES

All 50 U.S. states mandate that children be vaccinated against certain diseases before they enter school. Children who have health conditions that could be exacerbated by vaccination can seek to be exempted. And, except for Mississippi, all states allow religious exemptions, while exemptions based on personal and moral beliefs are allowed in 20 states.

THE CONSEQUENCES OF MISINFORMATION

Vaccination rates are still high in the United States, but requests for exemptions have increased. Since the chances of contracting a vaccine-preventable infection are quite small in the United States, what is the risk?

The danger lies in clusters of communities in which like-minded anti-vaccination parents live. In 1991, a measles outbreak occurred in Philadelphia in schools run by fundamentalist churches. About 350 children attending these schools were not immunized, and the infection spread to 1,500 children, leading to nine fatalities.

Pockets of unvaccinated children exist around the nation, particularly in the states of California, Utah, Oregon, and Washington. Vaccine exemptions are particularly high in Washington, where some elementary schools have an exemption rate of 43 percent. Nevertheless, overall vaccination rates in these states remain relatively high.

Measles was declared to have been eliminated in the United States in the year 2000. But, in 2015, a measles outbreak occurred at Disneyland in California. It turned into a large-scale outbreak that spread to 13 states across the country and affected 147 people. The disease was determined to have been primarily carried by unvaccinated children whose parents put them and other children at risk by taking them to a crowded public place.

That the outbreak was contained serves as a testament to the success of vaccination programs. It also demonstrates that science by itself cannot totally overcome the detrimental effects of virulent misinformation. The risks of immunization are very negligible, while the advantages are great and the repercussions of not vaccinating are extremely high. Vaccines are backed by more than a century of scientific research and safeguards. They are rigorously tested, and effective systems ensure potency, purity, and safety. Children need to be protected against preventable diseases by ensuring vaccination. And this seems to be possible only if we inoculate ourselves with facts.

References

Myers, Martin G. and Pineda, Diego. "Misinformation about Vaccines," AutismTruths, 2009. Available online. URL: www.autismtruths.org/pdf/MisinformationAboutVaccines.pdf. Accessed August 18, 2023.

Parker, Laura. "The Anti-Vaccine Generation: How Movement Against Shots Got Its Start," National Geographic, February 6, 2015. Available online. URL: http://news.nationalgeographic.com/news/2015/02/150206-measles-vaccine-disney-outbreak-polio-health-science-infocus. Accessed August 18, 2023.

Patel, Kavita and Hart, Rio. "What the Anti-Vaxxers Are Getting Dangerously Wrong," Brookings, February 6, 2015. Available online. URL: www.brookings.edu/2015/02/06/what-the-anti-vaxxers-are-getting-dangerously-wrong. Accessed August 18, 2023.

Chapter 80 | Risks of Delaying or Skipping the Vaccines

While babies are born with some immunity, they have not yet built up the necessary defenses against the diseases that vaccines prevent. Delaying vaccines could leave your child vulnerable to disease when they are most likely to have serious complications.

PREVENT COMPLICATIONS

Think of vaccines like a helmet for your baby. Just like safety equipment protects them from serious injury, vaccinating on schedule protects them from potentially serious diseases.

Young babies are at highest risk of serious disease complications. For example, for you, whooping cough may mean a lingering cough for several weeks, but it can be very serious—even deadly—for babies less than a year old. If you delay vaccinations, your baby could be exposed to diseases such as whooping cough when they are most likely to have serious complications.

EARLY PROTECTION

It is best to vaccinate before your child is exposed to dangerous diseases. You would not wait until you are already driving down the road to put your baby in a car seat. You buckle him in every time, long before there is any chance he could be in a crash. Vaccines work the same way—your baby needs them long before he/she is exposed to a disease.

If you wait until you think your child could be exposed to a serious illness—such as when he starts daycare or during a disease outbreak—there may not be enough time for the vaccine to work. That is why the experts who set the schedule pay such careful attention to timing. They have designed it to provide immunity early in life before children are likely to be exposed to life-threatening diseases.

It can take weeks for a vaccine to help your baby make protective disease-fighting antibodies, and some vaccines require multiple doses to provide the best protection.

BEST PROTECTION

Your child is not fully protected if you cover just a few of the outlets she can reach around your home. Similarly, your baby will not have the best protection from vaccines until they have all the recommended doses.

Each vaccine is carefully developed to protect against a specific illness. Some require more than one dose to build strong enough immunity to protect your baby or to boost immunity that decreases over time. Others need additional doses to ensure your baby is protected in case the first dose did not produce enough antibodies. Your child needs the flu vaccine each year because the disease changes over time. Simply put, every recommended dose of each vaccine on the schedule is important.

LONG-TERM PROTECTION

Maternal antibodies and breastfeeding do not provide enough protection. Just as you help your child learn to walk, the protection (antibodies) you passed to your baby before birth will help protect your little one from diseases during the first months of life. And, just as your child needs to eventually walk on his own, his immune system eventually needs to fight diseases on its own. Vaccines help protect your child when your maternal antibodies wear off.

For example, when you get whooping cough and flu vaccines while you are pregnant, you can pass some protection to your baby before birth. However, you can only pass on protection from diseases that you have immunity to, and this can only protect your child in the first few months.

Breastfeeding provides important protection from some infections as your baby's immune system is developing. However, breast milk does not protect children against all diseases. Even for breastfed infants, vaccines are the most effective way to prevent many diseases. That is why it is so important to follow the immunization schedule. It ensures your baby's immune system gets the help it needs to protect your child long-term from preventable diseases.

SPREADING ILLNESS

Children who are not vaccinated on schedule are not only at risk of getting sick themselves, but they can also spread illness to others who are not protected, such as newborns who are too young for vaccines and people with weakened immune systems. By getting your child's vaccines on time, you are not only protecting your baby but also helping to protect your friends, family, and community, too.[1]

[1] "Reasons to Follow CDC's Immunization Schedule," Centers for Disease Control and Prevention (CDC), February 25, 2020. Available online. URL: www.cdc.gov/vaccines/parents/schedules/reasons-follow-schedule.html. Accessed on September 15, 2023.

Chapter 81 | Preventing Nosocomial Infections

Chapter Contents

Section 81.1 | Patient Tips to Prevent Health-Care-Associated Infections

PATIENT SAFETY: WHAT YOU CAN DO TO BE A SAFE PATIENT

You go to the hospital to get well, right? Of course, but did you know that you can get infections in the hospital while you are being treated for something else?

Time in the hospital can put you at risk for a health-care-associated infection (HAI), such as a blood, surgical site, or urinary tract infection.

Every day, patients get infections in health-care facilities while they are being treated for something else. These infections can have devastating emotional, financial, and medical effects. Worst of all, they can be deadly.

Health-care procedures can leave you vulnerable to germs that cause HAIs. These germs can be spread in health-care settings from patient to patient on unclean hands of health-care personnel or through the improper use or reuse of equipment.

These infections are not limited to hospitals. For example, in the past 10 years alone, there have been more than 30 outbreaks of hepatitis B and hepatitis C in nonhospital health-care settings, such as:

- outpatient clinics
- dialysis centers
- long-term care facilities

PROTECT YOURSELF AND YOUR FAMILY FROM HARMFUL GERMS THAT CAN CAUSE INFECTIONS

- Keep your hands clean. Regular hand cleaning is one of the best ways to remove germs, avoid getting sick, and prevent the spread of germs.
- Take antibiotics only when your provider thinks you need them. Ask if your antibiotic is necessary. If you take antibiotics when you do not need them, you are only exposing yourself to unnecessary risk of side effects and

potentially serious infections in the future. If you do need antibiotics, take them exactly as they are prescribed.

- Watch for signs of infection and its complications, such as sepsis. Get care right away—do not delay.
    - Tell your doctor if you think you have an infection or if your infection is not getting better or is getting worse.
- Watch out for life-threatening diarrhea caused by *Clostridium difficile*. If you have been taking an antibiotic, tell your doctor if you have three or more diarrhea episodes in 24 hours.
- Get vaccinated against flu and other infections to avoid complications.

BE A SAFE PATIENT IN THE HOSPITAL

- Tell your doctors if you have been hospitalized in another facility, have recently received health care outside of the United States, or have recently had an infection.
- Ask your health-care provider what they and the facility will do to protect you and your family from an antibiotic-resistant infection.
    - If you have a catheter, ask daily when it can be removed.
    - If you are having surgery, ask your doctor how they prevent infections. Also, ask how you can prepare for surgery to reduce your infection risk.
- Keep your hands clean. Make sure everyone cleans their hands before touching you. Remind health-care personnel and your visitors to clean their hands.
- Let your doctors check you for resistant germs if needed. Hospitals need to screen patients if they are exposed, and this helps protect you and those around you.
- Understand that if you have a resistant bacterium, health-care providers may use gowns and gloves when caring for you.
- Allow people to clean your room while you are in the hospital, even when it feels inconvenient for you.

- Environmental services workers are the people who clean patient rooms in the hospital, and they are important members of the health-care team.
- Allowing them to clean and disinfect your room helps keep you safe by reducing your risk of developing an infection—do not say, "Come back later."[1]

Section 81.2 | Prevention and Control of Influenza in Health-Care Settings

FUNDAMENTAL ELEMENTS TO PREVENT INFLUENZA TRANSMISSION

Preventing transmission of influenza virus and other infectious agents within health-care settings requires a multifaceted approach. Spread of the influenza virus can occur among patients, health-care personnel (HCP), and visitors; in addition, HCP may acquire influenza from persons in their household or community. The core prevention strategies include the following:

- administration of influenza vaccine
- implementation of respiratory hygiene and cough etiquette
- appropriate management of ill HCP
- adherence to infection control precautions for all patient-care activities and aerosol-generating procedures
- implementing environmental and engineering infection control measures.

Successful implementation of many, if not all, of these strategies is dependent on the presence of clear administrative policies and organizational leadership that promote and facilitate adherence to these recommendations among the various people within the health-care setting, including patients, visitors, and HCP.

[1] "Patient Safety: What You Can Do to Be a Safe Patient," Centers for Disease Control and Prevention (CDC), November 6, 2019. Available online. URL: www.cdc.gov/hai/patientsafety/patient-safety.html. Accessed July 10, 2023.

RECOMMENDATIONS

Promotion and Administration of Seasonal Influenza Vaccine

Annual vaccination is the most important measure to prevent seasonal influenza infection. Achieving high influenza vaccination rates of HCP and patients is a critical step in preventing health-care transmission of influenza from HCP to patients and from patients to HCP. According to current national guidelines, unless contraindicated, vaccinate all people aged six months and older, including HCP, patients, and residents of long-term care facilities.

Taking Steps to Minimize Potential Exposures

A range of administrative policies and practices can be used to minimize influenza exposures before arrival, upon arrival, and throughout the duration of the visit to the health-care setting. Measures include screening and triage of symptomatic patients and implementation of respiratory hygiene and cough etiquette. Respiratory hygiene and cough etiquette are measures designed to minimize potential exposures of all respiratory pathogens, including influenza virus, in health-care settings and should be adhered to by everyone—patients, visitors, and HCP—upon entry and continued for the entire duration of stay in health-care settings.

BEFORE ARRIVAL TO A HEALTH-CARE SETTING

- When scheduling appointments, patients and persons who accompany them are instructed to inform HCP upon arrival if they have symptoms of any respiratory infection (e.g., cough, runny nose, fever) and to take appropriate preventive actions (e.g., wear a face mask upon entry, follow triage procedure).
- During periods of increased influenza activity:
  - steps are taken to minimize elective visits by patients with suspected or confirmed influenza (For example, telephone consultation is provided to patients with mild respiratory illness to determine if there is a medical need to visit the facility.)

UPON ENTRY AND DURING A VISIT TO A HEALTH-CARE SETTING

- Take steps to ensure all persons with symptoms of a respiratory infection adhere to respiratory hygiene, cough etiquette, hand hygiene, and triage procedures throughout the duration of the visit. These might include the following:
    - posting visual alerts (e.g., signs, posters) at the entrance and in strategic places (e.g., waiting areas, elevators, cafeterias) to provide patients and HCP with instructions (in appropriate languages) about respiratory hygiene and cough etiquette, especially during periods when the influenza virus is circulating in the community. Instructions should include the following:
        - How to use face masks or tissues to cover the nose and mouth when coughing or sneezing and to dispose of contaminated items in waste receptacles.
        - How and when to perform hand hygiene.
    - implementing procedures during patient registration that facilitate adherence to appropriate precautions (e.g., at the time of patient check-in, inquire about the presence of symptoms of a respiratory infection and, if present, provide instructions)
- Face masks are provided to patients with signs and symptoms of respiratory infection.
- Supplies are provided to perform hand hygiene to all patients upon arrival to the facility (e.g., at entrances of the facility, waiting rooms, at patient check-in) and throughout the entire duration of the visit to the health-care setting.
- Enough space is provided and persons with symptoms of respiratory infections are encouraged to sit as far away from others as possible.
- During periods of increased community influenza activity, triage stations are set up that facilitate rapid screening of patients for symptoms of influenza and separation from other patients.

Adhering to Standard Precautions

During the care of any patient, all HCP in every health-care setting should adhere to standard precautions, which are the foundation for preventing the transmission of infectious agents in all health-care settings. Standard precautions assume that every person is potentially infected or colonized with a pathogen that could be transmitted in the health-care setting. Elements of standard precautions that apply to patients with respiratory infections, including those caused by the influenza virus, are as follows.

HAND HYGIENE

- The HCP should perform hand hygiene frequently, including before and after all patient contact, contact with potentially infectious material, and before putting on and upon removal of personal protective equipment, including gloves. Hand hygiene in health-care settings can be performed by washing with soap and water or using alcohol-based hand rubs. If hands are visibly soiled, use soap and water, not alcohol-based hand rubs.
- Health-care facilities would ensure that supplies for performing hand hygiene are available.

GLOVES

- Wear gloves for any contact with potentially infectious material. Remove gloves after contact, followed by hand hygiene. Do not wear the same pair of gloves for the care of more than one patient. Do not wash gloves for the purpose of reuse.

GOWNS

- Wear gowns for any patient-care activity when contact with blood, body fluids, secretions (including respiratory), or excretions is anticipated. Remove the gown and perform hand hygiene before leaving the patient's environment. Do not wear the same gown for the care of more than one patient.

Adhering to Droplet Precautions

- Droplet precautions are implemented for patients with suspected or confirmed influenza for seven days after illness onset or until 24 hours after the resolution of fever and respiratory symptoms, whichever is longer, while a patient is in a health-care facility. In some cases, facilities may choose to apply droplet precautions for longer periods based on clinical judgment, such as in the case of young children or severely immunocompromised patients, who may shed influenza virus for longer periods of time.
- Patients with suspected or confirmed influenza are placed in a private room or area. When a single patient room is not available, consultation with infection control personnel is recommended to assess the risks associated with other patient placement options (e.g., cohorting (i.e., grouping patients infected with the same infectious agents together to confine their care to one area and prevent contact with susceptible patients), keeping the patient with an existing roommate)
- If a patient under droplet precautions requires movement or transport outside of the room:
    - the patient should wear a face mask, if possible, and follow respiratory hygiene, cough etiquette, and hand hygiene

Managing Visitor Access and Movement within the Facility

Visitors are limited for patients in isolation for influenza to persons who are necessary for the patient's emotional well-being and care. Visitors who have been in contact with the patient before and during hospitalization are a possible source of influenza for other patients, visitors, and staff.

For persons with acute respiratory symptoms, facilities have developed visitor restriction policies that consider the location of the patient being visited (e.g., oncology units) and circumstances, such as end-of-life situations, where exemptions to the restriction may be considered at the discretion of the facility. Regardless of the restriction policy, all visitors should follow the precautions listed in the respiratory hygiene and cough etiquette section.

- Visits to patients in isolation for influenza are scheduled and controlled to allow for screening visitors for symptoms of acute respiratory illness before entering the hospital.
- Facilities will provide instruction, before visitors enter patients' rooms, on hand hygiene, limiting surfaces touched, and use of personal protective equipment (PPE) according to current facility policy while in the patient's room.
- Visitors should not be present during aerosol-generating procedures.
- Visitors will be instructed to limit their movement within the facility.
- If consistent with facility policy, visitors will be advised to contact their health-care provider for information about influenza vaccination.

Training and Educating Health-Care Personnel

Health-care administrators will ensure that all HCP receive job- or task-specific education and training on preventing transmission of infectious agents, including influenza, associated with health care during orientation to the health-care setting. This information would be updated periodically during ongoing education and training programs. Competency will be documented initially and repeatedly, as appropriate, for the specific staff positions. A system will be in place to ensure that HCP employed by outside employers meet these education and training requirements through programs offered by the outside employer or by participation in the health-care facility's program.

Key aspects of influenza and its prevention that should be emphasized to all HCP include the following:

- influenza signs, symptoms, complications, and risk factors for complications (HCP should be made aware that if they have conditions that place them at higher risk of complications, they should inform their

health-care provider immediately if they become ill with an influenza, so they can receive early treatment if indicated.)
- central role of administrative controls such as vaccination, respiratory hygiene and cough etiquette, sick policies, and precautions during aerosol-generating procedures
- appropriate use of personal protective equipment, including respirator fit testing and fit checks
- use of engineering controls and work practices, including infection control procedures to reduce exposure

Administering Antiviral Treatment and Chemoprophylaxis of Patients and Health-Care Personnel When Appropriate

The current recommendations on the use of antiviral agents for treatment and chemoprophylaxis are available on the CDC website (www.cdc.gov/flu/professionals/antivirals/). Both HCP and patients should be reminded that persons treated with influenza antiviral medications continue to shed the influenza virus while on treatment. Thus, hand hygiene, respiratory hygiene, and cough etiquette practices should continue while on treatment.[2]

[2] "Influenza (Flu)," Centers for Disease Control and Prevention (CDC), May 13, 2021. Available online. URL: www.cdc.gov/flu/professionals/infectioncontrol/healthcaresettings.htm. Accessed July 10, 2023.

Chapter 82 | **Public Health Measures for Contagious Diseases**

Chapter Contents

Section 82.1 | Health-Care-Associated Infections

The U.S. Department of Health and Human Services (HHS) released targets for the national acute care hospital metrics for the National Action Plan to Prevent Health Care-Associated Infections: Road Map to Elimination (HAI Action Plan) in October 2016. The targets used data from the calendar year 2015 as a baseline and were in effect for a five-year period from 2015 to 2020. The HHS is currently working to update this plan with new indicator targets and data, new research and intervention efforts, and a review of the impact of the COVID-19 public health emergency on health-care-associated infections (HAIs). The measures track population-based harm from HAIs at the national level. These measures address the following goals from the HAI Action Plan:

- Reduce central-line-associated bloodstream infections (CLABSI) in intensive care units and ward-located patients.
- Reduce catheter-associated urinary tract infections (CAUTI) in intensive care units and ward-located patients.
- Reduce the incidence of invasive health-care-associated methicillin-resistant *Staphylococcus aureus* (MRSA) infections.
- Reduce hospital-onset MRSA bloodstream infections.
- Reduce hospital-onset *Clostridioides difficile* infections (CDIs).
- Reduce the rate of *C. diff* hospitalizations.
- Reduce surgical site infections (SSI).

Progress in reducing HAIs, as assessed by National Healthcare Safety Network (NHSN) data, is tracked using a standardized infection ratio (SIR). The SIR compares the number of HAIs observed to the predicted number of infections. The predicted number is a risk-adjusted estimate that is determined using national baseline data. Health-care facilities, state and local health departments, and federal agencies, such as the Centers for Medicare and Medicaid Services (CMS), can use NHSN data to identify problem areas and target HAI prevention efforts within specific facilities, regions, and states.

Progress in reducing *C. diff* hospitalizations is tracked using Healthcare Cost and Utilization Project (HCUP) State Inpatient Databases of the Agency for Healthcare Research and Quality (AHRQ), beginning in 2010 (the date at which complete data was available for whether the data was present on admission). A description of the HCUP data, methodology, and progress toward eliminating CDIs in nonfederal short-term general and other specialty hospitals can be found in AHRQ's report on Adult, Nonmaternal Inpatient Stays Related to *Clostridioides difficle*: National Trends, 2011-2016 and 2019.

The CDC publishes data reports to help track progress and target areas that need further assistance. The CDC data comes from two complementary HAI surveillance systems, the NHSN and the Emerging Infections Program Healthcare-Associated Infections–Community Interface (EIP-HAIC). NHSN data are used to generate the CDC's annual HAI national and state progress reports. EIP-HAIC data is used to help track the national burden of certain HAIs and track MRSA infections and CDIs inside and outside of health-care settings. Additional HAI and antibiotic stewardship metrics are located on the CDC's Antibiotic Resistance and Patient Safety Portal (AR & PSP; https://arpsp.cdc.gov). Additional information on the CDC's HAI prevention efforts and HAI-AR metrics can be found on the CDC's website (www.cdc.gov/hai).[1]

[1] "National HAI Targets & Metrics", U.S. Department of Health and Human Services (HHS), September 2, 2021. Available online. URL: www.hhs.gov/oidp/topics/health-care-associated-infections/targets-metrics/index.html.

Section 82.2 | **Quarantine and Isolation Measures**

ISOLATION AND QUARANTINE

Isolation and quarantine help protect the public by preventing exposure to people who have or may have a contagious disease.

- Isolation separates sick people with a quarantinable communicable disease from people who are not sick.
- Quarantine separates and restricts the movement of people who were exposed to a contagious disease to see if they become sick.

In addition to serving as medical functions, isolation and quarantine are also "police power" functions, derived from the right of the state to take action affecting individuals for the benefit of society.

Federal Isolation and Quarantine Are Authorized for These Communicable Diseases

- cholera
- diphtheria
- infectious tuberculosis
- plague
- smallpox
- yellow fever
- viral hemorrhagic fevers
- severe acute respiratory syndromes
- flu that can cause a pandemic
- measles

Federal isolation and quarantine are authorized by the executive order of the president. The president can revise this list by executive order.

FEDERAL LAW

The federal government derives its authority for isolation and quarantine from the Commerce Clause of the U.S. Constitution.

Under Section 361 of the Public Health Service Act (42 U.S. Code § 264), the U.S. Secretary of Health and Human Services is authorized to take measures to prevent the entry and spread of communicable diseases from foreign countries into the United States and between states.

The authority for carrying out these functions on a daily basis has been delegated to the Centers for Disease Control and Prevention (CDC).

ROLE OF THE CENTERS FOR DISEASE CONTROL AND PREVENTION

Under 42 Code of Federal Regulations Parts 70 and 71, the CDC is authorized to detain, medically examine, and release persons arriving in the United States and traveling between states who are suspected of carrying these communicable diseases.

As part of its federal authority, the CDC routinely monitors persons arriving at U.S. land border crossings and passengers and crew arriving at U.S. ports of entry for signs or symptoms of communicable diseases.

When alerted about an ill passenger or crew member by the pilot of a plane or captain of a ship, the CDC may detain passengers and crew as necessary to investigate whether the cause of the illness on board is a communicable disease.

STATE, LOCAL, AND TRIBAL LAW

States have police power functions to protect the health, safety, and welfare of persons within their borders. To control the spread of disease within their borders, states have laws to enforce the use of isolation and quarantine.

These laws can vary from state to state and can be specific or broad. In some states, local health authorities implement state law. In most states, breaking a quarantine order is a criminal misdemeanor.

Tribes also have police power authority to take actions that promote the health, safety, and welfare of their own tribal members. Tribal health authorities may enforce their own isolation and quarantine laws within tribal lands if such laws exist.

WHO IS IN CHARGE?

The Federal Government

- acts to prevent the entry of communicable diseases into the United States (Quarantine and isolation may be used at U.S. ports of entry)
- is authorized to take measures to prevent the spread of communicable diseases between states
- may accept state and local assistance in enforcing federal quarantine
- may assist state and local authorities in preventing the spread of communicable diseases

State, Local, and Tribal Authorities

- enforce isolation and quarantine within their borders

It is possible for federal, state, local, and tribal health authorities to have and use all at the same time separate but coexisting legal quarantine power in certain events. In the event of a conflict, federal law is supreme.

ENFORCEMENT

If a quarantinable disease is suspected or identified, the CDC may issue a federal isolation or quarantine order.

Public health authorities at the federal, state, local, and tribal levels may sometimes seek help from police or other law enforcement officers to enforce a public health order.

U.S. Customs and Border Protection (CBP) and U.S. Coast Guard (USCG) officers are authorized to help enforce federal quarantine orders.

Breaking a federal quarantine order is punishable by fines and imprisonment.

Federal law allows the conditional release of persons from quarantine if they comply with medical monitoring and surveillance.

In the rare event that a federal order is issued by the CDC, those individuals will be provided with an order for quarantine or isolation. An example of a Quarantine Order for Novel

Coronavirus (www.cdc.gov/quarantine/pdf/Public-Health-Order_Generic_FINAL_02-13-2020-p.pdf) is provided. This document outlines the rationale of the federal order as well as information on where the individual will be located, quarantine requirements including the length of the order, the CDC's legal authority, and information outlining what the individual can expect while under federal order.

FEDERAL QUARANTINE RARELY USED

Large-scale isolation and quarantine were last enforced during the influenza ("Spanish flu") pandemic in 1918–1919. In recent history, only a few public health events have prompted federal isolation or quarantine orders.

SPECIFIC LAWS AND REGULATIONS GOVERNING THE CONTROL OF COMMUNICABLE DISEASES

The Secretary of the Department of Health and Human Services has statutory responsibility for preventing the introduction, transmission, and spread of communicable diseases in the United States. Under its delegated authority, the Division of Global Migration and Quarantine works to fulfill this responsibility through a variety of activities, including the following:

- the operation of quarantine stations at ports of entry
- establishment of standards for medical examination of persons destined for the United States
- administration of interstate and foreign quarantine regulations, which govern the international and interstate movement of persons, animals, and cargo

The legal foundation for these activities is found in Titles 8 and 42 of the U.S. Code and relevant supporting regulations.

Legal Authorities for Isolation and Quarantine

The federal government derives its authority for isolation and quarantine from the Commerce Clause of the U.S. Constitution.

U.S. Federal Laws and Regulations for Control of Communicable Diseases

U.S. CODE

The U.S. Code is a consolidation and codification by subject matter of the general and permanent laws of the United States. Sections 264–272 of the following portion of the code apply: Title 42: The Public Health and Welfare, Chapter 6A: Public Health Service, Subchapter II: General Powers and Duties, and Part G: Quarantine and Inspection.

CODE OF FEDERAL REGULATIONS

The Code of Federal Regulations (CFR) is the official and complete text of the general and permanent rules published in the Federal Register. These regulations are established by the executive departments and agencies of the federal government. The CFR is divided into various titles that represent broad subject areas of federal regulation. The CDC's regulations fall under Title 42: Public Health, Chapter 1: Public Health Service, Department of Health and Human Services.

EXECUTIVE ORDERS

Executive orders specify the list of diseases for which federal quarantine is authorized, which is required by the Public Health Service Act. On the recommendation of the HHS Secretary, the president may amend this list whenever necessary to add new communicable diseases, including emerging diseases that are a threat to public health. The most recent executive order added measles to the list of quarantinable communicable diseases.

IMPORTATION OF HUMAN REMAINS INTO THE UNITED STATES FOR BURIAL, ENTOMBMENT, OR CREMATION

The CDC requirements for importing human remains depend on the purpose of importation, whether the body has been embalmed or cremated, and if the person died from a quarantinable communicable disease.

When a U.S. citizen or lawful permanent resident dies outside the United States, the deceased person's next of kin or legal representative should:

- notify U.S. consular officials at the Department of State:
  - Consular personnel are available 24 hours a day, seven days a week, to provide assistance to U.S. citizens for overseas emergencies.
  - If the deceased person's next of kin or legal representative is in a different country from that of the deceased person, they should call the Department of State's Office of Overseas Citizens Services in Washington, D.C., from 8 a.m. to 5 p.m. Eastern time, Monday through Friday, at 888-407-4747 (toll-free) or 202-501-4444.
  - For emergency assistance after working hours or on weekends and holidays, call the Department of State switchboard at 202-647-4000 and ask to speak with the Overseas Citizens Services duty officer.
  - In addition, the U.S. embassy or consulate closest to or in the country where the U.S. citizen or lawful permanent resident died may provide assistance.
- work with consular officials to obtain:
  - country export clearance requirements where death occurred (such as death certificate, autopsy report*)
  - U.S. import documents (such as death certificate, consular mortuary certificate, Affidavit of Foreign Funeral Director and Transit Permit, and CDC import permit in the case of a quarantinable communicable disease)
  - packaging (such as urn for cremation, casket, and body transfer case)
  - assistance with transportation (such as local transportation and international airline)

**While the CDC does not require an autopsy before the remains of a person who died overseas are returned to the United States,* *depending on the circumstances surrounding the death, some countries may require an autopsy before exportation.*

There likely will need to be an official identification of the body and official documents issued by the consular office.

Authority and Guidance

The CDC's regulatory authority under 42 CFR §71.55 Importation of Human Remains governs the importation of the remains of a person intended for burial, entombment, or cremation ("final resting"). This authority applies to the whole body or body portion of a deceased human being, including internal or external body parts, being consigned directly to a licensed mortuary, cemetery, or crematory for immediate and final preparation before final resting. This provision explains that if imported remains undergo a medical examination or autopsy, the remains must be consigned directly to an entity authorized to perform such functions under the laws of the applicable jurisdiction prior to final resting.

42 CFR §71.55 also indicates that certain human remains may require a permit under 42 CFR §71.54 Import regulations for infectious biological agents, infectious substances, and vectors. Human remains imported for any purpose other than final resting (such as research, training, education, ceremonial, and collectible) or those remains of a person who died from a quarantinable communicable disease unless embalmed fall under the authority of 42 CFR §71.54 and may require a CDC import permit.

Permits for the importation of the remains of a person known or suspected to have died from a quarantinable communicable disease such as COVID-19 may be obtained through the CDC Division of Global Migration and Quarantine by calling the CDC Emergency Operations Center at 770-488-7100 or emailing dgmqpolicyoffice@cdc.gov.

There are no requirements for the importation of human remains consisting entirely of:

- clean, dry bones or bone fragments; human hair; teeth; fingernails; or toenails
- a deceased human body and portions thereof that have already been fully cremated before importation

DEATH CERTIFICATE

Except for cremated or embalmed remains, human remains intended for final resting after entry into the United States must be accompanied by a death certificate stating the cause of death. A death certificate is an official government document that certifies a death has occurred and provides identifying information about the deceased, including (at a minimum) name, age, and sex. The document must also certify the time, place, and cause of death (if known).

If the official death certificate is not written in English, then it must include an English language translation of the official government document. A person licensed to perform acts in legal affairs in the country where the death occurred, such as a notary, must attest to the document's authenticity. In lieu of a death certificate, a copy of the consular mortuary certificate and the Affidavit of Foreign Funeral Director and Transit Permit shall together constitute acceptable identification of human remains. If a death certificate is not available in time for returning the remains, the U.S. embassy or consulate should provide a consular mortuary certificate stating whether the person died from a disease classified as quarantinable in the United States.

LEAK-PROOF CONTAINERS

All non-cremated remains must be fully contained within a leak-proof container that is packaged and shipped in accordance with all applicable legal requirements. Germs that can cause disease could be present in the blood or other body fluids of a deceased person even if the stated cause of death is not a contagious disease. Such germs include human immunodeficiency virus (HIV), hepatitis B virus, hepatitis C virus, and other germs that can be present in body fluids.

The requirement for leak-proof containers is based on medical standard precautions to prevent exposure to infectious diseases carried in the blood and other body fluids. This requirement is intended to protect the public as well as federal, airline, and airport employees from potential exposure to blood and other body fluids during transportation, inspection, or storage of human remains.

This guidance does not apply to these items addressed under other U.S. federal regulations:

- patient specimens or diagnostic specimens
- human tissue or products intended for research, education, training, or other purposes (such as ceremonial or collectible)
- tissues or organs legally imported into the United States for the purpose of transplantation that are regulated by the Food and Drug Administration
- all other infectious biological agents, infectious substances, and vectors covered by 42 CFR §71.54
- passengers or crew members who die during travel[2]

Section 82.3 | Viral Hepatitis Prevention

The Viral Hepatitis National Strategic Plan for the United States: A Roadmap to Elimination 2021–2025 (www.hhs.gov/hepatitis/viral-hepatitis-national-strategic-plan/national-viral-hepatitis-action-plan-overview/index.html), released on January 7, 2021, is a new phase in the fight against viral hepatitis in the United States. Building on three prior National Viral Hepatitis Action Plans over the past 10 years, the Viral Hepatitis National Strategic Plan is the first to aim for the elimination of viral hepatitis as a public health threat in the United States.

The Viral Hepatitis Plan sets forth a clear vision for how the United States will be a place where new viral hepatitis infections are prevented, every person knows their status, and every person with viral hepatitis has high-quality health care and treatment and lives free from stigma and discrimination. In support of this vision, it includes five major goals, objectives and strategies to achieve these goals, and indicators with measurable targets to monitor progress.

[2] "Quarantine and Isolation," Centers for Disease Control and Prevention (CDC), September 17, 2021. Available online. URL: www.cdc.gov/quarantine/aboutlawsregulationsquarantineisolation.html. Accessed July 11, 2023.

Coordinated by the Office of the Assistant Secretary for Health (OASH) through the Office of Infectious Disease and HIV/AIDS Policy (OIDP), the Viral Hepatitis Plan was developed collaboratively by more than 20 federal agency partners. Stakeholders and the public had significant input into the development of this plan, through a variety of opportunities for public comment. The Viral Hepatitis Plan is a whole-of-nation plan. It is intended to serve as a comprehensive, data-driven roadmap for federal and other stakeholders to reverse the rates of viral hepatitis, prevent new infections, improve care and treatment, and ultimately eliminate viral hepatitis as a public health threat in the United States. Its success depends on the active participation and coordinated action from a broad mix of stakeholders from various sectors, both public and private.

The OIDP will continue to lead the coordination of the federal implementation of the Viral Hepatitis Plan. Other stakeholders are encouraged to develop implementation plans for viral hepatitis-related issues within their purview.

WHAT IS THE VIRAL HEPATITIS NATIONAL STRATEGIC PLAN?

The Viral Hepatitis National Strategic Plan: A Roadmap to Elimination 2021–2025 (www.hhs.gov/sites/default/files/Viral-Hepatitis-National-Strategic-Plan-2021-2025.pdf) provides a framework to eliminate viral hepatitis as a public health threat in the United States by 2030. The Viral Hepatitis Plan focuses on hepatitis A, hepatitis B, and hepatitis C—the three most common hepatitis viruses that have the most impact on the health of the nation. The Viral Hepatitis Plan is necessary as the nation faces unprecedented hepatitis A outbreaks, progress in preventing hepatitis B has stalled, and hepatitis C rates nearly tripled from 2011 to 2018. The Viral Hepatitis Plan provides goal-oriented objectives and strategies that can be implemented by a broad mix of stakeholders at all levels and across many sectors, both public and private, to reverse the rates of viral hepatitis, prevent new infections, improve care and treatment, and ultimately eliminate viral hepatitis as a public health threat in the United States.

The Viral Hepatitis Plan builds on three prior National Viral Hepatitis Action Plans, which covered the periods of 2011–2020.

The Viral Hepatitis National Strategic Plan: A Roadmap to Elimination 2021–2025 is the first plan to aim for the elimination of viral hepatitis as a public health threat in the United States.

The Viral Hepatitis Plan was developed under the direction of the Office of Infectious Disease and HIV/AIDS Policy (OIDP) in the Office of the Assistant Secretary for Health (OASH), the U.S. in collaboration with subject matter experts from across the federal government and with input from a wide range of stakeholders including the public.

WHY DO WE NEED A VIRAL HEPATITIS NATIONAL STRATEGIC PLAN?

Viral hepatitis is a significant public health threat that puts people who are infected at an increased risk for serious disease and death. The Viral Hepatitis Plan is necessary as the nation faces unprecedented hepatitis A outbreaks, progress in preventing hepatitis B has stalled, hepatitis C rates nearly tripled from 2011 to 2018, and, as of 2016, an estimated 3.3 million people were chronically infected with hepatitis B and hepatitis C. Viral hepatitis is associated with substantial health consequences, stigma, and discrimination. It takes a large toll on individuals as well as communities, many of which are disproportionately impacted. Collectively, viral hepatitis costs people, health systems, states, and the federal government billions of dollars each year.

Despite the availability of effective clinical interventions, including vaccines, diagnostic tests, and therapeutics, new or acute viral hepatitis infections have increased in recent years.

- From 2014 to 2018, the rate of new hepatitis A cases increased by 850 percent; the rate of acute hepatitis B increased by 11 percent; and the rate of acute hepatitis C cases increased by 71 percent.
- As of 2016, nearly 3.3 million people in the United States were living with chronic viral hepatitis—an estimated 862,000 with hepatitis B and 2.4 million with hepatitis C.

Surveillance data (www.cdc.gov/hepatitis/statistics/2018surveillance/index.htm) collected by the Centers for Disease Control and Prevention (CDC) reveal the following trends:

- **Hepatitis A**. The hepatitis A incidence rate decreased by greater than 95 percent from 1996 to 2011. However, the rate of new cases increased by 850 percent from 2014 (0.4 cases per 100,000) to 2018 (3.8 cases per 100,000) primarily because of large person-to-person outbreaks among people who use drugs and people experiencing homelessness. Hepatitis A is preventable by a safe and effective vaccine.
- **Hepatitis B**. Despite the availability of a safe and effective vaccine, the rate of acute hepatitis B cases increased by 11 percent from 2014 (0.9 per 100,000) to 2018 (1.0 per 100,000). The rate of infection increased even more dramatically in states the hardest hit by the opioid crisis. Injection drug use (IDU) and sexual transmission are risk factors associated with rising acute hepatitis B cases in the United States.
- **Hepatitis C**. The rate of acute hepatitis C cases increased 71 percent from 2014 (0.7 per 100,000) to 2018 (1.2 per 100,000), with two-thirds of cases occurring among persons aged 20–39 years, the age group most impacted by the opioid crisis.

All three viral hepatitis infections disproportionately impact certain populations, many of which experience other significant health and social inequities. The escalation of hepatitis B and hepatitis C infections is correlated with an increase in substance use disorders (SUDs) and injection drug use (IDU).

VIRAL HEPATITIS NATIONAL STRATEGIC PLAN

Vision

The United States will be a place where new viral hepatitis infections are prevented, every person knows their status, and every person with viral hepatitis has high-quality health care and treatment and lives free from stigma and discrimination.

This vision includes all people, regardless of age, sex, gender identity, sexual orientation, race, ethnicity, religion, disability, geographic location, or socioeconomic circumstance.

Goals

Five high-level goals frame the Viral Hepatitis Plan:

- Prevent new viral hepatitis infections.
- Improve viral hepatitis-related health outcomes of people with viral hepatitis.
- Reduce viral hepatitis-related disparities and health inequities.
- Improve viral hepatitis surveillance and data usage.
- Achieve integrated, coordinated efforts that address the viral hepatitis epidemics among all partners and stakeholders.

Each of the goal areas presents evidence-based objectives and strategies that stakeholders can use that are most likely to contribute toward achieving national goals to eliminate the public health threat of viral hepatitis.

Scope

The Viral Hepatitis Plan covers the most common types of viral hepatitis: hepatitis A, hepatitis B, and hepatitis C—the hepatitis viruses that most significantly impact the health of the nation. The plan provides a framework to control the viral hepatitis epidemics and eliminate viral hepatitis as a public health threat in the United States by 2030. Elimination is defined in the plan and by the World Health Organization (WHO) as a 90 percent reduction in new chronic infections and a 65 percent reduction in mortality, compared to a 2015 baseline, although the Plan uses 2017 data as a baseline. The Viral Hepatitis Plan is designed to facilitate a whole-person health perspective and whole-of-nation response to achieve the elimination of viral hepatitis as a public health threat.

The Viral Hepatitis Plan emphasizes viral hepatitis as part of a syndemic, which occurs when health-related problems—such as viral hepatitis, human immunodeficiency virus (HIV), sexually transmitted infections (STIs), and SUDs—cluster by person, place, or time and interact synergistically. The syndemic also includes social determinants of health, stigma, discrimination, and mental health. This complex, multifactorial environment must be addressed to eliminate viral hepatitis in the United States.

The Viral Hepatitis Plan provides a roadmap to integrate prevention, screening, and linkage to care for all components of the syndemic to meet people where they are with no wrong point of entry to health-care and related systems.

The Viral Hepatitis Plan recognizes the importance of addressing social determinants of health to improve health outcomes for racial, ethnic, sexual, and gender minority populations. By working to establish policies and programs that positively influence social and economic conditions and by supporting changes in individual behavior, health can be improved and sustained, and disparities reduced.

Priority Populations

Although viral hepatitis affects millions of Americans nationwide from all social, economic, racial, and ethnic groups, it disproportionately impacts certain populations and communities. Viral hepatitis prevention and treatment efforts can be more efficient and effective by identifying and focusing efforts on populations that bear a disproportionately higher burden of infection and disease, referred to in the Viral Hepatitis Plan as priority populations.

The Viral Hepatitis Plan uses nationwide surveillance data to determine the priority populations. Focusing on the priority populations will reduce health disparities and put the nation on the path toward the elimination of viral hepatitis. This approach should not diminish efforts to increase awareness, prevention, treatment, and integration of viral hepatitis efforts more generally for all populations. Stakeholders are encouraged to analyze the data for the populations and communities they serve to determine their priority populations.

National incidence, prevalence, and mortality rates were used to identify a small number of groups most impacted by each type of viral hepatitis (see Table 82.1).

Table 82.1. Priority Populations by Hepatitis Type and Measure

Type	Incidence (Acute)	Prevalence (Chronic)	Mortality
Hepatitis A	• People who use drugs • People experiencing homelessness	Not applicable	
Hepatitis B	• People who inject drugs	• Asian and Pacific Islander • Black, non-Hispanic	• Asian and Pacific Islander • Black, non-Hispanic
Hepatitis C	• People who inject drugs • American Indian/ Alaska Native	• People who inject drugs • Black, non-Hispanic • People born between 1945 and 1965 • People with HIV	• American Indian/ Alaska Native • Black, non-Hispanic • People born between 1945 and 1965

Other Key Elements of the Viral Hepatitis Plan

The Viral Hepatitis Plan:

- aims to increase uptake of hepatitis vaccination among populations for whom vaccination is recommended; increase access to harm reduction services, substance use treatment, and peer navigation; and utilize a treatment as a prevention approach
- seeks to implement universal hepatitis C screening guidelines, hepatitis B testing, and linkage to care in a range of settings and expand the capacity of the public health and provider workforce to provide viral hepatitis prevention, testing, care, and treatment services
- seeks to implement strategies and promote policies to enhance collaborative, integrated, patient-centered models of care
- focuses on opportunities to expand research and development of a hepatitis C vaccine, point of care testing, and improved diagnostics and therapeutics
- focuses on implementation research to put into practice evidence-based interventions, as effective interventions to improve prevention, testing, and treatment are identified

- aims to improve viral hepatitis surveillance data collection, management, and analysis, including interoperability of data and data sharing, to understand the true scope, level of public health threat, and opportunities to address viral hepatitis

Indicators

The Viral Hepatitis Plan establishes indicators, as well as baseline measures and quantitative targets, to help measure progress toward the plan's goals. Eight core indicators will be used to measure progress in preventing new infections and improving viral hepatitis-related health outcomes of people with viral hepatitis. Five of the core indicators are stratified by one or more of the priority populations to measure progress toward reducing disparities.

The Viral Hepatitis Plan recommends the development of five additional indicators, referred to as developmental indicators. Data for these developmental indicators are not currently collected and doing so would fill critical gaps in measuring the nation's efforts to eliminate the viral hepatitis epidemic.

Although focused on the years 2021–2025, the Viral Hepatitis Plan includes annual targets through 2030 because it will take more than five years to eliminate viral hepatitis as a public health threat in this nation. Establishing 2030 targets aligns with other national plans such as Healthy People 2030, the HIV National Strategic Plan: A Roadmap to End the Epidemic 2021–2025, the STI National Strategic Plan 2021–2025, and global targets established by the World Health Organization (WHO).

WHAT IS NEXT?

Implementation and Accountability

In 2021, federal partners will collaborate to develop an implementation plan that will set forth federal partners' commitments to policies, initiatives, and activities to meet the goals and objectives of the Viral Hepatitis Plan. The implementation plan will be published for transparency and accountability.

Federal agency partners have committed to serve on a viral hepatitis implementation working group. This working group will meet regularly to coordinate activities across agencies and departments, including with other components of the syndemic; implement lessons learned from epidemiological data and research findings; monitor progress toward the indicator targets; course correct as needed; and report on national progress.

Stakeholders are encouraged to use the Viral Hepatitis Plan to build their own roadmap to reduce viral hepatitis and viral hepatitis-related health disparities and inequities and to eliminate the viral hepatitis epidemics among the populations and communities they serve.

Stakeholders should consider adopting the vision and goals of the Viral Hepatitis Plan; examining challenges from a health equity lens; implementing the objectives and strategies relevant to their role, population, and community; applying other evidence-based objectives and strategies; using available data to identify where their resources will have the most impact; and identifying indicators and targets to measure their progress.[3]

Section 82.4 | **Sexually Transmitted Infections**

In the United States, recent data show that rates of sexually transmitted infections (STIs) reached an all-time high in 2021 among both females and males and all racial and ethnic groups. According to the Centers for Disease Control and Prevention (CDC), the number of combined cases of gonorrhea, syphilis, and chlamydia was more than 2.54 million in 2021 up from 2.4 million in 2020; racial/ethnic and sexual minority groups remain disproportionately affected.

The current rise of STIs is a serious public health concern that requires immediate attention. If left untreated, STIs can lead to severe health complications, including pelvic inflammatory disease (PID), increased risk of getting human immunodeficiency virus (HIV), certain cancers, and even infertility.

[3] "Viral Hepatitis National Strategic Plan," U.S. Department of Health and Human Services (HHS), January 4, 2021. Available online. URL: www.hhs.gov/hepatitis/viral-hepatitis-national-strategic-plan/index.html. Accessed July 11, 2023.

The Office of the Assistant Secretary for Health (OASH) through the Office of Infectious Disease and HIV/AIDS Policy (OIDP) has coordinated, along with other federal partners, the development of an inaugural Sexually Transmitted Infections National Strategic Plan (STI National Strategic Plan). Stakeholders and the public had significant input into the development of this plan, through a variety of opportunities for public comment. The STI National Strategic Plan was released on December 17, 2020, and provides a roadmap for prevention, diagnosis, treatment, and care designed to meet significant measurable goals. The aim is for federal agencies and stakeholders to work together to reverse the alarming increase in STI rates and improve our nation's health.

The OIDP will continue to lead the coordination of federal implementation of the STI National Strategic Plan. Other stakeholders are encouraged to develop implementation plans for STI-related issues within their purview.

WHAT IS THE SEXUALLY TRANSMITTED INFECTIONS NATIONAL STRATEGIC PLAN?

The STI National Strategic Plan is a groundbreaking, first-ever, five-year plan that aims to reverse the recent dramatic rise in STIs in the United States. The STI National Strategic Plan sets a vision as well as goals, objectives, and strategies to respond to this STI epidemic. It also includes indicators with measurable targets to track progress.

The STI National Strategic Plan aims to provide a roadmap for a broad range of stakeholders—including public health, health care, government, community-based organizations, educational institutions, researchers, private industries, and academia—to develop, enhance, and expand STI prevention and care programs at the local, state, tribal, and national levels over the next five years.

WHY DO WE NEED A SEXUALLY TRANSMITTED INFECTIONS NATIONAL STRATEGIC PLAN?

The STI epidemic affects the health of people and communities and is costly to the health-care system. When left untreated, STIs can lead to long-term health problems such as chronic pelvic pain, infertility, and poor birth outcomes, including death of newborns. STIs can also increase the risk of getting HIV and giving HIV to others. Additionally, human papillomavirus (HPV) infection causes about 35,000 cases of cancer each year, even though there is a safe and highly effective vaccine that prevents the cancer-causing strains of HPV. STIs affect the quality of life for millions of Americans and cost the health-care system billions of dollars annually.

The STI rates have risen dramatically. From 2014 to 2018, the rates of reported cases of primary and secondary syphilis, congenital syphilis, gonorrhea, and chlamydia rose 71, 185, 63, and 19 percent, respectively. The HPV, the most common STI, accounts for 14 million new infections each year.

The impact of the STI epidemic does not fall equally across all populations and regions. Adolescents and young adults, men who have sex with men, and pregnant women are disproportionately impacted by STIs. Social determinants of health contribute to an unequal burden of STIs in Black, American Indian/Alaska Native, and Hispanic communities. In addition, people living in the Southern and Western regions of the United States are disproportionately affected.

SEXUALLY TRANSMITTED INFECTIONS NATIONAL STRATEGIC PLAN

Vision

The United States will be a place where STIs are prevented and where every person has high-quality STI prevention, care, and treatment while living free from stigma and discrimination.

This vision includes all people, regardless of age, sex, gender identity, sexual orientation, race, ethnicity, religion, disability, geographic location, or socioeconomic circumstance.

Goals

The STI National Strategic Plan has five high-level goals:

- Prevent new STIs.
- Improve the health of people by reducing adverse (harmful) outcomes of STIs.
- Accelerate progress in STI research, technology, and innovation.

- Reduce STI-related health disparities and health inequities.
- Achieve integrated, coordinated efforts that address the STI epidemic.

Each of the goals has a set of objectives and strategies to help steer federal partners and other stakeholders toward achieving them. The objectives and strategies are evidence- and science-based, flexible, integrated, and innovative approaches.

Scope

The STI National Strategic Plan's goals, objectives, and strategies apply equally to most STIs although it highlights four of the STIs that have the greatest impact on the health of the nation: chlamydia, gonorrhea, syphilis, and HPV. It also identifies populations and geographic regions that experience the highest burden of STIs based on nationwide data so that federal agencies and other stakeholders can focus their resources to have the greatest impact. Stakeholders are encouraged to use the data for the jurisdiction or population(s) they serve to identify where their resources may have the greatest impact.

Priority Populations

The STI National Strategic Plan is designed to meet the prevention and treatment needs of everyone in the United States—but the plan recognizes that some groups of people and some communities and regions are more impacted by STIs than others. These specific groups are called "priority populations." Based on national-level data, they are:

- adolescents and young adults
- men who have sex with men
- pregnant women

Within these populations, the plan also notes that certain racial and ethnic minority communities (Black, American Indian/Alaska Native, and Hispanic) and geographic regions (Southern and

Western regions of the United States) are more impacted by STIs than others.

OTHER KEY ELEMENTS OF THE SEXUALLY TRANSMITTED INFECTIONS NATIONAL STRATEGIC PLAN

The STI National Strategic Plan strongly emphasizes the need to address stigma, discrimination, and social determinants of health in order to reverse the rise in STI rates. Another theme interwoven in the STI National Strategic Plan is the need to integrate STI prevention and control into other public health efforts to prevent and treat HIV, viral hepatitis, and substance use disorders.

The plan notes that we can improve and sustain people's health and reduce health inequities by working to establish policies and programs that improve the conditions in which we live, learn, work, and play. These actions will ultimately create a healthier population and society.

Progress Indicators

The STI National Strategic Plan identifies indicator measures and sets targets for each indicator. These will be used to track progress toward achieving the plan's goals. There are seven core indicators to measure progress for the entire plan. Some core indicators are also used to measure progress in addressing disparities in STIs among the priority populations and subpopulations (i.e., disparities indicators). The STI National Strategic Plan also offers recommendations for developing additional indicators to improve our nation's ability to measure progress in reducing STIs.

For each core and disparities indicator, the STI National Strategic Plan begins with a baseline measurement and establishes annual quantitative targets through 2030 because STIs will continue to pose a threat to the public's health past 2025. The indicators use existing national data sources that:

- generate data regularly and consistently, making it possible to do nationwide, cross-year comparisons
- allow for breaking down the information by age, geographic region, race, ethnicity, and sex, and, when available, sex of sex partners

NEXT STEPS: FEDERAL SEXUALLY TRANSMITTED INFECTIONS IMPLEMENTATION PLAN

Federal partners will collaborate to develop an implementation plan that supports the STI National Strategic Plan's goals and suggested action steps. This Federal Implementation Plan will spell out federal partners' specific commitments to developing policies, initiatives, and activities to meet the goals of the STI National Strategic Plan. The Department of Health and Human Services (HHS) will publish this implementation plan to ensure transparency and accountability.

As part of their ongoing commitment to reduce STIs in the United States, federal partners have committed to serve on an STI National Strategic Plan implementation working group. This group will meet regularly to coordinate activities across agencies and departments, monitor progress toward the indicator targets, implement lessons learned from data and research findings, change course when necessary, and report on national progress.[4]

Section 82.5 | Ending the HIV Epidemic

WHAT IS "ENDING THE HUMAN IMMUNODEFICIENCY VIRUS EPIDEMIC IN THE UNITED STATES"?

Ending the Human Immunodeficiency Virus Epidemic in the United States (EHE) is a bold plan announced in 2019 that aims to end the HIV epidemic in the United States by 2030. Agencies across the U.S. Department of Health and Human Services (HHS) developed an operational plan to pursue that goal accompanied by a request for additional annual funding.

The plan leverages critical scientific advances in human immunodeficiency virus (HIV) prevention, diagnosis, treatment, and outbreak response by coordinating the highly successful programs,

---

[4] "Sexually Transmitted Infections (STIs)," U.S. Department of Health and Human Services (HHS), June 7, 2023. Available online. URL: www.hhs.gov/programs/topic-sites/sexually-transmitted-infections/index.html. Accessed July 11, 2023.

resources, and infrastructure of many HHS agencies and offices. Initially, the initiative focuses on areas where HIV transmission occurs most frequently, providing 57 geographic focus areas with an infusion of additional resources, expertise, and technology to develop and implement locally tailored EHE plans.

GOAL

The initiative seeks to reduce the number of new HIV infections in the United States by 75 percent by 2025, and then by at least 90 percent by 2030, for an estimated 250,000 total HIV infections averted.

HUMAN IMMUNODEFICIENCY VIRUS IN AMERICA

The HIV has cost America too much for too long and remains a significant public health issue:

- More than 700,000 American lives have been lost to HIV since 1981.
- More than 1.1 million Americans are currently living with HIV, and many more are at risk of HIV infection.
- While new HIV diagnoses have declined significantly from their peak, progress on further reducing them has stalled with an estimated 38,000 Americans being newly diagnosed each year. Without intervention, nearly 400,000 more Americans will be newly diagnosed over 10 years despite the availability of tools to prevent transmissions.
- The U.S. government spends $20 billion in annual direct health expenditures for HIV prevention and care.
- There is a real risk of an HIV resurgence due to several factors, including trends in injection and other drug use; HIV-related stigma; homophobia and transphobia; lack of access to HIV prevention, testing, and treatment; and a lack of awareness that HIV remains a significant public health threat.

RIGHT DATA AND RIGHT TOOLS

Data tell us that most new HIV infections occur in a limited number of counties and among specific populations, giving us the information needed to target our efforts to those locales that will make the biggest impact on ending the HIV epidemic. Furthermore, today we have the tools available to end the HIV epidemic. Landmark biomedical and scientific research advances have led to the development of many successful HIV treatment regimens, prevention strategies, and improved care for persons living with HIV. Notably:

- Thanks to advances in antiretroviral therapy, the medicine used to treat HIV, people with HIV who take HIV medicine as prescribed and, as a result, maintain, get, and keep an undetectable viral load can live long and healthy lives and will not transmit HIV to an HIV-negative partner through sex.
- We have proven models of effective HIV care and prevention based on more than two decades of experience engaging and retaining patients in effective care.
- Pre-exposure prophylaxis (PrEP), a daily regimen of two oral antiretroviral drugs in a single pill, has proven to be highly effective in preventing HIV infection for individuals at high risk, reducing the risk of acquiring HIV by up to 97 percent. A long-acting injectable form of PrEP has also been approved by the U.S. Food and Drug Administration (FDA).
- Syringe services programs (SSPs) dramatically reduce HIV risk and can provide an entry point for a range of services to help stop drug use, overdose deaths, and infectious diseases.
- New laboratory and epidemiological techniques allow us to pinpoint where HIV infections are spreading most rapidly, so health officials can respond swiftly with resources to stop the further spread of new transmissions and support those newly diagnosed.

With these powerful data and tools, we have a once-in-a-generation opportunity to end the HIV epidemic.

THE U.S. DEPARTMENT OF HEALTH AND HUMAN SERVICES LEADERSHIP

This initiative is leveraging critical scientific advances in HIV prevention, diagnosis, treatment, and care by coordinating the highly successful programs, resources, and infrastructure of many HHS agencies and offices, including the:

- Centers for Disease Control and Prevention (CDC)
- Health Resources and Services Administration (HRSA)
- Indian Health Service (IHS)
- National Institutes of Health (NIH)
- Office of the Assistant Secretary for Health (OASH)
- Substance Abuse and Mental Health Services Administration (SAMHSA)

The HHS OASH is coordinating this cross-agency initiative.

WHOLE-OF-SOCIETY INITIATIVE

Achieving EHE's goals will require a whole-of-society effort. In addition to the coordination across HHS agencies, the success of this initiative will also depend on dedicated partners from all sectors of society working together, including people with HIV or at risk for HIV; city, county, tribal, and state health departments and other agencies; local clinics and health-care facilities; health-care providers; providers of medication-assisted treatment for opioid use disorder; professional associations; advocates; community- and faith-based organizations; and academic and research institutions, among others. The engagement of the community in developing and implementing jurisdictional EHE plans as well as in the planning, designing, and delivering local HIV prevention and care services is vital to the initiative's success.

PRIORITY JURISDICTIONS

Initially, the EHE initiative will focus on 57 priority jurisdictions, including 48 counties; Washington, DC; and San Juan, Puerto Rico, where more than 50 percent of new HIV diagnoses occurred in 2016 and 2017, and also seven states with a disproportionate occurrence of HIV in rural areas. Subsequently, efforts will expand more widely across the nation to reduce new infections by 90 percent by 2030. Ultimately, intensive case management will be implemented to maintain the number of new infections at fewer than 3,000 per year.

KEY STRATEGIES

The EHE initiative focuses on four key strategies that, implemented together, can end the HIV epidemic in the United States: diagnose, treat, prevent, and respond.

FUNDING

Congress approved some additional HIV resources in fiscal years 2020, 2021, and 2022 to support this multiyear initiative focused on ending the HIV epidemic in America by 2030.

CHALLENGES

Despite the game-changing developments in HIV prevention and treatment tools, not everyone is benefiting equally from these advances. New infections are highly concentrated among men who have sex with men; minorities, especially African Americans, Hispanics/Latinos, American Indians, and Alaska Natives; and those who live in the southern United States.

Furthermore, analysis from the CDC shows the vast majority (about 80%) of new HIV infections in the United States in 2016 were transmitted from nearly 40 percent of people with HIV who either did not know they had HIV or had been diagnosed but were not receiving HIV care. These data underscore the impact of undiagnosed and untreated HIV in the nation and also the critical need to expand HIV testing and treatment in the United States. And stigma—which can be a debilitating barrier preventing people with or at risk for HIV from receiving the health care, services, and respect they need and deserve—still tragically surrounds HIV. Responding to HIV is not just a biomedical issue but also a social challenge.

Effective interventions have driven the number of new HIV infections down to approximately 35,000 per year—the lowest level ever. However, recent data show that our progress in reducing the number of new HIV infections has plateaued. Now there are new threats to the progress we have made, the most significant being the opioid crisis: One in 10 new HIV infections occurs among people who inject drugs.

OUR OPPORTUNITY

Our nation faces an unprecedented opportunity once thought impossible. The most powerful HIV prevention and treatment tools in history are now available. Areas where HIV transmission is occurring most rapidly can also be identified. By deploying those tools swiftly and to the greatest effect, the HIV epidemic in America can end. The time to act is now.[5]

Section 82.6 | **Combating COVID-19**

COVID-19 PREVENTION ACTIONS

There are many ways your actions can help protect you, your household, and your community from severe illness from COVID-19. The COVID-19 hospital admission levels of the Centers for Disease Control and Prevention (CDC; www.cdc.gov/coronavirus/2019-ncov/your-health/covid-by-county.html) provide information about the amount of severe illness in the community where you are located to help you decide when to take action to protect yourself and others.

[5] HIV.gov, "About Ending the HIV Epidemic in the U.S.," U.S. Department of Health and Human Services (HHS), August 1, 2023. Available online. URL: www.hiv.gov/federal-response/ending-the-hiv-epidemic/overview. Accessed September 1, 2023.

PREVENTION ACTIONS TO USE AT ALL COVID-19 COMMUNITY LEVELS

In addition to basic health and hygiene practices, such as handwashing, the CDC recommends some prevention actions at all COVID-19 hospital admission levels, which include the following.

Staying Up to Date with COVID-19 Vaccines

COVID-19 vaccines help your body develop protection from the virus that causes COVID-19. Although vaccinated people sometimes get infected with the virus that causes COVID-19, staying up to date on COVID-19 vaccines significantly lowers the risk of getting very sick, being hospitalized, or dying from COVID-19. The CDC recommends that everyone stay up to date on their COVID-19 vaccines, especially people with weakened immune systems.

Improving Ventilation and Spending Time Outdoors

Improving ventilation (moving air into, out of, or within a room) and filtration (trapping particles on a filter to remove them from the air) can help prevent virus particles from accumulating in indoor air. Improving ventilation and filtration can help protect you from getting infected with and spreading the virus that causes COVID-19. Spending time outside when possible instead of inside can also help: Viral particles spread between people more readily indoors than outdoors.

Actions that can improve ventilation and filtration include the following:

- bringing in as much outdoor air as possible—for example, opening windows
- increasing air filtration in your heating, ventilation, and air conditioning (HVAC) system, such as by changing filters frequently and using filters that are properly fitted and provide higher filtration
- using portable high-efficiency particulate air (HEPA) cleaners

- turning on exhaust fans and using other fans to improve airflow
- turning your thermostat to the "ON" position instead of "AUTO" to ensure your HVAC system provides continuous airflow and filtration

The CDC's interactive ventilation tools can help you see how much you can improve ventilation in your home or school.

Moving Indoor Activities Outdoors

You are less likely to be infected with COVID-19 during outdoor activities because virus particles do not build up in the air outdoors as much as they do indoors. As the COVID-19 hospital admission level rises, consider increasing the number of group activities you move outside.

Getting Tested for COVID-19

Get tested if you have COVID-19 symptoms. A viral test tells you if you are infected with the virus that causes COVID-19. If you have COVID-19 symptoms, you should get tested for COVID-19 immediately. If you have been exposed to COVID-19 and do not have symptoms, you should test five full days after your exposure. If you do not test at the right time, you are more likely to get an inaccurate test result.

You may choose to get a polymerase chain reaction (PCR) test at a testing site or health-care facility. PCR tests are more likely to detect the virus compared to antigen tests. Rapid antigen tests provide results quickly and are available at testing sites or for use at home. The U.S. Food and Drug Administration (FDA) recommends two negative antigen tests (if you have symptoms) or three negative antigen tests (if you do not have symptoms), performed two days (48 hours) apart to be confident that you do not have COVID-19.

Even when you do not have symptoms or recent exposure to COVID-19, testing may help you make informed decisions about your health and your risk of spreading COVID-19 to others, especially those who are at higher risk of severe illness.

Following Recommendations for What to Do If You Have Been Exposed

If you were exposed to someone with COVID-19, you may have been infected with the virus. Follow the CDC's recommendations for what to do if you are exposed. This includes wearing a high-quality mask when indoors around others (including inside your home) for 10 days, testing, and monitoring yourself for symptoms.

Staying Home When You Have Suspected or Confirmed COVID-19

If you have COVID-19, you can spread it to others, even if you do not have symptoms. If you have symptoms, get tested and stay home until you have your results. If you have tested positive (even without symptoms), follow the CDC's isolation recommendations (www.cdc.gov/coronavirus/2019-ncov/your-health/quarantine-isolation.html). These recommendations include staying home and away from others for at least five days (possibly more, depending on how the virus affects you) and wearing a high-quality mask when indoors around others for a period of time.

Seeking Treatment If You Have COVID-19 and Are at High Risk of Getting Very Sick

Effective treatments are now widely available and free, and you may be eligible.

- Contact your health-care provider, health department, or community health center (CHC) to learn about treatment options.
- Do not delay! Treatment must be started within a few days after you first develop symptoms to be effective.
- If you do not have timely access to a health-care provider, check if a Test to Treat location (https://covid-19-test-to-treat-locator-dhhs.hub.arcgis.com) is in your community. You can get tested, receive a prescription from a health-care provider (either onsite or by telehealth), and have it filled all at one location.

Avoiding Contact with People Who Have Suspected or Confirmed COVID-19

Avoiding contact with people who have COVID-19, whether or not they feel sick, can reduce your risk of catching the virus from them. If possible, avoid being around a person who has COVID-19 until they can safely end home isolation. Sometimes, it may not be practical for you to stay away from a person who has COVID-19 or you may want to take care of them. In those situations, use as many prevention strategies as you can, such as practicing hand hygiene, consistently and correctly wearing a high-quality mask, improving ventilation, and keeping your distance, when possible, from the person who is sick or who tested positive.

PREVENTION ACTIONS TO ADD AS NEEDED

There are some additional prevention actions that may be done at any level, but the CDC especially recommends considering in certain circumstances or at medium or high COVID-19 hospital admission levels.

Wearing Masks or Respirators

Masks are made to contain droplets and particles that you breathe, cough, or sneeze out. A variety of masks are available. Some masks provide a higher level of protection than others.

Respirators (e.g., N95) are made to protect you by fitting closely on the face to filter out particles, including the virus that causes COVID-19. They can also block droplets and particles you breathe, cough, or sneeze out, so you do not spread them to others. Respirators (e.g., N95) provide higher protection than masks.

When wearing a mask or respirator (e.g., N95), it is most important to choose one that you can wear correctly, that fits closely to your face over your mouth and nose, that provides good protection, and that is comfortable for you.

Increasing Space and Distance

Small particles that people breathe out can contain virus particles. The closer you are to a greater number of people, the more likely you are to be exposed to the virus that causes COVID-19. To avoid this possible exposure, you may want to avoid crowded areas or keep a distance between yourself and others. These actions also protect people who are at high risk of getting very sick from COVID-19 in settings where there are multiple risks for exposure.[6]

[6] "How to Protect Yourself and Others," Centers for Disease Control and Prevention (CDC), July 6, 2023. Available online. URL: www.cdc.gov/coronavirus/2019-ncov/prevent-getting-sick/prevention.html. Accessed July 11, 2023.

Part 7 | **Additional Help and Information**

Chapter 83 | Glossary of Terms Related to Contagious Diseases

acute: A short-term, intense health effect.

adjuvant: A substance included in some vaccine formulations to enhance the immune-stimulating properties of the vaccine.

adverse events: Undesirable experiences occurring after immunization that may or may not be related to the vaccine.

antibiotics: Medicines that can damage or kill bacteria and are used to treat bacterial diseases.

antibodies: Molecules (also called "immunoglobulins") produced by a B cell in response to an antigen. When an antibody attaches to an antigen, it destroys the antigen.

antigen: A substance or molecule recognized by the immune system. The molecule can come from foreign materials such as bacteria or viruses.

antitoxin: Antibodies capable of destroying toxins generated by microorganisms, including viruses and bacteria.

artificially acquired immunity: Immunity provided by vaccines, as opposed to naturally acquired immunity, which is acquired from exposure to a disease-causing organism.

asthma: A chronic medical condition where the bronchial tubes (in the lungs) become easily irritated.

This glossary contains terms excerpted from documents produced by several sources deemed reliable.

attenuated vaccine: A vaccine in which a live virus is weakened through chemical or physical processes in order to produce an immune response without causing the severe effects of the disease.

B cells: Small white blood cells crucial to the immune defenses. These are also known as "B lymphocytes."

bone marrow: A soft tissue located within bones that produce all blood cells, including the ones that fight infection.

booster shot: An additional dose of a vaccine, usually smaller than the first dose, given to maintain immunity.

cell: The smallest unit of life.

chronic health condition: A long-lasting health condition (e.g., cancer, asthma) that persists over an extended period.

communicable disease: An infectious disease that is contagious and which can be transmitted from one source to another by infectious bacteria or viral organisms.

computed tomography (CT): A procedure for taking x-ray images from many different angles and then assembling them into a cross-section of the body. This technique is generally used to visualize bone.

conjugate vaccine: A vaccine in which proteins that are easily recognizable to the immune system are linked to the molecules that form the outer coat of disease-causing bacteria to promote an immune response.

contagious disease: A highly communicable disease capable of spreading rapidly from one person to another through contact or close proximity.

contraindication: A condition in a recipient that is likely to result in a life-threatening problem if a vaccine were given.

diphtheria: A bacterial disease marked by the formation of a false membrane, especially in the throat, which can cause death.

disease: A state in which a function or part of the body is no longer in a healthy condition.

deoxyribonucleic acid (DNA): A complex molecule found in the cell nucleus that contains an organism's genetic information.

DNA vaccine: A vaccine that uses a microbe's genetic material, rather than the whole organism or its parts, to stimulate an immune response.

encephalitis: Inflammation of the brain caused by a virus. Encephalitis can result in permanent brain damage or death.

encephalopathy: A general term describing brain dysfunction.

endemic: The continual, low-level presence of disease in a community.

epidemic: A disease outbreak that affects many people in a region at the same time.

exposure: Contact with infectious agents (bacteria or viruses) in a manner that promotes transmission and increases the likelihood of disease.

genes: Units of genetic material (DNA) that carry the directions a cell uses to perform a specific function.

genetic material: Molecules of deoxyribonucleic acid (DNA) or ribonucleic acid (RNA) that carry the directions that cells or viruses use to perform a specific function, such as making a particular protein molecule.

genomes: All of an organism's genetic material. A genome is organized into specific functional units called "genes."

herpes zoster: A disease characterized by painful skin lesions that occur mainly on the trunk (back and stomach) of the body but which can also develop on the face and in the mouth. It is also known as the "shingles."

hives: The eruption of red marks on the skin that is usually accompanied by itching.

immune globulin: A protein found in the blood that fights infection. It is also known as "gamma globulin."

immune response: Reaction of the immune system to foreign invaders such as microbes.

immune system: A complex network of specialized cells, tissues, and organs that defends the body against attacks by disease-causing microbes.

immunity: Protection from germs.

inactivated vaccine or killed vaccine: A vaccine made from a whole virus or bacteria inactivated with chemicals or heat.

incubation period: The time from contact with infectious agents (bacteria or viruses) to onset of disease.

infection: A state in which disease-causing microbes have invaded or multiplied in body tissues.

infectious agents: Organisms capable of spreading disease (e.g., bacteria or viruses).

intussusception: A type of bowel blockage that happens when one portion of the bowel slides into the next, much like the pieces of a telescope.

jaundice: Yellowing of the skin and eyes. This condition is often a symptom of hepatitis infection.

lesion: An abnormal change in the structure of an organ, due to injury or disease.

live, attenuated vaccine: A vaccine made from microbes that have been weakened in the laboratory so that they cannot cause disease.

lupus: A disease characterized by inflammation of the connective tissue (which supports and connects all parts of the body).

lymph node: A small bean-shaped organ of the immune system, distributed widely throughout the body and linked by lymphatic vessels.

lymphocyte: A white blood cell central to the immune system's response to foreign microbes. B cells and T cells are lymphocytes.

macrophage: A large and versatile immune cell that devours and kills invading microbes and other intruders.

magnetic resonance imaging (MRI): A noninvasive procedure that uses magnetic fields and radio waves to produce three-dimensional computerized images of areas inside the body.

memory cells: A group of cells that help the body defend itself against disease by remembering prior exposure to specific organisms (e.g., viruses or bacteria). Therefore, these cells are able to respond quickly when these organisms repeatedly threaten the body.

molecule: A building block of a cell. Some examples are proteins, fats, and carbohydrates.

mutate: To change a gene or unit of hereditary material that results in a new inheritable characteristic.

naturally acquired immunity: Immunity produced by antibodies passed from mother to fetus (passive) or by the body's own antibody and cellular immune response to a disease-causing organism (active).

orchitis: A complication of mumps infection occurring in males (who are beyond puberty).

otitis media: A viral or bacterial infection that leads to inflammation of the middle ear.

outbreak: Sudden appearance of a disease in a specific geographic area (e.g., neighborhood or community) or population (e.g., adolescents).

pandemic: An epidemic occurring over a very large geographic area.

parasites: Plants or animals that live, grow, and feed on or within another living organism.

pathogens: Organisms (e.g., bacteria, viruses, parasites, and fungi) that cause disease in human beings.

petechiae: A tiny reddish or purplish spot on the skin or mucous membrane, commonly part of infectious diseases such as typhoid fever.

placebo: A substance or treatment that has no effect on human beings.

pneumonia: Inflammation of the lungs characterized by symptoms such as fever, cough, shortness of breath, and chest pain.

polysaccharide: A long, chain-like molecule made up of a linked sugar molecule. The outer coats of some bacteria are made of polysaccharides.

potency: A measure of strength.

quarantine: The isolation of a person or animal who has a disease (or is suspected of having a disease) in order to prevent further spread of the disease.

recombinant: Of or resulting from new combinations of genetic material or cells.

Reye syndrome: Encephalopathy (general brain disorder) in children following an acute illness, such as influenza or chickenpox. Symptoms include vomiting, agitation, and lethargy. This condition may result in coma or death.

serology: Measurement of antibodies and other immunological properties in the blood serum.

strain: A specific version of an organism. Many diseases, including human immunodeficiency virus (HIV)/acquired immune deficiency syndrome (AIDS) and hepatitis, have multiple strains.

subunit vaccine: A vaccine that uses one or more components of a disease-causing organism, rather than the whole, to stimulate an immune response.

T cell or T lymphocyte: A white blood cell that directs or participates in immune defenses.

tetanus: A toxin-producing bacterial disease marked by painful muscle spasms.

thimerosal: A mercury-containing preservative used in some vaccines and other products since the 1930s.

tissue: A group of similar cells joined to perform the same function.

titer: The detection of antibodies in blood through a laboratory test.

toxin: Agent produced by plants and bacteria, normally very damaging to cells.

toxoid: A toxin such as those produced by certain bacteria that have been treated by chemical means, heat, or irradiation and are no longer capable of causing disease.

toxoid vaccine: A vaccine containing a toxoid, used to protect against toxins produced by certain bacteria.

vaccine: A product that stimulates immunity, protecting the body from a particular disease. Vaccines are administered through injections, oral means, or aerosols.

virus: A tiny organism that multiplies within cells and causes diseases such as chickenpox, measles, mumps, rubella, pertussis, and hepatitis. Viruses are not affected by antibiotics, the drugs used to kill bacteria.

x-ray: A type of radiation used in the diagnosis and treatment of cancer and other diseases. In low doses, x-rays are used to diagnose diseases by making pictures of the inside of the body.

yoga: An ancient system of practices used to balance the mind and body through exercise, meditation (focusing thoughts), and control of breathing and emotions. Yoga is being studied as a way to relieve stress and treat sleep problems in cancer patients.

Chapter 84 | Directory of Organizations Providing Information about Contagious Diseases

GOVERNMENT AGENCIES

Administration for Strategic Preparedness and Response (ASPR)
200 Independence Ave.
Washington, DC 20201
Website: aspr.hhs.gov

Agency for Healthcare Research and Quality (AHRQ)
5600 Fishers Ln.
7th Fl. Rockville, MD 20857
Phone: 301-427-1364
Website: www.ahrq.gov

Centers for Disease Control and Prevention (CDC)
1600 Clifton Rd.
Atlanta, GA 30329-4027
Toll-Free: 800-232-4636
Toll-Free TTY: 888-232-6348
Website: www.cdc.gov
Email: cdcinfo@cdc.gov

Resources in this chapter were compiled from several sources deemed reliable; all contact information was verified and updated in October 2023.

Eunice Kennedy Shriver National Institute of Child Health and Human Development (NICHD)
P.O. Box 3006
Rockville, MD 20847
Toll-Free: 800-370-2943
Toll-Free Fax: 866-760-5947
Website: www.nichd.nih.gov
Email: NICHDInformation ResourceCenter@mail.nih.gov

Federal Trade Commission (FTC)
600 Pennsylvania Ave., N.W.
Washington, DC 20580
Phone: 202-326-2222
Website: www.ftc.gov

Genetics Home Reference (GHR)
8600 Rockville Pike
Bethesda, MD 20894
Website: medlineplus.gov/about/general/genetics/aboutmedlineplusgenetics

Health Resources and Services Administration (HRSA)
5600 Fishers Ln.
Rockville, MD 20857
Toll-Free: 800-221-9393
Phone: 301-443-3376
Toll-Free TTY: 877-897-9910
Website: www.hrsa.gov
Email: press@hrsa.gov

Healthfinder®
1101 Wootton Pkwy
Rockville, MD 20852
Website: health.gov/myhealthfinder
Email: healthfinder@hhs.gov

MedlinePlus
8600 Rockville Pike
Bethesda, MD 20894
Toll-Free: 888-346-3656
Phone: 301-594-5983
Website: www.medlineplus.gov

National Cancer Institute (NCI)
9609 Medical Center Dr.
Rockville, MD 20850
Toll-Free: 800-422-6237
Website: www.cancer.gov
Email: NCIinfo@nih.gov

National Center for Complementary and Integrative Health (NCCIH)
9000 Rockville Pike
Bethesda, MD 20892
Toll-Free: 888-644-6226
Website: nccih.nih.gov
Email: info@nccih.nih.gov

National Heart, Lung, and Blood Institute (NHLBI)
31 Center Dr. Bldg. 31
Bethesda, MD 20892
Toll-Free: 877-645-2448
Website: www.nhlbi.nih.gov
Email: nhlbiinfo@nhlbi.nih.gov

National Institute of Allergy and Infectious Diseases (NIAID)
5601 Fishers Ln. MSC 9806
Bethesda, MD 20892-9806
Toll-Free: 866-284-4107
Phone: 301-496-5717
Toll-Free TDD: 800-877-8339
Fax: 301-402-3573
Website: www.niaid.nih.gov
Email: ocpostoffice@niaid.nih.gov

National Institute of Diabetes and Digestive and Kidney Diseases (NIDDK)
9000 Rockville Pike
Bethesda, MD 20892
Toll-Free: 800-860-8747
Website: www.niddk.nih.gov
Email: healthinfo@niddk.nih.gov

National Institute of Neurological Disorders and Stroke (NINDS)
P.O. Box 5801
Bethesda, MD 20824
Toll-Free: 800-352-9424
Website: www.ninds.nih.gov
Email: InformationOffice4@mail.nih.gov

National Institute on Aging (NIA)
P.O. Box 8057
Gaithersburg, MD 20898
Toll-Free: 800-222-2225
Toll-Free TTY: 800-222-4225
Website: www.nia.nih.gov
Email: niaic@nia.nih.gov

National Institutes of Health (NIH)
9000 Rockville Pike
Bethesda, MD 20892
Phone: 301-496-4000
Toll-Free TTY: 301-402-9612
Website: www.nih.gov
Email: olib@od.nih.gov

National Prevention Information Network (NPIN)
P.O. Box 6003
Rockville, MD 20849-6003
Website: npin.cdc.gov
Email: npin-info@cdc.gov

National Women's Health Information Center (NWHIC)
1101 Wootton Pkwy.
Rockville, MD 20852
Toll-Free: 800-994-9662
Phone: 202-690-7650
Fax: 202-205-2631
Website: www.womenshealth.gov
Email: womenshealth@hhs.gov

NIH *News in Health*
9000 Rockville Pike
Bldg. 31, Rm. 5B52
Bethesda, MD 20892
Phone: 301-451-8224
Website: newsinhealth.nih.gov
Email: nihnewsinhealth@od.nih.gov

Office of Dietary Supplements (ODS)
6705 Rockledge Dr.,
Rm. 730 MSC 7991
Bethesda, MD 20817
Phone: 301-435-2920
Fax: 301-480-1845
Website: ods.od.nih.gov
Email: ods@nih.gov

U.S. Department of Health and Human Services (HHS)
200 Independence Ave., S.W.
Hubert H. Humphrey Bldg.
Washington, DC 20201
Toll-Free: 877-696-6775
Website: www.hhs.gov

U.S. Environmental Protection Agency (EPA)
1200 Pennsylvania Ave., N.W.
Washington, DC 20460
Phone: 202-564-4700
Website: www.epa.gov

U.S. Food and Drug Administration (FDA)
10903 New Hampshire Ave.
Silver Spring, MD 20993-0002
Toll-Free: 888-463-6332
Website: www.fda.gov

U.S. National Library of Medicine (NLM)
8600 Rockville Pike
Bethesda, MD 20894
Toll-Free: 888-346-3656
Phone: 301-594-5983
Website: www.nlm.nih.gov
Email: NLMCommunications@nih.gov

Vaccine Adverse Event Reporting System (VAERS)
P.O. Box 1100
Rockville, MD 20849-1100
Toll-Free: 800-822-7967
Toll-Free Fax: 877-721-0366
Website: www.vaers.hhs.gov
Email: info@vaers.org

PRIVATE AGENCIES

American Academy of Allergy, Asthma, & Immunology (AAAAI)
555 E. Wells St., Ste. 1100
Milwaukee, WI 53202-3823
Phone: 414-272-6071
Website: www.aaaai.org
Email: info@aaaai.org

American Academy of Family Physicians (AAFP)
11400 Tomahawk Creek Pkwy.
Leawood, KS 66211-2680
Toll-Free: 800-274-2237
Phone: 913-906-6000
Fax: 913-906-6075
Website: www.aafp.org
Email: aafp@aafp.org

American Cancer Society (ACS)
3380 Chastain Meadows Pkwy., N.W., Ste. 200
Kennesaw, GA 30144
Toll-Free: 800-227-2345
Website: www.cancer.org

American Liver Foundation (ALF)
P.O. Box 299
West Orange, NJ 07052
Toll-Free: 800-465-4837
Website: www.liverfoundation.org
Email: info@liverfoundation.org

American Lung Association (ALA)
55 W. Wacker Dr., Ste. 1150
Chicago, IL 60601
Toll-Free: 800-586-4872
Website: www.lung.org
Email: info@lung.org

American Medical Association (AMA)
AMA Plz., 330 N. Wabash Ave., Ste. 39300
Chicago, IL 60611-5885
Toll-Free: 800-262-3211
Phone: 312-464-4782
Website: www.ama-assn.org

American Sexual Health Association (ASHA)
P.O. Box 13827
Research Triangle Park, NC 27709
Phone: 919-361-8400
Fax: 919-361-8425
Website: www.ashasexualhealth.org
Email: info@ashasexualhealth.org

Association for the Advancement of Blood & Biotherapies (AABB)
4550 Montgomery Ave., Ste. 700
North Twr.
Bethesda, MD 20814
Phone: 301-907-6977
Fax: 301-907-6895
Website: www.aabb.org

National Foundation for Infectious Diseases (NFID)
7201 Wisconsin Ave., Ste. 750
Bethesda, MD 20814
Phone: 301-656-0003
Website: www.nfid.org

National Organization for Rare Disorders (NORD)
1900 Crown Colony Dr., Ste. 310
Quincy, MA 02169
Phone: 617-249-7300
Website: www.rarediseases.org

National Patient Advocate Foundation (NPAF)
1100 H St., N.W., Ste. 710
Washington, DC 20005
Phone: 202-347-8009
Website: www.npaf.org

The Nemours Foundation/ KidsHealth®
10140 Centurion Pkwy., N. Jacksonville, FL 32256
Toll-Free: 800-472-6610
Website: www.kidshealth.org

Pfizer Inc.
235 E. 42nd St.
New York, NY 10017
Toll-Free: 800-879-3477
Website: www.pfizer.com

Scleroderma Research Foundation (SRF)
220 Montgomery St., Ste. 484
San Francisco, CA 94104
Toll-Free: 800-441-2873 (800-441-CURE)
Phone: 415-834-9444
Website: https://srfcure.org
Email: info@srfcure.org

Sepsis Alliance
3180 University Ave., Ste. 310
San Diego, CA 92104
Phone: 619-232-0300
Website: www.sepsis.org
Email: info@sepsis.org

Sjögren's Foundation
10701 Parkridge Blvd., Ste. 170
Reston, VA 20191
Phone: 301-530-4420
Fax: 301-530-4415
Website: https://sjogrens.org
Email: info@sjogrens.org

INDEX

INDEX

Page numbers followed by "n" refer to citation information; by "t" indicate tables; and by "f" indicate figures.

A

B

Index

C

Index

D

E

I

J

K

L

M

N

O

P

Q

R

S

T

U

V